Laparoscopic Biliary Surgery

Laparoscopic Biliary Surgery

ALFRED CUSCHIERI
MD, ChM, FRCSEd, FRCSEng, FIBiol

and

GEORGE BERCI
MD, FACS

With contributions by:

MARGARET PAZ-PARTLOW
MA, MFA

L.K. NATHANSON
FRACS

JONATHAN SACKIER
MD, FRCS

SECOND EDITION
REVISED AND EXTENDED

WITH THE COMPLIMENTS OF
KARL STORZ

OXFORD
BLACKWELL SCIENTIFIC PUBLICATIONS
LONDON EDINBURGH BOSTON
MELBOURNE PARIS BERLIN VIENNA

Editorial Offices:
Osney Mead, Oxford OX2 0EL
25 John Street, London WC1N 2BL
23 Ainslie Place, Edinburgh EH3 6AJ
238 Main Street, Cambridge
Massachusetts 02142, USA
54 University Street, Carlton
Victoria 3053, Australia

Other Editorial Offices:
Librairie Arnette SA
2, rue Casimir-Delavigne
75006 Paris
France

Blackwell Wissenschafts-Verlag
Meinekestrasse 4
D-1000 Berlin 15
Germany

Blackwell MZV
Feldgasse 13
A-1238 Wien
Austria

First published 1990
Reprinted 1991

French edition 1991
Spanish edition 1991
German edition 1991
Japanese edition 1992

Second edition 1992

Set by Semantic Graphics, Singapore
Printed in Italy by
Vincenzo Bona srl, Turin
and bound in France by
SIRC, Marigny-le-Châtel

DISTRIBUTORS

Marston Book Services Ltd
PO Box 87
Oxford OX2 0DT
(*Orders*: Tel: 0865 791155
Fax: 0865 791927
Telex: 837515)

USA
Blackwell Scientific Publications, Inc.
238 Main Street
Cambridge, MA 02142
(*Orders*: Tel: 800 759-6102
617 876-7000)

Canada
Times Mirror Professional Publishing, Ltd.
5240 Finch Avenue East
Scarborough, Ontario M1S 5A2
(*Orders*: Tel: 800 268-4178
416 298-1588)

Australia
Blackwell Scientific Publications
(Australia) Pty Ltd
54 University Street
Carlton, Victoria 3053
(*Orders*: Tel: 03 347-0300)

A catalogue record for this title is available from the British Library

ISBN 0-632-03277-4

Library of Congress
Cataloging-in-Publication Data

Cuschieri, A. (Alfred)
Laparoscopic biliary surgery/
Alfred Cuschieri and George Berci,
with contributions by Margaret Paz-Partlow,
L.K. Nathanson, Jonathan Sackier.—2nd ed.
p. cm.
Includes index.
ISBN 0-632-03277-4
1. Biliary tract—Endoscopic surgery.
2. Gallbladder—Endoscopic surgery.
3. Laparoscopic surgery. I. Berci, George, 1921–
II. Title.
[DNLM: 1. Bile Duct Diseases—surgery.
2. Cholecystectomy—methods.
3. Peritoneoscopy—methods.
WI 750 C984L]
RD546.C873 1992
617.5′56059—dc20
DNLM/DLC
for Library of Congress

Contents

Introduction

The second edition of *Laparoscopic Biliary Surgery* has been prompted by the rapid and unprecedented progress in the field since the publication of the first edition. Undoubtedly the new surgery has caught the imagination of surgeons worldwide, and has ushered in a wave of innovative effort within the medical profession which has contributed in a large measure to the remarkable progress in such a short time. The message is now clear—cholecystectomy remains the standard treatment for symptomatic gallstone-related disease, and is best performed in the vast majority of patients through the laparoscopic approach. The advantages of laparoscopic cholecystectomy over the open procedure include reduced postoperative ileus and discomfort and an accelerated recovery, with early return to full activity. In addition, it virtually abolishes all wound-related complications, both early and late. In relation to a commonly performed operation such as cholecystectomy, the cost advantages to the health service of any country, irrespective of its nature, are evident. The viability of this approach, however, depends on the safety of such a procedure and its general applicability to patients with symptomatic gallstone disease requiring treatment.

Since the publication of the first edition, laparoscopic cholecystectomy has become firmly established as the treatment of choice for symptomatic gallstone disease. Analysis of several substantive reports from various centres worldwide indicates that this operation *when performed by the fully trained* is safe and accompanied by a low morbidity. With experience, it is applicable to about 95% of patients and carries significant advantages in terms of early recovery and absence of wound complications. There are still some unresolved issues, such as the need or otherwise for routine peroperative cholangiography, the place of intraoperative ultrasound, and the optimal way of managing patients with ductal calculi. These and other problems can only be resolved by well planned and executed prospective clinical studies.

The clinical relevance of the other treatment modalities has changed drastically as a result of the development of laparoscopic cholecystectomy. This applies particularly to extracorporeal shock-wave lithotripsy (ESWL). Although this has been an undoubted significant advance in the treatment of renal calculi, the promise of the early reports of its value in gallstone disease has not materialized, since it has now been demonstrated that ESWL is applicable to only 15–20% of patients with gallstone disease. Furthermore, in those patients in whom stone fragmentation and clearance is achieved, recurrence of stones is high, averaging 10% per annum with a plateau of 50% at 5 years, despite oral bile-salt maintenance therapy. These considerations, together with prohibitive cost of long-term oral bile-salt therapy, indicate that there is no place for ESWL in the treatment of gallstones, although it is useful when used in conjunction with endoscopic sphincterotomy in the treatment of large ductal calculi, especially in the elderly and poor-risk patients.

Even the established role of endoscopic sphincterotomy and stone extraction is being challenged, in some instances with good reason and judgment. The problem has to be addressed in two quite distinct situations: ductal stones discovered preoperatively, where endoscopic extraction is advisable in some (elderly high-risk patients, cholangitis) but not all patients prior to laparoscopic cholecystectomy; and unsuspected stones discovered during cholecystectomy, when laparoscopic removal is a sensible and often rewarding approach.

Percutaneous or laparoscopic stone extraction (cholecystolithotomy) with or without stone fragmentation (lithotripsy) or chemical dissolution with methyl tert-butyl ether (MTBE) has been used in patients with chronic symptoms. There is still a place for this approach in poor-risk or elderly patients with symptomatic gallstone disease. Another indication for laparoscopic cholecystolithotomy concerns patients who develop gallstones after vagotomy and drainage, as the removal of a functioning gallbladder in these patients often precipitates severe explosive diarrhoea.

Cholecystectomy remains the treatment of choice for patients who develop acute biliary colic/cholecystitis or gallstone-associated acute pancreatitis. However, although the safety record of this operation in the fit adult is undoubted, it carries an appreciable mortality in the elderly, in patients with co-existent cardiorespiratory disease, and in cirrhotic individuals, the risk being particularly high for emergency cholecystectomy. In these high-risk groups, percutaneous or laparoscopic cholecystostomy of the severely inflamed gallbladder or empyema is a sensible option of proven benefit, which tides the poor-risk patient over the critical episode.

Chemical sclerosis of the gallbladder after the removal of stones is attractive. Experimentally, several sclerosants have been investigated in both small and large animals. There are, however, problems with this approach which must be overcome before the method can be used clinically. The important ones include the availability of a safe sclerosant with a high LD_{50}, such that toxicity is minimal subsequent to absorption into the bloodstream, a safe and reliable method of temporary occlusion of the cystic duct, total consistent full-thickness destruction of the gallbladder mucosa, and the absence of regeneration. At present there is no chemical ablation technique which meets all these criteria. Regeneration of the gallbladder mucosa from the cystic duct lining may turn out to be the most difficult aspect to resolve. There are also fears concerning the risk of malignant change following sclerosant-induced fibrosis of the gallbladder in the long term. At present, therefore, chemical cholecystectomy must be regarded as experimental.

In the second edition of *Laparoscopic Biliary Surgery*, all the chapters have been extensively revised and extra chapters have been included to cover the new surgical advances in the field: laparoscopic treatment of ductal calculi (extraction through the cystic duct and supraduodenal exploration of the common duct), laparoscopic staging of pancreatic malignancy and bilioenteric anastomosis for advanced inoperable disease, drainage of hepatic and perihepatic abscesses, and deroofing of simple hepatic cysts.

Although necessitating the acquisition of advanced laparoscopic techniques, the coelioscopic palliative biliary drainage procedures impart an undoubted benefit to patients with malignant jaundice due to inoperable pancreatic cancer, as they abolish the complications inherent to endoscopic stenting, such as encrustation and cholangitis. These laparoscopic procedures provide a one-off treatment with early discharge, enabling these unfortunate patients to spend the remainder of their limited life with their families and friends, without the need for further hospitalization.

1 : Training for laparoscopic biliary surgery

In the USA, surgical training usually consists of a well-structured 5- or 6-year programme, during which residents learn the principles of procedures and graduate from observer to assistant to surgeon. In the UK, although not so pragmatically structured, a similar technique of 'apprenticeship' leads to training in 10–15 years.

When a young surgeon is able to perform open cholecystectomy safely and competently, it is a significant moment in training, as this procedure is an excellent exercise in surgical anatomy and technique. The operation requires retraction, exposure and dissection—all of which continue to be important in the laparoscopic operation.

Until the early 1980s endoscopy in the USA was all but ignored by surgeons, until the American Board demanded that it become part of residency programmes. Despite this, many programmes continued to exclude endoscopy and therefore most surgeons who have graduated, even in the last 10 years, are not accomplished endoscopists. The situation in Europe, including the UK, is different in that endoscopy is practised by many general surgeons on a wide scale and forms an integral part of the surgical training programme. However, until recently, laparoscopy was practised in only a few surgical departments within the UK and mainland Europe.

Therefore, there are two aspects of training for laparoscopic biliary surgery that require consideration. Firstly, the education of surgeons who are out of residency and in practice and, secondly, incorporating laparoscopic training into the years of residency training.

However, gaining laparoscopy skills is not a simple matter. Certainly some procedures will be performed laparoscopically that have no corollary in open surgery, but even without this there are certain aspects that demand attention. These include the absence of tactile sensation, altered hand–eye coordination due to the length and design of instruments, and the absence of depth perception due to two-dimensional representation of the three-dimensional abdominal cavity.

Requirements for safe laparoscopic surgery

There are a number of considerations which will help to ensure that laparoscopic surgery is performed safely.

1 The individual must be a fully trained and accredited general surgeon.

2 He or she must have practical experience in diagnostic laparoscopy.

3 He or she must acquire the basic skills of operating from a distance with a TV image of the operating field. This is achieved by practice with bench-top trainers.

4 He or she must practise the procedure in suitable animal models, because manipulations are more difficult *in vivo* owing to respiratory movements and oozing of blood during dissection. Obviously this is not always possible due to local constraints on the use of animals, but accommodation may be made in training boxes.

5 He or she must observe, or preferably assist, at clinical laparoscopic procedures in centres where these operations are established.

6 A system of quality assurance and peer review in the institution will ensure that technical problems are identified early and corrected.

7 Continuing education in new techniques and the problems of others will be of value.

Training of qualified surgeons

As stated above, it is vital that laparoscopic operations such as cholecystectomy are performed only by fully trained and accredited abdominal surgeons. The reason for this is that a laparoscopic operation should always be considered by both patient and physician as a trial inspection/dissection in the first instance. If the procedure is considered technically not feasible, or complications are encountered during the course of the operation which cannot be dealt with safely by the laparoscopic approach, the operation is simply converted to a standard incision. Only an established surgeon is in a position to deal with this eventuality.

Training in diagnostic laparoscopy

Prior to attempting any major laparoscopic intervention, the general surgeon should become familiar with the basic steps of laparoscopy, such as the establishment of pneumoperitoneum, the introduction of trocars and the manipulation of instruments, by performing diagnostic procedures. Initially this may be done by scrubbing with a gynaecologist or other laparoscopic general surgeon.

Laparoscopy is extremely useful in the elective situation, where it may be used to gauge the nature and extent of liver disease, ascites, abdominal masses, organomegaly, the patient with malignancy and the patient with pyrexia of unknown origin.

In the emergency situation, laparoscopy is valuable for the assessment of patients with right iliac fossa or obscure abdominal pain, the evaluation of the trauma patient, or defining the window of opportunity for treating elderly patients with possible mesenteric ischaemia.

This initiation into laparoscopy will give the surgeon an insight into the problems alluded to above, such as hand–eye coordination and depth perception, especially when an accessory trocar is introduced either for a blunt probe to move tissue, or for a coagulation probe. This will enable the surgeon to overcome the problems of overshooting targets, and learn how to manipulate instruments and prevent the frustration of seeing devices waving around in the abdomen in a seemingly meaningless fashion. Quite apart from gaining a slow and safe introduction to laparoscopy, the surgeon's confidence will not be shattered by some of the early exasperating instances during a 20-minute diagnostic procedure, rather than during a 3- or 4-hour difficult cholecystectomy.

Bench trainers

These devices are ideal in assisting the surgeons to gain skill in manipulating long laparoscopic instruments, either with monocular or television image. A number of training devices are available (Fig. 1.1) which may be used by one doctor working alone, in which case the camera is held in a 'goose-neck' grasper. Obviously, two or three surgeons may work together on coordinated tasks. The trainer shown in Fig. 1.1 has been modified to include a white base, which provides better illumination. Other boxes are available that have a clear plastic top, but this encourages the surgeon to 'cheat'.

If financial constraints prevent the purchase of such a bench trainer, an inverted cardboard box may be used, with holes punched in the top. The box demonstrated in Fig. 1.1 has four rubber gaskets, corresponding to the positions of the trocars which are inserted during laparoscopic cholecystectomy. The sides of the box are occluded, and on two sides the occlusion is by means of a rubber curtain which is fastened with Velcro tape which can be peeled off to expose the interior of the box. Above the 'subcostal' trocar there are positions for suspending objects, which therefore come to lie within the body of the trainer. A number of tasks are available for the surgeon training on this device:

1 Suspend a bunch of grapes within the cavity and, with assistants, identify a given grape and remove it from the bunch with scissors, without damaging any other grapes (Fig. 1.2).

2 Suspend a tangerine and carefully peel given areas, which are marked

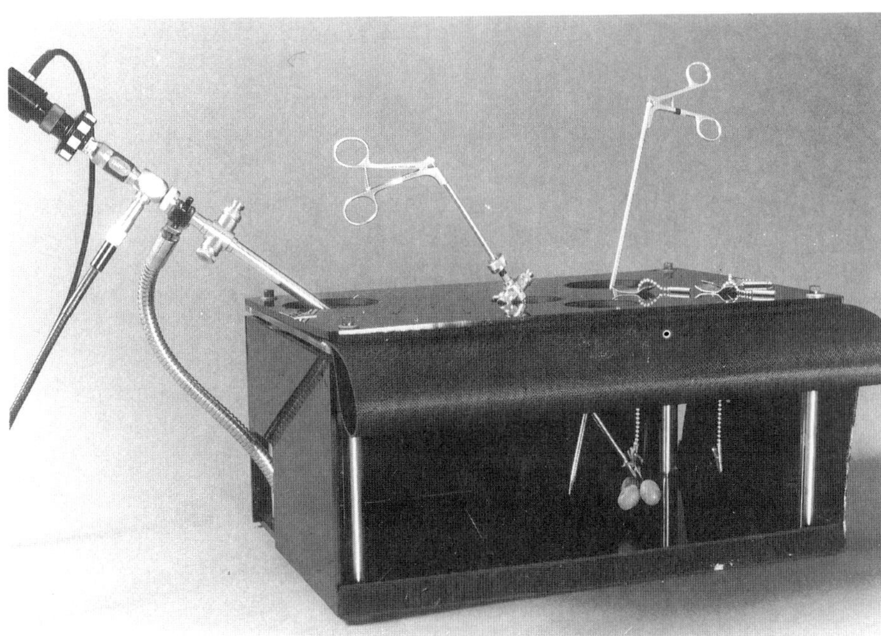

Fig. 1.1 The laparoscopic training box is constructed of black perspex except for two sides of rubber which may be raised to gain access to the interior.

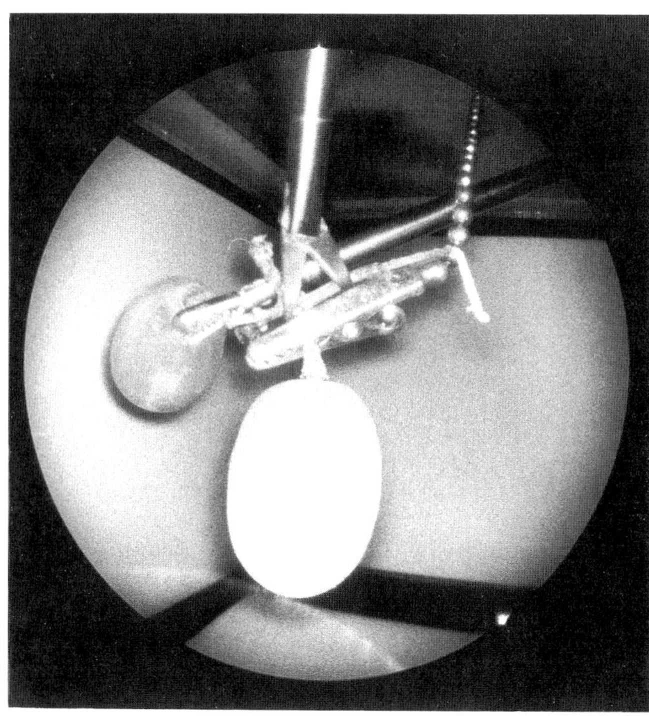

Fig. 1.2 A bunch of grapes may be suspended inside the box and a selected grape is carefully cut free.

before positioning in the box. Either sharp dissection with scissors can be used, or the electrocautery device once a grounding plate has been applied to the tangerine.

3 Suspend a piece of cooked chicken breast and carefully dissect the skin away from the flesh.

4 Insert a foam model of the gallbladder with partially separated cystic duct and artery. These can be divided between clips or tied using Roeder loops.

5 Suspend a foam structure with multiple loops within the box, and then clip or tie and divide these loops.

6 Where it is impossible to perform live-animal experimentation, an *ex-vivo* porcine liver/gallbladder preparation may be placed inside the training box and an electrocautery earthing plate underneath this. The gallbladder may then be removed in the standard fashion, as described later, from the liver.

Suturing

Once basic laparoscopic techniques have been mastered in the training box, the surgeon should turn to developing the skills of intracorporeal and extracorporeal knotting and suturing. Initially the coordination and orchestration of hand movements is so complex, that to incorporate this together with video-imaging is extremely frustrating. Therefore, it is preferable to first perform the suturing in an open cardboard box with direct visualization. Once this has been mastered the surgeon may go on to suturing under laparoscopic control in a bench trainer. A good model for practising such

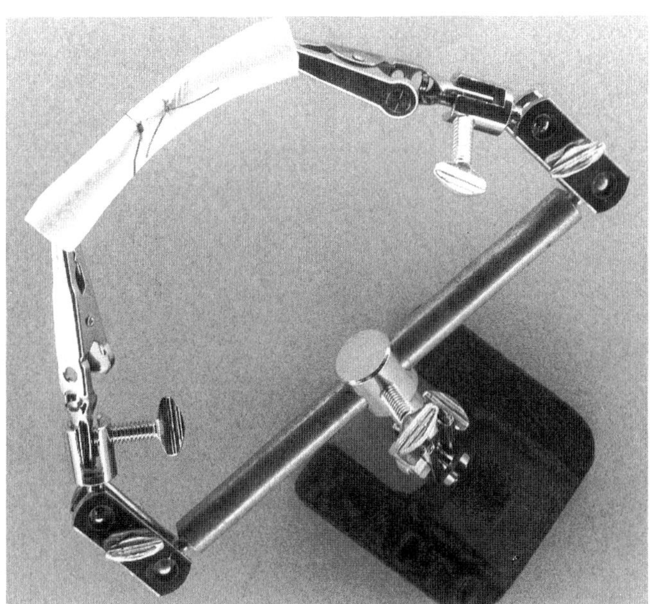

Fig. 1.3 A rig may be placed inside the training box. This device holds a vascular graft which is used to practise suturing.

skills is a mount, which holds a piece of vascular graft with a slit which may then be sutured (Fig. 1.3).

Depth perception

One of the most common problems in learning laparoscopic skills is orientating instruments with the target. Usually, a surgeon will wave the instrument around in a circular fashion and having struck the target, then attempt to grasp it. This is not only time-consuming but it is dangerous, as organs may be caught and damaged. Additionally, the surgeon may become frustrated by failure to achieve the given task.

Training courses

It is vital that a surgeon should attend a well-structured and preferably endorsed training course, which will assist in gaining privileges according to the requirements of the hospital credential committees. However, attendance at a course is no substitute for a thorough background in practical procedures and assistance with the first few cases. In the early days of laparoscopic cholecystectomy there were a number of ill-conceived courses, with training on inappropriate or small animal species. This did not provide any constructive education for the course participants.

A suitable course should consist of: (i) didactic sessions on laparoscopy (including all safety aspects); (ii) patient selection for laparoscopic cholecystectomy; (iii) instrumentation; (iv) performance of the technique of laparoscopic cholecystectomy; (v) indications and contraindications; and (vi) possible pitfalls and future developments. Videotapes or live performances of the operations should be incorporated at some stage. Thereafter, training on live animals should be given if possible.

Setting up a clinical programme

Once a surgeon has gained a background in diagnostic laparoscopy, worked on a bench trainer, attended a course and has had experience with animal experimentation, he or she is then ready to start work on humans. At this stage skills may be further enhanced by using the training box to iron out any technical problems that may have been encountered during the later stages of training. It is highly desirable that a surgeon trained and experienced in laparoscopic cholecystectomy in humans should act as first assistant and proctor on the first few patients, and the wise and humble surgeon will select thin and uncomplicated patients for his or her initial experience with this procedure.

As concerns about quality assurance become more prominent around the world, the surgical profession should develop a formula for certifying surgeons to perform new procedures. Obviously it is difficult to define strict criteria in a field that is changing as rapidly as endoscopic surgery. There is no doubt that the major surgical organizations must take a lead and lay down basic guidelines for postgraduate training. These guidelines should be generic, so that new techniques are not disseminated and practised until they have a proven place and are not deemed to be experimental. This obviously raises the question as to what is experimental? One definition that may be acceptable is that any surgical procedure that has been published in the peer review literature, presented at scientific fora and that has an established place in clinical practice — that is, one not requiring a human subjects committee's approval — would be considered non-experimental. Previously, all new treatments have undergone the acid test of prospective randomized clinical trials, but this has not occurred with laparoscopic cholecystectomy. It is vital therefore that the profession should insist upon diligent personal and institutional peer review in order to identify potentially dangerous practices and correct them.

Training in animals

The use of live animals for experimentation has always been an emotionally contentious issue, but it seems that there is no other equivalent way for the surgeon to learn the requisite skills. Training in animal models is desirable because it provides the opportunity of executing the steps of the operation under conditions which closely resemble those encountered in clinical practice. The most appropriate animal for mastering the technique of laparoscopic cholecystectomy is the adult pig, preferably the Large White/ Landrace cross-breed. Ideally, surgeons should work in teams of three, preferably from the same institution. Each participant should gain experience on at least two and preferably three, pigs, as primary surgeon, first assistant and camera operator.

Anatomy

The use of female pigs is to be preferred, as in the male the penis is on the anterior abdominal wall, which interferes with trocar placement. The anatomy of the hepatobiliary tract of this animal is similar to that of the human. The liver is large and floppy, and is divided into four principal lobes, with the bulk of the hepatic parenchyma being to the right of the midline. There is no falciform ligament and usually no ligamentum teres. The gallbladder is comparatively large and has a bluish coloration. It is attached by loose areolar tissue to the undersurface of the right lateral lobe, with its fundus projecting beyond the margin of the lobe as in the human, although it does tend to be rather more intraparenchymal. The cystic duct is long and narrow, and joins the common bile duct high up in the porta hepatis. The cystic artery runs in intimate contact with the cystic duct and the relative position of these structures is variable, but the artery usually lies anterior to the duct, dividing into a medial and a lateral branch (Fig. 1.4). Although the cystic duct is usually no more than 1 mm across and the artery is considerably less, after careful training the diligent surgeon is usually able to separately isolate and clip or tie and divide both branches of the artery, separately isolate, cannulate and then divide the cystic duct, and remove the gallbladder intact. In the pig, the common bile duct lies in the free edge of the lesser omentum, but because it is covered with fat it is very difficult to identify, especially because it lacks the blue tinge of the normal human bile duct.

Anaesthesia

Laparoscopic cholecystectomy in the pig has to be performed under general anaesthesia. The animal should be starved for at least 12 hours and then premedicated. An ideal technique is to mix in one syringe ketamine 20 mg/kg, acepromazine 0.5 mg and atropine 0.05 mg/kg, and give this as an intramuscular injection. The animal is then somnolent and may be taken to

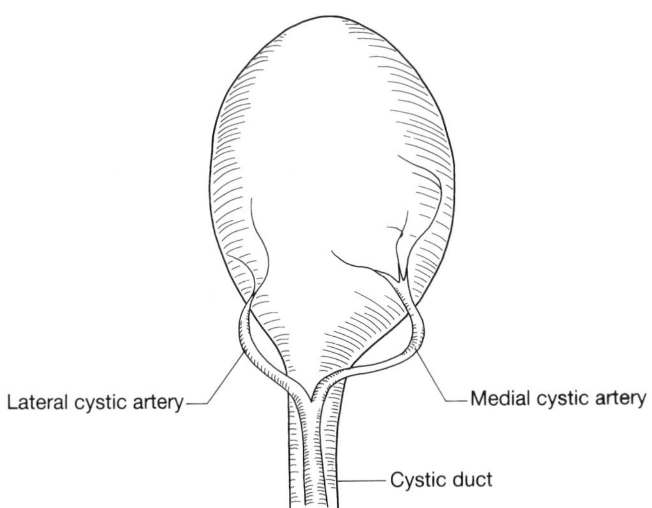

Fig. 1.4 The porcine gallbladder is similar to the human in certain respects. However, the cystic artery usually overlies the cystic duct and then divides into medial and lateral branches.

the animal operating room. An alternative technique is to use Hypnorm (Janssen Pharmaceuticals) and then hold the animal in a restraining cage and induce anaesthesia with halothane delivered via a mask from a Boyles machine. A useful index of the depth of anaesthesia is the position of the eyes. During safe and deep anaesthesia the eyes of the pig roll down, exposing the white sclera. In deeply anaesthetized animals the eyes roll back, exposing the pupils. The latter stage should be avoided, and if and when encountered necessitates the temporary cessation of anaesthesia. The anaesthetized animal is then transferred to the operating table for endotracheal intubation. This may be difficult unless approached methodically, as the epiglottis of this animal is long and normally overlies the larynx. The steps for safe endotracheal intubation of the pig are as follows:

1 Introduction of a laryngoscope with a long blade (10 cm), which is initially used to depress the tongue. This reveals the closed epiglottis.

2 The laryngoscope blade is used to lift the folded epiglottis.

3 The epiglottis is held down with the laryngoscope to reveal the larynx, which should be wide open if the animal is deeply anaesthetized.

4 The endotracheal tube is inserted into the trachea and the balloon inflated.

The most important causes of failure to intubate are insufficient depth of anaesthesia and failure to lift the epiglottis off the larynx. If the first attempt is not successful, it is wise to sedate the animal further or administer more halothane before further attempts at intubation are made.

If problems are encountered intubating the pig in the supine position, it may be rolled prone and the snout lifted up into the 'sniffing the morning air' position. Particular care should be taken not to injure the fingers, as the hard palate of the pig is rather sharp and painful cuts may be sustained.

Endotracheal anaesthesia is maintained with a mixture of halothane, nitrous oxide and oxygen, using a rebreathing circuit (including carbon dioxide absorbent) with the animal breathing spontaneously. In the authors' experience the use of muscle relaxants is not necessary. Some prefer to use intermittent injections of barbiturate to maintain the depth of anaesthesia. The animal should be monitored with an electrocardiogram during anaesthesia, and a warming blanket should be placed over the thorax as these animals are sensitive to hypothermia, especially for long procedures. It is important to carefully shave an area for application of the electrocautery plate, or good contact will not be made. To make the procedure more palatable for the surgeons, delousing powder should be applied to the pig at some stage, although the surgeon should not be too concerned as pig lice are unable to survive on human skin.

Cholecystectomy in the pig

The surgeon should initially master a safe technique for insufflation of the peritoneal cavity with carbon dioxide using an electronic insufflator. The Veress needle is introduced into the midline, three-quarters of the way down in sows and 2 cm proximal to the penis in boars, or alternatively in the left iliac fossa in the male. The peritoneal cavity is insufflated to a preselected pressure of 12–15 mmHg. The Veress needle is then withdrawn and the wound enlarged and deepened by an artery forceps and an 11 mm trocar introduced. It is useful for the student to practise the technique of open laparoscopy, whereby a mini-laparotomy is made, stay sutures are placed and a blunt trocar is introduced and held in place by the stays.

The prewarmed telescope attached to the camera is then inserted and used to visualize the peritoneal cavity and identify the gallbladder. Often this is obscured because of the multilobed nature of the pig's liver. Not infrequently the stomach is found to be distended with swallowed air. As this obscures the operative field it should be deflated, although it is extremely difficult to place a nasogastric tube in the pig. Therefore, the Veress needle may be introduced through a separate incision into the pig's stomach, with the awareness that this is a thick-walled organ and that force will be necessary. The gas can then be suctioned out. Although it is more difficult to use the 30° forward oblique telescope, it is worthwhile gaining experience with this early in the introduction to laparoscopic surgery.

The accessory cannulae are then introduced under visual control as follows:

1 An 11 mm trocar/cannula in the midline just below the lower margin of the liver.

2 A 5 mm cannula on the right side of the lateral edge of the rectus, just below the level of the subxiphisternal trocar.

3 A further 5 mm trocar/cannula well laterally in the right paracolic gutter, almost on the level with the cannula through which the telescope is introduced (Fig. 1.5).

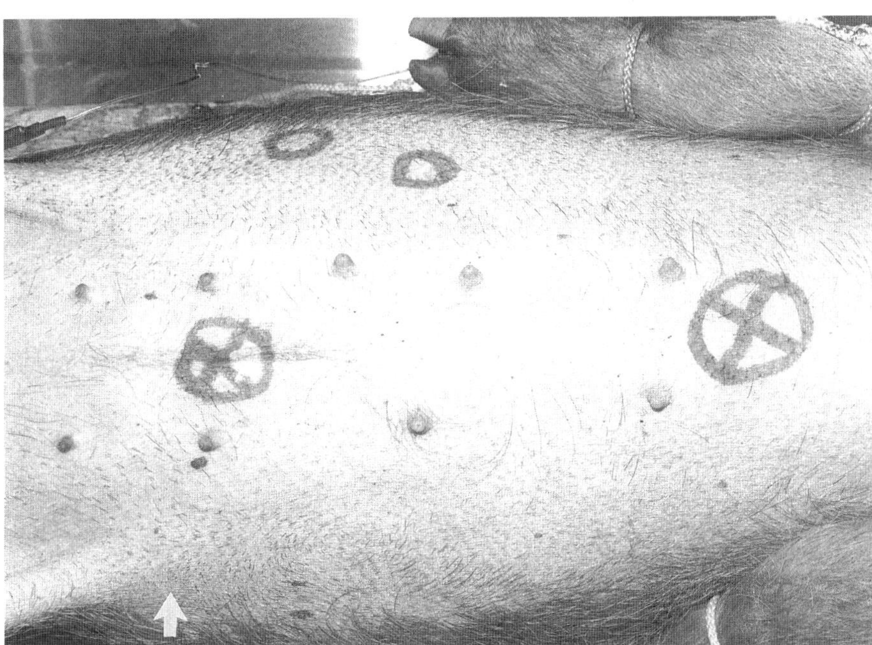

Fig. 1.5 The trocar insertion sites for porcine cholecystectomy. ⊗ = 10/11 mm; ○ = 5 mm. In the male, the left iliac fossa is preferable for the trocar which houses the laparoscope (arrowed).

Two graspers are introduced through the 5 mm cannulae. The lateral one is used to grasp the fundus of the gallbladder, thus putting the organ on a stretch in a cephalic direction. The medial grasper is applied to the neck of the gallbladder, which is tilted upwards thus exposing the cystic pedicle.

It is vital that the telescope follows the introduction and exit of every surgical instrument as this prevents inadvertent injury. Because good camera work is vital for the completion of the operation and a tendency to wander is frequent, it is useful to draw a square on the television screen with a white wax pencil. The camera operator is then charged with maintaining the target area within the white square, which helps to concentrate his or her mind on the task at hand.

The dissecting instrument (electrosurgical hook, blunt-nose scissors) is inserted through the 11 mm cannula after the prior insertion of a reducer tube or seal. When using a clip applier this is obviously introduced through the same 11 mm cannula without the reducer.

It is initially very useful to divide the loose areolar connections between Hartmann's pouch and the liver, first on the lateral and then on the medial side of the gallbladder. The cystic arteries may then be carefully freed both medially and laterally, and either clipped or tied and then divided in turn. Using blunt dissection the junction of the cystic duct and gallbladder may then be isolated, and early in the experience clipped, although later an extracorporeal tie may be used here.

The surgeon should then grasp Hartmann's pouch from the substernal portal and incise the cystic duct with the curved microscissors making an oblique cut. He or she should attempt to cannulate the cystic duct using the 3 Fr. ureteric catheter, which may be facilitated by passing a guidewire through this. Thus the surgeon may practise the skill required to perform cholangiography. Once this has been accomplished, the gallbladder should again be grasped from the lateral portal and the cystic duct remnant clipped or tied.

Once Hartmann's pouch has been elevated from the hepatic parenchyma is useful to practise application of the pretied Roeder catgut loop, as described later in the book. The removal of the gallbladder from the liver bed is an excellent opportunity for the surgeons to practise teamwork, as by retracting the gallbladder laterally the medial aspect is exposed and by moving it medially the lateral aspect is available for dissection. Prior to complete removal of the gallbladder, the liver bed should be inspected and irrigated, and the cystic artery and duct stumps should be closely inspected. Once freely dissected, the cystic duct end of the gallbladder should be firmly grasped by the lateralmost portal.

As the parietal peritoneum is a pain-sensitive structure it may be anaesthetized with a local anaesthetic, and this may be practised by injecting saline through the abdominal wall until a wheal is raised in the peritoneum. The telescope should be moved to the substernal trocar cannula, and the gallbladder may be removed from the umbilical trocar site.

Electrosurgical safety

Many surgeons are unfamiliar with the characteristics of monopolar electrosurgical generators, and it will be useful for them to see the different tissue effects under laparoscopic control with a coagulation setting. For instance, if the entire surface area of the dissecting instrument is placed on the liver and a short coagulation burst applied, there will be gradual heating and desiccation seen. However, if just the tip of the instrument is applied, more of an arcing current is seen, as the same current is passed through a smaller surface area. This will enable the surgeon to modulate the tissue effect, which is of value in deciding how he or she wishes to dissect in laparoscopic surgery.

Problem solving

It is useful during the training course for the instructor to simulate problems which may arise in human surgery, and see how the students cope with them. The following are examples:

1 The instructor should surreptitiously turn off the gas supply. The students will learn to keep a close eye on the insufflator, as they will gradually lose visualization. The most common cause of loss of view during laparoscopic surgery is a failure of the pneumoperitoneum. The students should be taught how to change gas tanks, gaskets, etc.

2 A haemostat clamp may be placed on the insufflation cable. This will cause the insufflator to show a constant pressure but gradually the pneumoperitoneum will be lost. This will cause some consternation to the students, as they will be receiving conflicting information. This nicely simulates the circumstance where an innocent member of the operating room team stands on the insufflation cable, thereby obstructing it.

3 The instructor should pull a cable out of the television or video camera control unit and allow the students to re-establish appropriate linkages.

4 Bleeding should be created by severing the cystic artery, and the instructor may then demonstrate how control may be retained by moving the fundal grasper to Hartmann's pouch and using this to grasp the artery, which may then be safely clipped.

5 Gallstones may be placed inside the abdomen and may be gathered by the students in a fibroid scoop forceps, placed inside a laparoscopic bag and retrieved.

6 The gallbladder, once grasped after removal from the liver, should be deliberately dropped and the pig moved around. The student should then have to make a careful search for the displaced organ. In ideal circumstances fluoroscopy may be used to locate the clip placed on Hartmann's pouch.

7 Bleeding of the trocar insertion site may be implied, and the students should then learn to place a through-and-through purse-string suture with a straight needle and non-absorbable suture.

Common bile duct exploration

In order to prepare the neophyte laparoscopic surgeon for common duct surgery, he or she should initially work in a common bile duct phantom box, and this will teach the necessary skills to manipulate the 3.2 mm nephroure-throscope baskets and accessory instruments (Fig. 1.6). Once this has been mastered, the animal model is useful in two regards. First, the surgeon may use the same technique as would be used in the clinical setting, that is, to dilate the cystic duct with a ureteral dilation balloon over a guidewire and then insert the scope via an 11 Fr. Hickman line introducer. Alternatively, a loop of small bowel may be isolated and suspended from the abdominal wall by a polypropylene suture, which simultaneously occludes the lumen over a 10 cm length. This loop of bowel may then be incised and thereby represent the common bile duct. Stones may be placed into this prior to endoscopy. A combination of these techniques will prepare the student for laparoscopic common duct exploration.

Residency training

Initial experience in training residents in laparoscopic surgery suggests that the techniques that have always been used are equally appropriate to laparoscopic surgery. The resident should be exposed to didactic education and then should work on training boxes, just as their more senior colleagues will do. The apprentice technique of training is perfectly suitable, as the resident may initially become involved in cases as camera operator, and may then incorporate their hand–eye coordination skills from the training box by graduating to first assistant after a suitable number of cases. When simple elective cases present themselves to a resident who has experienced a

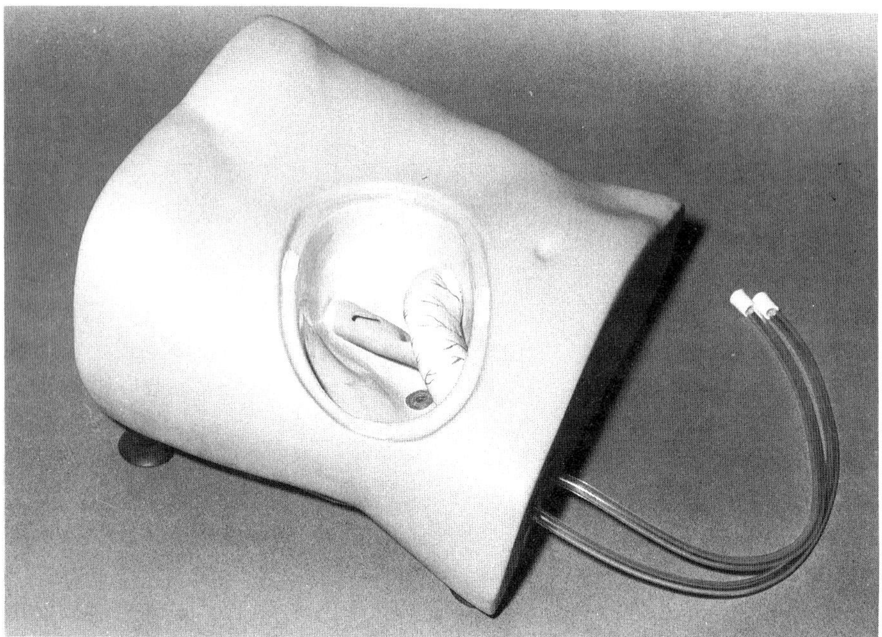

Fig. 1.6 The skills of choledochoscopy may be developed in a common duct trainer.

suitable number of cases as an assistant, they may work as primary surgeon as long as an experienced laparoscopist is available to teach.

In skilled hands, the operation of laparoscopic cholecystectomy flows smoothly with minimal blood loss and minimal scarring, and it is an extremely gratifying procedure to perform. The uninitiated may believe that the apparently untraumatized patient is representative of a minor procedure; however, such a degree of competence does not occur by accident but by careful and considered training. To this end high standards must be set for those wishing to become laparoscopic surgeons.

Future training techniques

As technology becomes increasingly incorporated into surgical practice, it is likely that this will affect surgical education. Initially we may see the development of superior phantom boxes, which instead of being manufactured from perspex will consist of a 'skin' which closely parallels the consistency of the human integument. Thus the techniques of pneumoperitoneum could be learnt and silastic organs could be dissected free inside such a box.

It is then likely that computer simulations will be developed, rather along the lines of driving or flight simulators which are interactive in nature. Thus, a surgeon could be exposed to a wide range of clinical presentations before ever touching a live patient.

Whatever developments visionary engineers and scientists make available, future surgeons will still need an excellent working knowledge of anatomy and all its varying presentations, and the principles of retraction, exposure and tissue manipulation, if he or she is to be a safe and competent laparoscopic surgeon.

2 : Imaging systems for laparoscopic surgery

Laparoscopic surgery is an outgrowth of the increasing combination of endoscopic and video-imaging systems, which enables more ambitious operative endoscopic undertakings than were possible without the addition of video co-observation [1]. These procedures are impossible to perform without the coordinated assistance that TV provides. The required presence of a video-imaging system with the addition of a recording medium permits the simultaneous boon of intraoperative documentation.

Advantages of video techniques

Television imaging is an integral part of these procedures in the following ways:

1 A common observed image enables the surgeon to correlate his movements with the assistant surgeon's help for more competent execution.

2 It permits the scrub nurse or technician to anticipate the surgeon's instrumentation needs.

3 It guarantees the safe introduction of instruments under visual control.

4 It aids in establishing anatomical orientation.

5 Pathology can be easily clarified to the screen's magnification.

6 The anaesthetist remains informed as to the procedure's progress.

7 A permanent record of the findings may be obtained, to be reviewed on subsequent occasions.

Perioperative considerations

This chapter cannot hope to encompass an extensive overview of all the equipment available for documentation. Instead, the system developed at the Cedars–Sinai Medical Center, Los Angeles, with its attendant advantages and limitations, will be described. Concise notes on some of the current technological developments will follow.

Laparoscopic surgery requires an optimal combination of telescope, camera, monitors and recording equipment, but it also demands skilled, knowledgeable workers. Once all the necessary equipment, from instruments and catheters to cameras and carts, has been acquired, operating-room staff have to be trained in its proper use. The authors are fortunate in possessing a surgical endoscopy unit staffed with technicians who have been specifically trained to perform endoscopic procedures and maintain endoscopic instrumentation. Even so, when totally new procedures, such as laparoscopic cholecystectomy and appendectomy for example, are introduced, repeated training sessions are held, both didactic and practical in content. The staff are also monitored during cases until all parties have established a predetermined level of competence at their new assignments. This is also true for registered nurses and operating room technicians who scrub in on the cases.

One very special position is that of the camera operator, because regardless of whether the telescope is held by the scrub nurse or the second assistant, that person becomes the surgeon's eyes and his or her performance is crucial to operative success. The second assistant must be shown in advance how to focus, white-balance and orientate the camera to the telescope. In this way a smooth running procedure can be ensured. At the authors' teaching hospital, house staff begin their operating-room training in laparoscopic surgery as second assistants, a position that affords them an excellent opportunity to assimilate anatomy and surgical expertise in the front ranks, so to speak, rather than blindly holding a retractor, as in open surgery.

The operating theatre's physical setup has to be considered, and an arrangement designed that is most comfortable for the operating team yet does not interfere with the aseptic field. The placement of other ancillary equipment (xenon light, insufflator, irrigation pump, etc.) has to be integrated into the available floor space while keeping in mind the logistic requirements of an adequate traffic flow pattern.

For laparoscopic cholecystectomy for example, we are at present utilizing a two-monitor approach, one placed on each side of the patient. The main TV cart, which holds a 48.3 cm high-resolution monitor, a 12 mm VHS recorder, a 19 mm recorder, and at times a video printer, stands on the patient's right close to the anaesthesia cart. This angle provides the operator with a comfortable straightforward view. The first assistant works from a 33 cm high-resolution monitor placed at the head of the table, on the patient's left. In an effort to consolidate carts and save space within the operating theatre, this monitor sits on the top shelf of the insufflator stand, which also holds a small irrigation pump. A larger monitor would compel the use of an additional cart, thus taking up precious floor space. These two monitors are looped together, with an additional ceiling-mounted monitor at the back of the room which allows the support staff to follow the case (Fig. 2.1).

Basic optical concepts

When the surgeon looks at an organ, light reflected from that organ passes through the cornea and aqueous humour, on through the pupil of the iris and into the lens, which is clear and is shaped and orientated something like a camera. In order for the image to come into focus, the light must be bent so that the rays converge at the fovea, the retina's centre. Visual sensation occurs when the retina is stimulated by a type of radiant energy called light. Night vision is achromatic vision. Similarly, a typical half-inch camera will lose colour as light is diminished. Visual perception may depend on the concurrent processing of multiplexed temporal messages from all visual areas [2]. By affording surgeons a well-illuminated binocular—albeit two-dimensional—video image from which to carry out a procedure, we improve upon the endoscope's monocular view and the viewer's visual adaptation

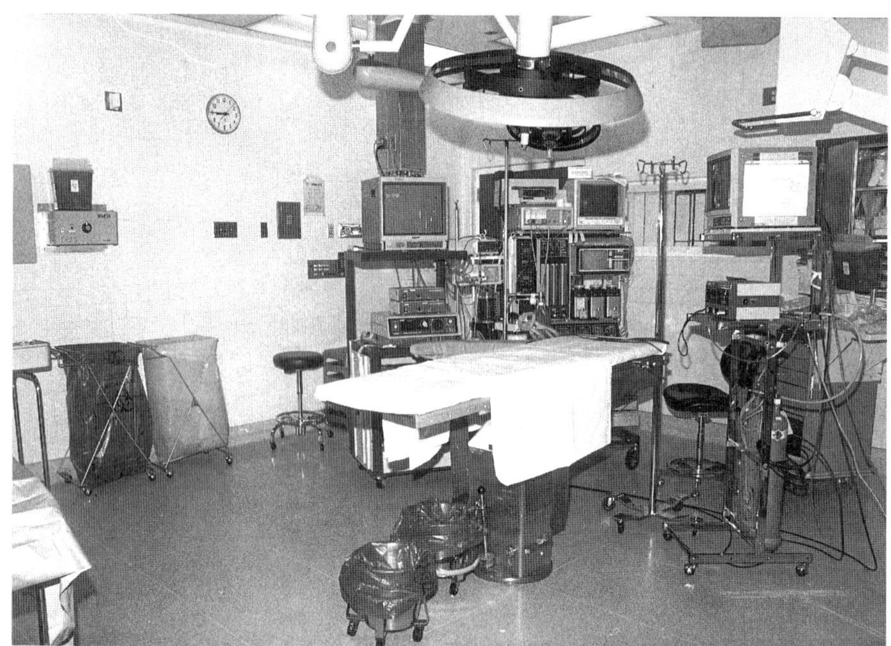

Fig. 2.1 The typical room arrangement for laparoscopic biliary surgery.

and perception by furnishing a binocular picture at an optimal viewing distance from an appropriately bright screen.

Equipment

Documentation is only useful if it is well performed, and in the operating room successful chronicling of significant events must be achieved by the simplest, most efficient method possible. The equipment chosen for our laparoscopic surgery carts has consistently functioned well, delivering high-quality results with regularity. Additionally, with proper training, its operation is not so complex that operating-room technicians and nurses are intimidated by it and thus reluctant to use it. A brief description of each piece and its function follows, along with comments on some of the emerging new technology.

Light source

To fulfil the physician's needs for permanent endoscopic records which are both easy to procure and of excellent quality, the development of new illumination sources has had to go hand-in-hand with new instrumentation. In instruments, the approach to increasing light has been the design of larger endoscopes incorporating more fibres. Halogen lamps, various flash bulbs and high-intensity light sources have culminated in the present standard, an automatic xenon high-intensity light source. This light unit, with its 300 W lamp is still the brightest, most dependable unit available for use with rigid endoscopes. The lamp combines xenon short-arc technology with special ceramic-to-metal sealing techniques. The internal reflector is prealigned, and results in a large collection angle around the arc, thus maximizing output efficiency. Further, it has excellent transmission from the ultraviolet to the infrared. As has previously been reported [3], this unit provides automatic light control for TV while also acting as a flash generator suitable for still photography (35 mm slides).

Monitors

The dependence of the operative team on the video image during all aspects of the procedure demands that the monitor on which this image is viewed should be of the highest quality. The picture should be flicker-free, with sufficient contrast and resolution. Currently, we employ a 48.3 cm high-resolution colour video monitor opposite the primary surgeon, and a 33 cm version of the same monitor for the assistant. Both monitors furnish approximately 700 lines of horizontal resolution, contrasted with only 350 lines on a standard monitor. In a room dedicated to laparoscopic surgery, monitors might be ceiling-mounted on rotating fixtures to allow positioning anywhere around the table. New portable digital X-ray units obviate the need for fixed room installations, and thus free up the ceiling for video.

Cameras

Essential to any endoscopic procedure is a lightweight, well-constructed camera which may be gas-sterilized or soaked in preparation for the daily caseload. The silicon charge-couple device (CCD) is the hub of all CCD imaging systems [4]. Conforming in a tightly packed grid of photocell receptors, each receptor generates a pixel (the smallest picture element unit of an image). The number of pixels that can fit on a chip determines its resolution. The average chip used in solid-state cameras today contains 250 000 – 380 000 pixels.

Because microtechnology is escalating so rapidly, we no longer use the cameras that only last year were considered state of the art. A new 16 mm CCD chip is the basis of our current model, combining the light sensitivity necessary in the upper abdomen with superior colour interpretation. The sensor is an 8.8×6.6 mm interline transfer CCD chip containing approximately 379 000 pixels. Its horizontal resolution is listed as greater than 450 lines and it has a signal-to-noise ratio of 47 dB. It is offered as a detachable camera with a built-in zoom lens that ranges from 25 to 38 mm. The camera head measures 34 mm in diameter by 86 mm in length, and weighs 4.5 ounces. This camera offers an automatic shutter feature which is more accurate than those we have tried in the past. The camera head and connecting cable may be cold-soaked or gas-sterilized. This is the camera model we routinely use on almost all procedures with satisfactory results as we continue to search for improved products (Fig. 2.2).

In addition to the 16 mm chip camera, we have recently evaluated 3-CCD cameras, which show great potential. They consist of three interline transfer

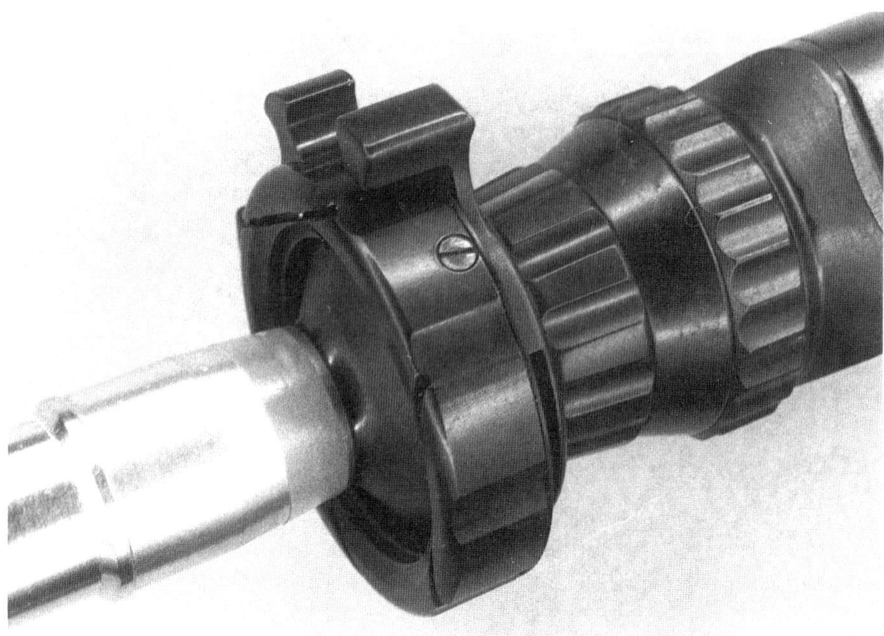

Fig. 2.2 A video camera's endocoupler attached to a laparoscope's eyepiece in close-up.

CCDs and an F5.6 ultraminiature primary colour (RGB) separation system. Endoscopic lenses in fixed focal lengths ranging from 22 mm to 40 mm are available, but a zoom lens encompassing all focal lengths has not yet been developed for these cameras. The sensing area measures 8.8 mm × 6.6. mm, which is equivalent to the 16 mm optical format. Each colour channel has 768(H) × 493(V) picture elements for a total of 1 135 782 pixels in the American NTSC format, and 1 369 998 pixels in the PAL European format. According to the manufacturer's specifications, horizontal resolution (luminance) is > 600 lines. When the camera's automatic gain control is switched on, shutter speed selection is reasonably fast and accurate. When coupled to an RGB monitor, three CCD cameras give a remarkably clear, bright, crisp image.

Unfortunately, three-chip cameras have proven, in their original configuration, to be too sensitive to overheating and chip displacement. Significant engineering redesign has been required before they could be used routinely in the field. The camera head weighs considerably more than that of a single-chip head and can become uncomfortable for the camera operator. A unit's costs is approximately two or three times that of most one-chip cameras, therefore its potential benefits must be carefully weighed against its drawbacks. The ideal solution would be a single-chip camera that could deliver an image comparable with that of three-chip cameras.

Several manufacturers are offering cameras that dispense with the traditional eyepiece, coupling the sensor to the ocular 'glass to glass', and eliminating a space where condensation and subsequent fogging might occur. It can also present a crisper, brighter image. Among the models we have used to conduct clinical trials, our preference lies with a variation in which camera and ocular are hermetically sealed within a hand grip. Using a fixed-focus lens, focus and exposure are automatic, freeing the second assistant from constant zoom adjustment and refocusing.

In some instances, such as laparoscopic common duct exploration, it is desirable to employ a second camera on the flexible choledochoscope, while retaining the abdominal image through the laparoscope for dilatation, scope introduction and orientation. As an alternative to having yet another cart in the operating room, a digital mixer can be used, which can split the screen and bring in the two video images side by side. Once programmed, the mixer's joystick allows the viewer to see both images or only one as needed. There are also some control units that power two camera heads simultaneously, but only one camera image at a time can be viewed.

One major manufacturer has introduced a flexible laparoscope aimed primarily at thoracoscopy, as they continue developing a videoscope similar to those used by gastroenterologists. Within the thoracic cavity's limited space, the ability to flex the scope's tip over 100° could be advantageous. They couple this model with their 1.2 mm chip camera for added light sensitivity. Several versions of a video laparoscope with a CCD imaging chip at the distal end are being marketed. Although adequate videotapes have been generated with these new models, our personal clinical experience with early prototypes suggested that additional time needed to be spent in their design to facilitate ease of operation. This is an area in which industry has been very active, and new, improved models are to be expected within the next 2 years.

At the prototype stage is a new high-definition camera system with an endoscopic adapter which may be coupled with standard endoscopes. The 1125-line HDTV display can provide horizontal resolution about five times that of standard video output. Some limited, promising clinical trials have been performed. A closed-circuit environment, such as an operating room, might actually be using HDTV quite soon given the pace of development. Already available for computerized design applications are workstations that incorporate HDTV display with almost 2 million pixels-worth of information, more than six times the relative size of standard NTSC television or VGA graphics.

A new development in solid-state imaging is a hole accumulator diode (HAD) sensor which tenders broader dynamic range and lower dark current, along with a new electronic shutter which executes charge separation within each individual pixel. This new HAD sensor can accommodate light levels up to 600% of normal exposure. Endoscopically, this would mean a clean noiseless view of pericolic gutters, while simultaneously controlling excessive highlights from the falciform ligament or stomach without blooming. In the newest version, HyperHAD, each pixel is capped with its own convex lens. Almost 100% of the light reaches the sensor's imaging area, thus augmenting sensitivity one full f-stop. Because OCL focuses almost all incident light, stray light reflection from insensitive imager elements is reduced, practically eliminating vertical smear [5].

In a remarkable feat of engineering, Sony has further miniaturized pixel size, so that the 1.2 mm HyperHAD chip carries the same number as their earlier 16 mm chip—378 624 (768 × 493).

Prototypes for one-chip and three-chip cameras based on these new sensors already exist. They provide sharper images, with over two stops' increased light sensitivity. Further design modifications include edge enhancement, which, to the observer, dramatically sharpens the image by straightening the edges on the picture elements. When the image from a single-chip prototype with edge enhancement was compared visually with that of a three-chip (also HyperHAD) prototype, observers unilaterally decided in favour of the one-chip camera. Final models are expected later this year.

Permanent records

Images can be stored on film in an analogue form, on still video disks, or on videotape. Images can also be digitized for storage on magnetic or optical media. It would be possible to store patients' records, X-rays, and specimen or operating-room photographs on photo CDs, thus creating an integrated database. Once on CD, images may be displayed on computer or video screens, transmitted over phone lines, and hard copies made using electronic or digital printers. They can be utilized in video conferences for consultation and education. A present limitation for us with the three-chip cameras is our current video-recording arrangement. We routinely record procedures for teaching, lecture and consultation on 19 mm U-matic format. Our laboratory is equipped with a cuts-only 19 mm videotape editing suite which allows us to prepare lecture tapes at short notice, as postproduction work prints in preparation for final editing at outside facilities. This system has a resolution of approximately 270 lines and is not capable of recording an RGB signal, through which the three-chip camera delivers its best pictures.

We are therefore faced with the additional expense of adding Super-VHS, ED Beta or Hi-band 8 mm video recorders to our carts, which would allow us to record at a horizontal resolution of over 400 lines. Additionally, a complete new editing suite would have to be purchased to enable us to work with these high-resolution tapes. Then, when lecturing outside our institution, there would be the concomitant problem of finding compatible machines in a lecture hall. For example, while regular VHS tapes may be played on a Super-VHS machine, the reverse is not true. The 19 mm U-matic format has the current advantage of being almost universally available.

Videotape recorders

Videotape recording is a common documentation method. It is possible to record either an entire procedure or selected highlights. The videotape record may be analysed at length, and may be edited for lectures and presentations. Our video carts are equipped with two videotape recorders interconnected into the system, so that either may be used without any need for repatching coaxial cables. The first videocassette recorder is a Sony VO-5800 19 mm U-matic recorder which is employed whenever a good resolution recording is desired for subsequent editing, particularly for teaching tapes. Since a 1-hour 19 mm U-matic cassette costs about four times the price of a 2-hour VHS cassette, requires more than twice the storage space and must be played back on a more expensive, less readily available 19 mm system, we have also obtained a Panasonic AG-6300 12 mm VHS recorder for routine applications. These tapes are retained by the individual surgeons, most of whom have access to standard equipment. Both machines are professional models with real-time counters and variable visual search. A momentary-contact footswitch has been attached to both recorders to enable the surgeon to control the pause function during recording. The 19 mm videotapes have also been improved. For example, the Sony BRS and XBR series deliver superior performance, with a higher signal-to-noise ratio, fewer dropouts and enhanced audio performance. However, to maintain a video library consumes both time and space, requiring review, cataloguing, storage location and the personnel to accomplish these tasks.

A digital tape system was first introduced in 1986, mainly designed to capture computer graphics without any signal degradation. It did away with one of the worst liabilities of analogue tape, the significant loss of signal quality over several generations. Analogue video is a continuous electronic signal that fluctuates with the brightness (luminance) and colour (chrominance) of the video signal. In contrast, digital recording converts the analogue signal to a bitstream of 1 s and 0 s, then processes this stream into a low bandwidth signal for recording. The digital video recorder virtually eliminates dropouts because its method of error correction is superior to that used for analogue video. Digital recording overcomes most of the performance limitations that have always plagued magnetic and optical recording, and its performance levels are much more consistent. Given the many advantages of a digital system, the choice between it and analogue would seem obvious. However, digital equipment is still very expensive; operating it and even building a facility within a medical centre to accommodate it would cost considerably more than using analogue equipment, thereby placing it beyond the reach of most hospitals today.

Scanners

Scanning technology now serves as a gateway through which photographic images can enter the digital arena. It changes printed material to an electronic signal that computers can comprehend. As well as the scanner, processing software and a compatible computer in which to store images are needed. The scanning unit consists of a light source that transmits and reflects a narrow strip of the page being scanned by the scan head (optical sensor). Intercepting light as it passes over the item, the head then relays to the unit's CCDs. Each CCD's electrical charge is then converted from analogue to digital, so that it may be stored and processed.

One rapid film scanner can digitize and display representative colour images in 18 seconds from any 35 mm source, colour negative, colour transparency or black-and-white negative. Compression technology can achieve ratios up to 24:1, so that up to 300 images can be stored on an 80 megabyte hard drive.

Flatbed scanners with better linear arrays use new microlenses, increasing the resolution and colour depth of the electronic images. They are capable of scanning both reflective and transmissive copy in varying sizes. An inexpensive overhead video unit has a 300 000 pixel, 12 mm CCD sensor head positioned over the baseboard by a single column.

The digital image is not degraded by copying or duplicating, as is the analogue video recording. Therefore, digital image copies will be as good in resolution as the original exposure. The question of analogue versus digital is probably the most important single issue in the outlook of electronic still imaging, along with the final storage medium. The more quickly electronic information is converted to digital signals, the less opportunity other parts of the electronic image environment have to introduce image-degrading signals.

Perhaps the most prominent value of digital imaging is that the image data can be processed, manipulated, enhanced, sharpened, cleaned up and enlarged in a way that is inconceivable with analogue images.

Disk recorders

Disk recorders utilizing either floppy or optical disks provide an effective alternative way of storing endoscopic images. The highest-quality recording media available are optical-memory disk recorders which record stills onto a laser disk with a horizontal resolution of approximately 580 lines. Both Panasonic and Sony offer laser disk systems, but there is currently no compatible hardcopy device. Sony and Canon also make floppy disk recorders which allow up to 25 video frames or 50 fields (2 fields = 1 frame) to be recorded on a two-sided floppy disk. Disks take up far less storage space and retrieving stored data from earlier examinations is simple and quick. Images stored on disk may be previewed after a procedure, and specific frames selected and printed using a still video printer. At many institutions, physicians show these prints to patients and relatives directly after an examination, to explain findings graphically before inserting them in the chart [6,7].

As camera sensors slowly begin to approach silver-image quality however, the 2″ floppy disk may not be able to pack all the necessary electronic information for higher-resolution images into a required disk sector. It may be possible to reduce the number of exposures on one disk and enlist several disk sectors into one image, or to use electronic data-compression techniques to crowd more information into less space. Alternatively, one firm has designed a system which permits the recording of 14 000 high-resolution still images on a single 2-hour S-VHS tape.

Still video printers

Outstanding high-resolution hardcopy devices are expensive, prices beginning at \$20 000. More economical, lower-resolution colour hardcopy printers are available, differing in technique and price, from inkjets and dye-transfer thermal to dry electrostatic-charge printers. As with chip technology, printers have progressed through various generations, each fine-tuning and refining the printing process. At present, the most promising affordable unit is manufactured by Sony. The Mavigraph is an inkjet printer with a built-in laminator. An image can be printed full size (166.7 × 121 mm) or the sheet can be divided into 4–9 smaller spaces containing progressive stages and/or complementary stored data, such as X-ray or ultrasound scans, and inserted into the patient's chart. This printer has been reduced in dimension and cost, making it a more attractive package. We examined various printers in detail before making our final choice. Recently, a less expensive, more compact model which offers a more basic service has been introduced by the same manufacturer.

A new digital continuous-tone printer produces photo-quality full-colour or black-and-white prints from digital sources. It transfers cyan, yellow and magenta from its ribbon to the thermal medium. Individual heating elements control each pixel's dye density by modulating electrical impulses. This results in a true continuous-tone print.

By coupling a solid-state camera to an endoscope, we simplify not only the questions of operator performance and comfort, but also those of team participation and data storage. In more complex procedures, such as laparoscopic cholecystectomy, it is imperative that the assistant works from the same monitor image as the operator, thus ensuring accuracy of execution and expediting the procedure.

The future

At present imaging systems are adequate for the more basic surgical procedures, but more and more ambitious surgeries are envisaged. To further these aims, surgeon and staff training must become more continously intensive. Equally, the calibre of the instrumentation must improve to prevent the causing of unwitting injury. Research is already under way to furnish the surgical community with tools with which to work more unerringly in a remote fashion than is possible in open surgery today.

Our visual apprehension of the world is founded on two-dimensional images—flat patterns of varying light intensity and colour falling on a single plane of cells in the retina. Yet we come to preceive solidity and depth, because a number of cues about depth are available in the retinal image: shading, perspective, occlusion of one object by another and stereoscopic disparity. Using the right software, two cameras and new commercially available PC boards, stereoscopic video capability is now possible. Endoscopic images, when interpreted in 3-D stereo are easily discerned. The impact of stereopsis on enhanced viewer performance has been chronicled in several studies [8,9]. We refer here to field sequential stereoscopy, in which the display presents left and right perspectives, alternating rapidly (60 times per second per eye) so that each eye sees only its own viewpoint. The viewer must wear special glasses with high-performance liquid crystal lenses which are synchronized to the video field rate. These battery-powered glasses respond to an infrared emitter in the monitor which broadcasts the synchronization data. The system manifests a flickerless image for the viewer because it functions at twice the rate of traditional video arrays. One perceives a flicker-free stereoscopic image if each eye can behold 60 fields per second of its essential standpoint. Adapting stereoscopy to endoscopy is complicated by the need to maintain image orientation when the scope is rotated along its longitudinal axis. Nevertheless, prototype systems using laparoscopes are being bench tested already [10]. A true stereoscopic display would do away with the disorientation the surgeon feels when faced with a two-dimensional image on which he must operate. Computer simulation training modules have already been designed for gastroenterology [11]—can surgery be far behind?

From trying to improve the surgical milieu is it really so far-fetched for the next step to be that of creating a totally new environment in which surgeons may operate with a new freedom and acuity? Artificial realities allow users to interact with computers in an intuitive and direct format, and to increase the number of interactions per unit of time. The ultimate objective is to devise a simulated reality that not only seems as real as the reality it depicts, but allows us to go beyond reality to overcome problems which presently defeat us [12]. While more advanced work on surgical simulation is still being conceptualized, some 3-D treatment planning is being utilized to administer to patients [13]. Gloves that translate hand and finger movements into electrical signals exist today. Just as one day a robot outside a space station will be able to carry out complex manoeuvres and repairs by mimicking the hand movements of an astronaut inside the station, so will surgeons be able to operate within the body by deploying microrobots from a remote workstation [14]. Minimally invasive surgery, as well as imaging and recording methods, are currently in a state of flux which promises pivotal outcomes within the next decade.

References

1 Berci G, Brooks P, Paz-Partlow M. TV laparoscopy. *J Repro Med* 1986; **31**(7): 585–588.

2 McClurkin JW, Optican L, Richmond BJ, Gawne T. Concurrent processing and complexity of temporally encoded neuronal messages in visual perception. *Science* 1991; **253**: 675–677.

3 Paz-Partlow M. Documentation for laparoscopy. In: Berci G, Cuschieri A (eds) *Practical Laparoscopy*. Baillière Tindall, London 1986; pp. 19–32.

4 Boyle WS, Smith GE. Charged-couple semiconductor devices. *Bell Syst Tech J* 1970; **49**: 285–90.

5 Thorpe L, Dahlberg D. On-chip lens HyperHAD sensors for increased CCD sensitivity. *Adv. Im* 1991; **6**: 43–45.

6 Berci G, Paz-Partlow M. Electronic imaging in endoscopy. *Surg Endo* 1988; **2**: 227–233.

7 Stroehlein JR, Barrosso A, Giombicki A, Sachs I. Documentation of fluoroscopic and endoscopic images using a color video printer. *Gastrointest Endo* 1990; **36**(4): 392–394.

8 Wickens CD. Three-dimensional stereoscopic display implementation: guidelines derived from human visual capabilities. *SPIE* 1990; **1256**: 2–11.
9 Reinhart WF, Beaton RF, Snyder HL. Comparison of depth cues for relative depth judgements. *SPIE* 1990; **1256**: 307–311.
10 McLaurin AP, Jones ER, Mason JL. Three-dimensional endoscopy through alternating-frame technology. *SPIE* 1990; **1256**: 307–311.
11 Noar M. Endoscopy simulation. *Endo Rev* 1991; **8**(4): 8–28.
12 Foley JD. Interfaces for advanced computing. *Sci Am* 1987; **10**: 127–135.
13 Rheingold H. *Virtual Reality*. Summit, New York 1991; pp. 31–34.
14 Freedman DH. Invasion of the insect robots. *Disc* 1991; **3**: 42–50.

3 : Instruments and basic techniques for laparoscopic surgery

The surgeon skilled in open abdominal procedures will encounter three restrictions during the conduct of laparoscopic procedures. The first and major one is monocular/two-dimensional vision. When first experienced, this impairs automatic depth perception when viewing the operative field through the laparoscope or TV screen. Gradually, with practice and care, visual clues other than binocular vision allow the estimation of depth and accurate instrument coordination. Secondly, the perception of organ size is altered and this varies in accordance with distance from the viewing optics—the closer the optic the bigger the magnification. This requires their actual size to be assessed by reference to instruments or by a graduated probe introduced for this purpose. Thirdly, the movement of instrument tips, e.g. for cutting, grasping tissue and manipulating sutures, is limited because every manoeuvre is only possible through a fixed trocar sleeve, which allows mobility only around a fixed point. The range of movement of these instruments once inserted through the cannula is described by a cone (Fig. 3.1). Proficiency with the basic instrumentation, experience in diagnostic laparoscopy and manual dexterity are essential. Familiarity with a procedure at open operation is a prerequisite to its performance under these conditions. Furthermore, operative techniques should be perfected on a practice bench (trainer, phantom) which allows the realistic insertion of cannulae and instruments with practice tissue or substitutes placed underneath (see Chapter 1). Tissue manipulation, cutting, suturing and knot tying, both extracorporeal and intracorporeal, should all be practised. A good understanding of the limitations of these techniques will allow their safer use.

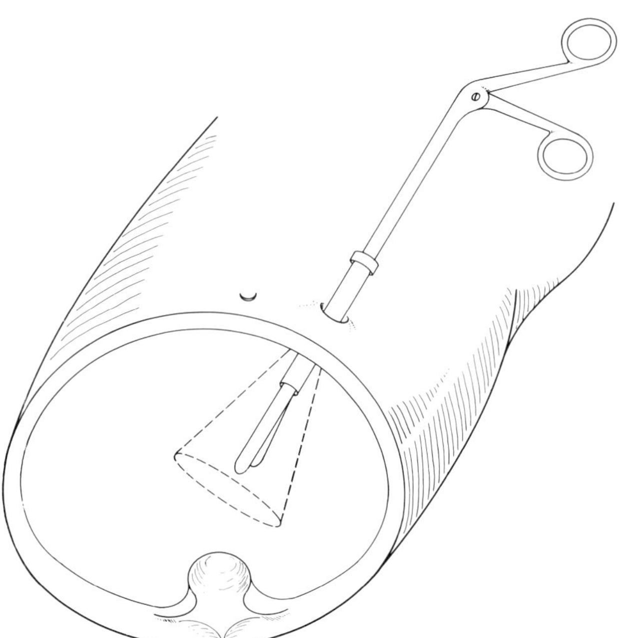

Fig. 3.1 The access port acts as a fixed point and the range of movement of the instruments inserted through it is described by a cone.

Many abdominal surgeons are uncomfortable during the initial phase of laparoscopic access into the peritoneal cavity, especially after previous laparotomy. It is for this reason that stress has been laid on the techniques of inducing a pneumoperitoneum and the insertion of the first cannula, especially when the presence of adhesions is suspected. With training, the right technique and the safe use of instruments, these procedures can be conducted with safety even in previously operated patients.

It is interesting to note that gynaecologists performing operative laparoscopy have noted a change in the trend of their surgery towards organ preservation, rather than ablation. In this respect, the avoidance of laparotomy (particularly repeated interventions) whenever possible is important in reducing morbidity from surgical treatment. Laparoscopy, by decreasing bowel handling and serosal drying, reduces the severity and duration of postoperative ileus. This, together with minimizing the extent of parietal wounds, is likely to decrease postoperative adhesion formation. In addition, the smaller, less painful wounds and smooth accelerated postoperative recovery render repeated intervention less problematic and more acceptable to the patient.

Exposure of peritoneal cavity and its contents

Patient position

The supine position is used for the creation of a pneumoperitoneum and manipulation of the small and large bowel. When a view is required of the stomach, liver and spleen, a head-up tilt of the table allows the bowel to move inferiorly by gravity. Conversely a good view of the pelvis is obtained by Trendelenburg tilt. If visualization of the bowel in the paracolic gutters is required, a lateral tilt (either left or right) is helpful. Care must be taken to stabilize the patient on the table during any tilting away from the horizontal. This is important to prevent pressure being exerted on unprotected limbs or bony points if a small amount of slipping occurs. Stabilization can be achieved by supports under the arms, stirrups or, better still, a safety belt that anchors the pelvis to the table. The head and arms are usually well supported by anaesthetic arm boards.

Nasogastric tube and indwelling urinary catheterization

Complete decompression of the stomach serves three purposes. During insufflation accidental penetration of the stomach is made less likely. Secondly, visualization of the liver, gallbladder and the free edge of the lesser sac is much easier. During reversal of anaesthesia, particularly during the danger period shortly after extubation, the risk of vomiting due to a stomach bloated with gas is minimized. In this respect the use of an adequate size nasogastric tube is important, i.e. Fr 14, to ensure adequate drainage. Duodenal air can impair the exposure of the cystic pedicle and common bile duct. This situation is remedied by the use of a Salem nasogastric sump tube, which is kept on low suction during the operation. The authors have found this simple manoeuvre to be particularly helpful in patients undergoing laparoscopic common bile duct exploration.

Catheterization of the bladder is a safe precaution during initial insufflation. This ensures that the extraperitoneal dome of the bladder lies inferiorly away from the periumbilical cannula insertion site. It is mandatory when pelvic procedures such as colectomy are contemplated.

Insufflation of the peritoneal cavity

Carbon dioxide is the standard gas used for most operative laparoscopy, largely because it does not support combustion. After absorption from the peritoneum, it is readily excreted via the lungs and if accidentally injected directly into a blood vessel, resulting in CO_2 embolism, this is more easily treated than air or nitrous oxide embolism (especially if the rate of insufflation is kept at 1.0 l/min). Of most importance in the setting of operative laparoscopy is the equipment used to deliver the CO_2 to the peritoneum. Optimum exposure is obtained with a constant pneumoperitoneum of 12.0–16.0 mmHg pressure. Operative laparoscopy entails the use of multiple cannulae and the frequent changing of instruments, with intermittent gas leakage throughout the procedure. The introduction of the automatic electronic insufflator (Fig. 3.2) has resolved this problem. This insufflator is capable of automatic flow rates of up to 8.0 l/min. Operative procedures without this machine are tedious and time-consuming. In addition, it provides good monitoring of the pressure within the abdomen, which can also be preselected and adjusted. Maintenance of a low intra-abdominal pressure is especially useful in women with lax abdominal walls following pregnancy, where very adequate visualization can be obtained with lower pressures of 10.0 mmHg. The benefit will be a decrease in postoperative shoulder-tip pain caused by diaphragmatic stretching.

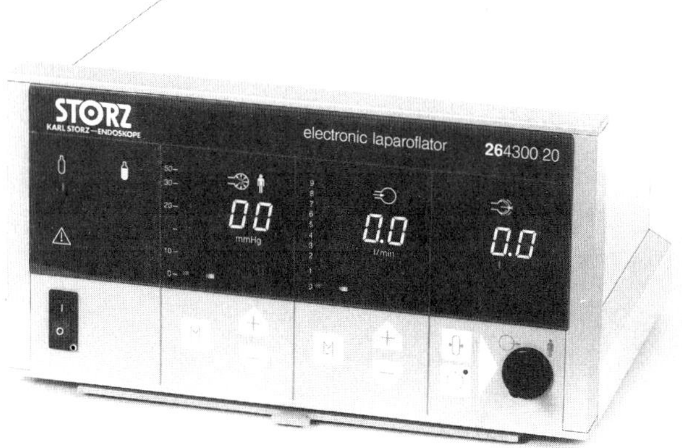

Fig. 3.2 Modern high-flow electronic pressure-controlled insufflator for laparoscopic surgery.

Placement of the Veress needle

The initial induction of the pneumoperitoneum is still most often performed with the Veress needle. The spring-loaded central trocar retracts as the needle encounters resistance, and retracts back on entering the peritoneal cavity. The function of the spring-loader snap mechanism should be confirmed prior to initial insertion, as should luminal patency, by checking the gas flow through it. The Veress needle is most often inserted at the subumbilical site, where the laparoscope trocar/cannula will be introduced. However, no hesitation should be felt in choosing a different site if subumbilical adhesions are suspected.

After the checks on the Veress needle, the *palpation test* is performed, to provide the surgeon with a clear idea of the depth required for insertion of the needle tip. This is achieved by finger-pressure palpation of the abdominal wall down to the aorta. This can be an alarmingly short distance in thin individuals.

The skin is then incised and the Veress needle inserted. The safest technique consists in holding the Veress needle along its shaft at a distance from the tip which is commensurate with the estimated abdominal wall thickness in the individual patient (Fig. 3.3). Held in this manner, the needle is 'threaded through' the parieties as the abdominal wall is lifted up. A definite click is felt as the rectus sheath is penetrated. More difficulty arises with judging parietal peritoneal penetration, as it tends to tent up with the needle. At this point clues to positioning are obtained as follows:

Aspiration test. A saline-filled syringe connected to the Veress needle is used next. Fluid instilled into the peritoneal cavity will flow away from the tip of the needle and cannot be aspirated back into the syringe. If fluid is aspirated back, an incorrect needle tip placement is likely. In addition if bowel content or blood is aspirated incorrect position of the needle tip is again obvious.

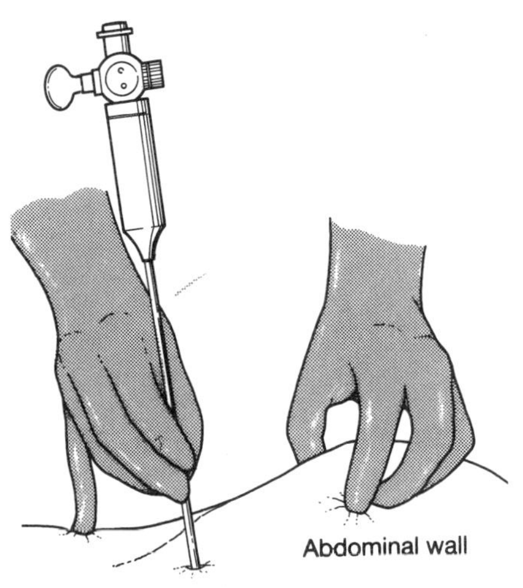

Fig. 3.3 Technique of safe insertion of the Veress needle. It is grasped along the shaft like a pencil and threaded through the parieties. Usually two 'gives' are felt — penetration of the anterior rectus sheath and penetration of the peritoneal lining.

Drop test. A more sensitive version of this manoeuvre is provided by the drop test. The tap on the Veress needle is closed and its terminal hub is filled with saline which forms a convex droplet due to its surface tension. This drop disappears down the shaft as soon as the tap is opened if the needle tip is lying free in the peritoneal cavity.

Negative pressure test. The tubing from the insufflator should next be connected to the Veress needle. Monitoring thc peritoneal pressure prior to any insufflation at this point will reveal a slight negative pressure easily accentuated by abdominal wall elevation.

Early insufflation pressures. The next clue to correct positioning is monitoring of the insufflation pressure, which should not exceed 8.0 mmHg at 1.0 l/min. The static pressure must not exceed 3.0 mmHg. Pressures greater than 15.0 mmHg with low or no flow of gas indicate incorrect needle tip position.

Some of the latest generation of electronic insufflators incorporate an automatic sensor system which signals the correct position of the needle tip when insufflation is commenced.

Volume test. In the average adult, the volume required to distend the peritoneum adequately and which creates a pressure of 10.0–12.0 mmHg is about 3.0 l of gas. If the static pressure as measured by the insufflator reaches these pressures with less than 1.0 l of gas, suspicion should arise that the needle tip is incorrectly placed. If this is extraperitoneal, it will often be accompanied by asymmetric anterior abdominal wall distension.

When using the electronic insufflator, once correct needle placement is assured and after a minimum of 1.0 l of gas has been insufflated, the machine can be switched to high flow to complete filling of the peritoneal cavity to approximately 10.0–15.0 mmHg pressure. At this point the Veress needle is withdrawn.

This sequence for insufflation, while not being essential in all cases, should be part of a routine carried out at every laparoscopy, be it diagnostic or operative. The establishment of a routine on the part of the operator and scrub nurse will lead to its rapid completion. Accidental misplacement of the needle leading to complications will then not be blamed on sloppy technique.

If during the induction of the initial pneumoperitoneum the needle tip is felt to be incorrectly positioned, the following steps should be taken. If the pressure test, volume test or aspiration test suggest extraperitoneal insufflation, the needle is simply withdrawn and reinserted. The number of passes required should be recorded in the operation notes. If blood is aspirated back then simple withdrawal of the needle and reinsertion is reasonable. However, if blood fountains back up the Veress needle, major vessel injury is likely and a laparotomy should be performed. If bowel content is aspirated, then the needle is withdrawn and reinserted in another site if local adhesions are suspected. In this event, it is important to inspect the area of bowel injury when the laparoscope is first introduced. If the hole in the bowel consists of a simple puncture, the administration of antibiotics and local lavage/suction followed by careful postoperative observation may be all that is required. More extensive injuries, for example when the bowel has been tangentially lacerated, require immediate suture repair either laparoscopically or by open operation.

In all cases an initial scan of the peritoneum and organs in the region of Veress needle insertion is mandatory. Any sign of retroperitoneal haemorrhage is suggestive of major vessel injury. Pneumo-omentum, CO_2 in the bowel mesentery or retroperitoneum can simply be left to resorb.

Safe induction of pneumoperitoneum in the presence of adhesions

This is an important consideration, as the risk of visceral and vascular injury is increased in the presence of intraperitoneal adhesions from previous surgical interventions. There is one simple preoperative test which is helpful. The preoperative detection and location of adhesions by ultrasound scanning, a simple and reliable technique, was developed by Sigel and colleagues [1] in Philadelphia. With the use of a 5.0 MHz linear probe, the 'visceral slide' is measured in the four quadrants of the abdomen. This consists of the movement of the bowel loops in relation to the abdominal wall with respiration and ballotment. Diminished slide at a particular spot indicates the presence of adherent bowel loops. The main aim of the test is to mark out exact spots which are free of adherent bowel loops. These represent 'safe sites' for insertion of the Veress needle. The efficacy and reliability of this technique was confirmed in a blind prospective study carried out at Ninewells Hospital [2]. The visceral slide test can be done preoperatively during the same session needed for ultrasound evaluation of the gallbladder and biliary tract, or in the operating theatre immediately before the start of the procedure.

The authors have found it extremely useful for the safe insertion of the Veress needle in patients with a scarred abdomen, and recommend its routine usage. In the absence of this facility, a quadrant away from the location of the scar is selected.

Insertion of initial trocar/cannula

The techniques used vary depending on the presence or absence of scars from previous surgery.

Intact abdomen

The site for insertion of the first trocar, which holds the laparoscope, is usually around the umbilicus. By preference, some use a disposable sheathed cannula (11.0 mm) for this purpose because of its alleged increased safety. However, care must be taken as injuries can still be caused by these cannulae due to the phenomenon of 'sheath drag' [3]. The use of the large 11.0 mm cannula (with 10.5 reducer flap) results in a wider space between the telescope and the inner wall of the cannula. This permits better gas flow and virtually guarantees the maintenance of an adequate pneumoperitoneum throughout the operation. All the other cannulae used are non-disposable, preferably of the flap-valve type.

Two approaches for the initial cannula insertion are possible: direct or 'Z' routes. However, if a pyramidal trocar is used this can only be introduced with safety directly through the linea alba. The 'Z' technique, which is only safe with the atraumatic conical system, entails advancement of the trocar/cannula through an initial subcutaneous path before passage of the instrument through the rectus abdominis. The advantages of the 'Z' technique include the avoidance of the weak linea alba and the creation of a shutter-type closure after withdrawal of the trocar. Its disadvantage in the context of laparoscopic cholecystectomy is enhanced difficulty of extraction of the gallbladder through the 'trap door', particularly when the stone load is large.

A direct tract through the linea alba is therefore preferable. In any event, the defect in the linea alba should be approximated by suture at the end of the procedure to decrease the risk of subsequent incisional hernia formation.

Scarred abdomen

In these patients special manoeuvres are needed. There are three options: the sounding test for adhesions prior to the insertion of cannulae, guided entry with a 5.5 mm cannula, or open laparoscopy.

Sounding test for adhesions (Fig. 3.4)

A 12.0 cm long 0.8 mm needle attached to a 50 ml syringe half-filled with saline is introduced perpendicularly through the abdominal wall in the region where initial trocar insertion is envisaged. As the needle is advanced, gas is slowly aspirated and continuous bubbling is observed in the syringe. This will stop suddenly when visceral peritoneum is touched. The level of the needle at the skin is then marked with a finger on the shaft, and the gas bubbling is observed as the needle is withdrawn until bubbling stops again. The distance the needle has been withdrawn to the point where bubbling stopped gives an accurate idea of the distance between visceral and parietal peritoneum. By repeating the procedure at 45° a mental picture of the underlying CO_2 cushion can be built up. The presence of omental or bowel adhesions is suggested by erratic variations in the size of the CO_2 cushion at different angles. This guide indicates an area for safe introduction of the laparoscope trocar.

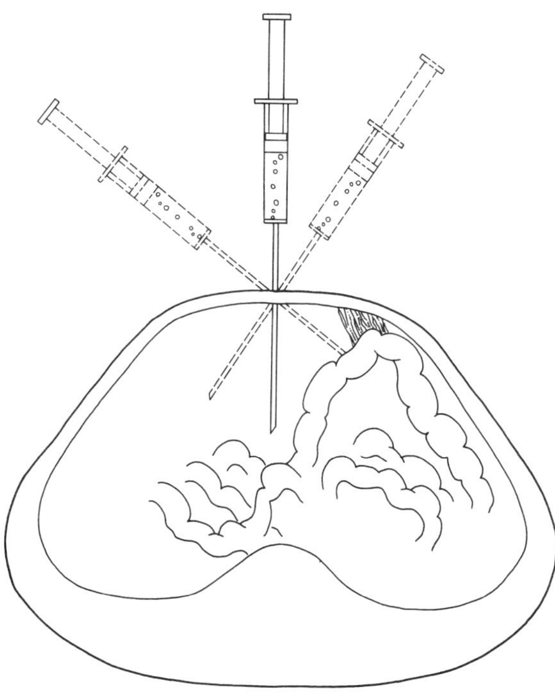

Fig. 3.4 Diagrammatic representation of the sounding test for adhesions. Constant bubbling ceases or becomes erratic once the needle tip impinges on adhesions, bowel or other tissue.

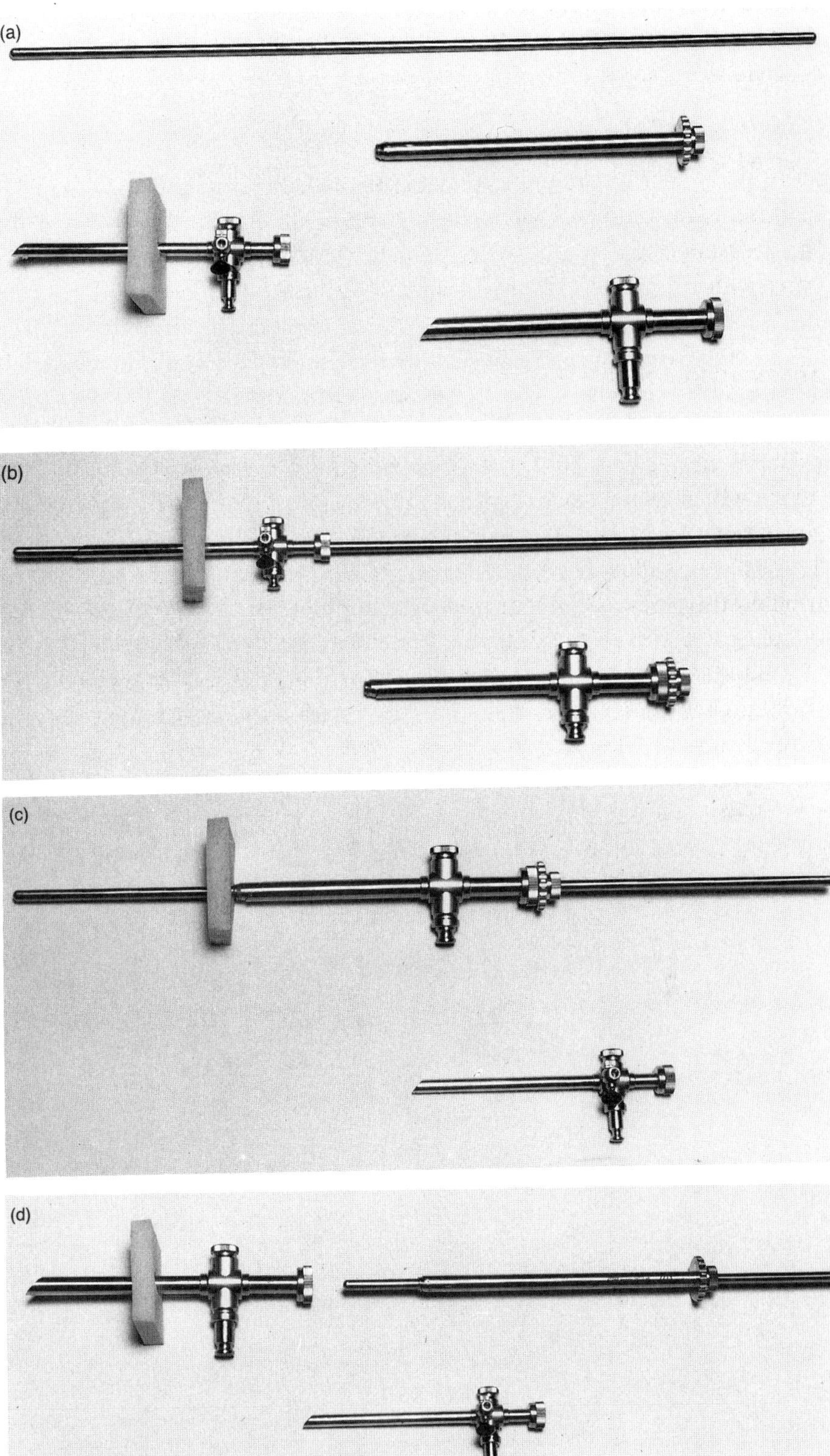

Fig. 3.5 Dilating system for replacing a 5.5 mm cannula with an 11.0 mm one. (a) Metal rod (5 mm); dilating tube (10 mm); 5.5 mm cannula in foam (representing abdominal wall; 11 mm cannula. (b) Metal rod inserted in 5.5 mm cannula; dilating tube inside 11 mm cannula. (c) The 5.5 mm cannula has been withdrawn over the rod and the dilating tube/11 mm cannula inserted over the rod. Using a rotational pushing movement, the assembly is threaded through the abdominal wall. (d) The rod and the dilating tube have been removed, leaving the 11 mm cannula *in situ*.

The risk and severity of organ trauma is further reduced if a 5.5 mm cannula is inserted in the first instance, and an initial scan of the underlying omentum, bowel and retroperitoneum is made to exclude injury. Once the surgeon is satisfied with the position, and the absence of iatrogenic damage, the small cannula is replaced by the 11.0 mm cannula using the trocar dilation system (Fig. 3.5).

Visually guided insertion

When the possibility of significant adhesions is high, as in patients who have had complicated or multiple previous surgical interventions, or when the sounding test suggests that bowel or omentum is adherent to the parietal peritoneum, insertion of the cannula tip should be done under vision (Fig. 3.6). This eminently safe technique, which is highly recommended in these difficult cases, is accomplished by the use of a 5.5 mm non-disposable cannula with a bevelled tip, which is inserted to just beyond the linea alba, such that its tip lies in the extraperitoneal fat if the direct route is used, or the rectus abdominis muscle if the 'Z' technique of insertion is adopted. The central trocar is then withdrawn and replaced with the 5.0 mm forward-viewing 0° telescope connected to the light source. Under vision and by gentle rotation, the cannula is advanced through the muscle and extraperitoneal fat until the peritoneum is reached. Intact peritoneum free of adhesions will appear as a translucent membrane with clearly visible small blood vessels on its surface. By contrast, in the presence of adherent bowel or omentum the peritoneum assumes an opaque appearance on transillumination with the

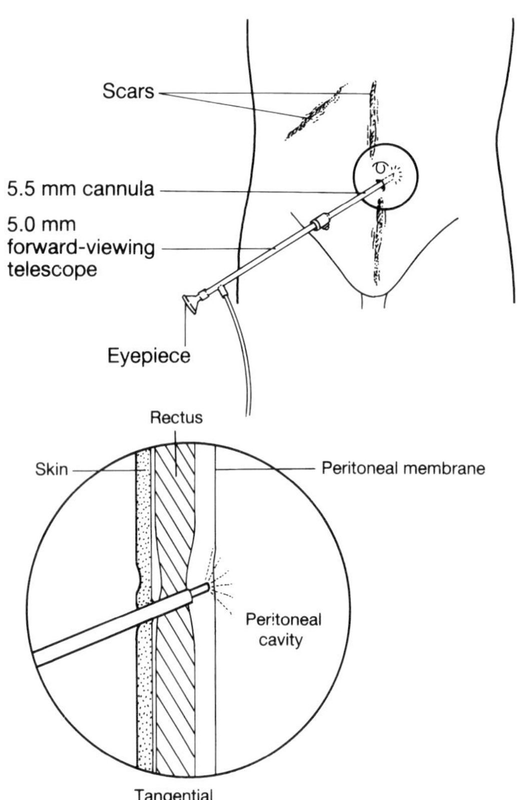

Fig. 3.6 Visually guided technique of safe insertion of 5.5 mm cannula into the peritoneal cavity in patients with multiple adhesions. The forward-viewing 5.0 mm telescope is used to transilluminate the peritoneal membrane. An opaque appearance indicates adhesions. A safe window through which the cannula can be inserted by rotation and wrist pressure is identified by a translucent appearance with fine leashes of blood vessels.

telescope. When this is encountered, the position of the cannula tip is altered until clear translucent peritoneum is visualized. This provides a 'safe window' for entry of the cannula into the peritoneal cavity. This is achieved by cannula rotation and gentle pressure from the wrist. Once the surgeon is satisfied that the 5.5mm cannula is correctly positioned, it may then be replaced with the 11.0 mm cannula using the trocar dilation technique.

Open laparoscopy

Finally, if the surgeon has no experience with the above techniques or when they cannot be used with safety, which is rare, open dissection down to the peritoneum should be considered—open laparoscopy.

Open laparoscopy

Open laparoscopy can be performed using an ordinary non-disposable cannula (without trocar) or, preferably, with the Hasson cannula first introduced in gynaecological laparoscopy in 1971 [4]. The modern version of this device (Fig. 3.7) has three components: a sliding olive which allows for variation in the length of the cannula inside the peritoneal cavity, fixation suture wings attached to the olive, and a blunt obturator.

There are some endoscopic surgeons who use open laparoscopy routinely in all cases, as it virtually abolishes the risk of major vascular injury,

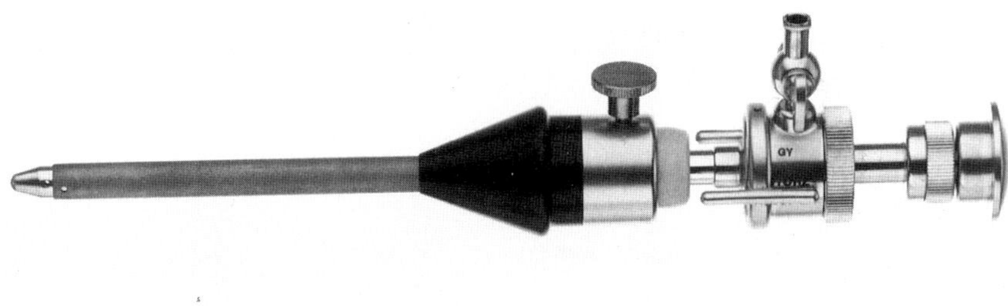

(a)

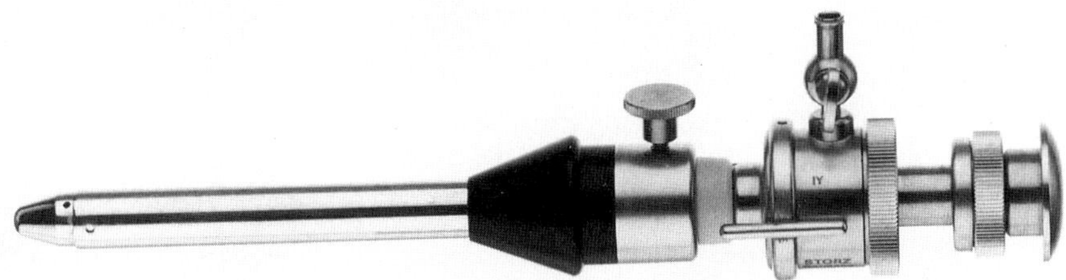

(b)

Fig. 3.7 Modern version of the Hasson cannula for open laparoscopy. (a) 8 mm; (b) 11 mm.

although injuries to the bowel may still occur. Others reserve it for difficult cases with adhesions. Either practice is perfectly acceptable, as the important consideration in endoscopic surgery is that the surgeon should practise what he is familiar with. Most of the criticisms, such as longer duration and higher incidence of umbilical wound complications (sepsis and hernia formation), are unfounded or unproven and its increased overall safety is unquestionable. Nonetheless, in the author's view it does have one disadvantage in patients with adhesions which has been overlooked. This concerns the siting of the incision in relation to the underlying adhesions. Problems are encountered if the exposure is made on top of or close to the adhesions. The division of these is then technically difficult unless the wound is enlarged. The insertion of a second trocar away from the site for endoscopic division of the adhesions is rendered difficult and dangerous. Thus the same considerations and tests to locate the position of adhesions and site the exposure accordingly are as important in open laparoscopy as they are in the closed procedure.

For the non-scarred abdomen, the standard site for insertion of the Hasson cannula is in the immediate subumbilical position through a vertical or horizontal wound (Fig. 3.8a). This is deepened to expose the umbilical raphe (Fig. 3.8b), which is then divided cleanly between two Allis forceps to open the peritoneal cavity. The peritoneal lining is adherent to the raphe in thin patients, but is separated from it by a layer of fat in obese patients. In these individuals care must be taken to avoid dissection between the peritoneal layer and the posterior rectus sheath. If an ordinary cannula is used a strong purse-string suture (00 polyamide or polydioxanone) is inserted around the fascial/peritoneal defect. This is tied firmly around the cannula after it is introduced into the peritoneal cavity without the inner trocar (Fig. 3.8c). Closure of the fascial defect is essential at the end of the procedure.

With the modified Hasson cannula, two interrupted sutures are placed at either end of the defect. After the cannula with blunt obturator is introduced into the peritoneal cavity, the sutures are tied to the wings attached to the side of the olive, which then seals the orifice (Fig. 3.8d). The olive's hold on the cannula is released and the cannula is slid inside the peritoneal cavity to the desired length before the hold is reapplied. At the end of the procedure, the retention sutures are tied to close the fascial defect.

In other sites away from the midline, the exposure entails division of the anterior rectus sheath, splitting of the muscle fibres and division of the posterior sheath. The purse-string (ordinary cannula) or interrupted sutures (modified Hasson cannula) are inserted in the anterior rectus sheath.

Sudden collapse of the patient

When the anaesthetist reports difficulties, a drop in blood pressure or sudden cardiac arrest, the surgeon should always consider the possibility of a major vascular injury. Although the mortality from laparoscopy is low (1 : 1000), a

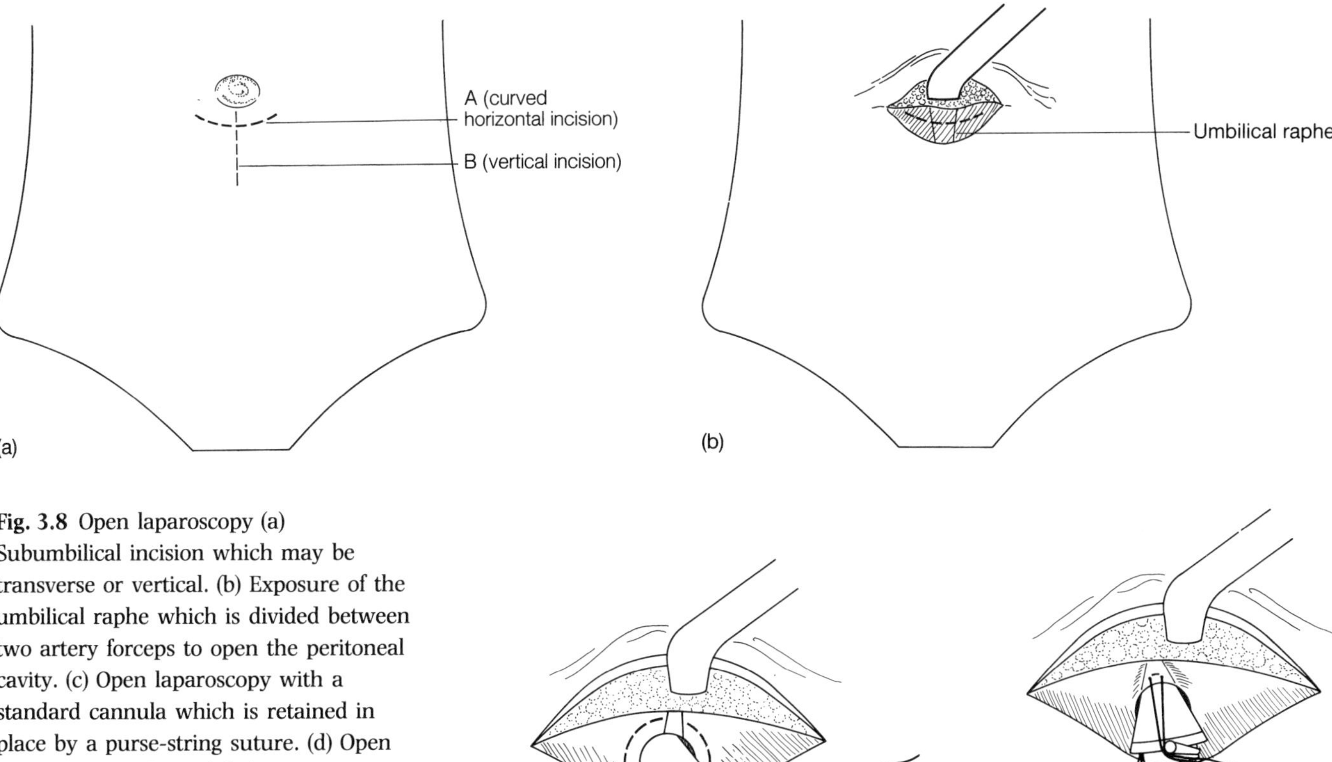

Fig. 3.8 Open laparoscopy (a) Subumbilical incision which may be transverse or vertical. (b) Exposure of the umbilical raphe which is divided between two artery forceps to open the peritoneal cavity. (c) Open laparoscopy with a standard cannula which is retained in place by a purse-string suture. (d) Open laparoscopy with modified Hasson cannula, the olive of which is used to plug the hole in the posterior rectus sheath and is retained in place by the two stay sutures which are tied to the fixation wings. These sutures are used to close the abdominal wall defect at the end of the procedure.

large proportion of these deaths are due to undiagnosed blood loss. The anaesthetist will naturally be preoccupied with the causes of the problem in his domain—drug reactions, myocardial arrhythmias, gas embolism, pneumothorax, etc. Retroperitoneal haemorrhage (the commonest site of bleeding caused by needles and instruments) is not apparent unless specifically looked for. Other causes of sudden collapse, i.e. cardiac arrhythmias, gas embolism, tension pneumothorax, require a completely different management. On the other hand immediate recognition of acute blood loss as the cause of the cardiovascular collapse, with prompt surgical intervention, is life-saving. The suggested steps in the event of sudden collapse are:

1 Discontinue gas insufflation immediately and reduce the intra-abdominal pressure to 8.0 mmHg.

2 Proceed immediately with 360° scan of the peritoneal cavity to rule out retroperitoneal bleeding.

3 If bleeding/expanding haematoma is documented, proceed to immediate long midline laparotomy and compress the aorta or injured vessels.

4 Aspirate blood, expose and control the injured vessel with a vascular clamp. When necessary, control the bleeding by simple pressure alone until

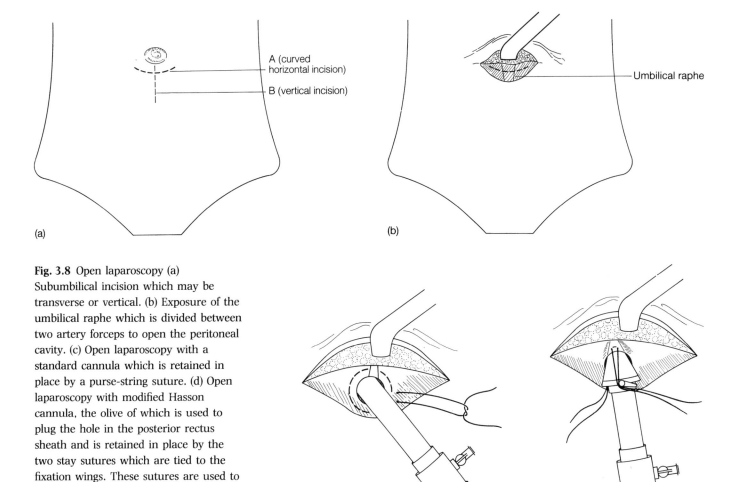

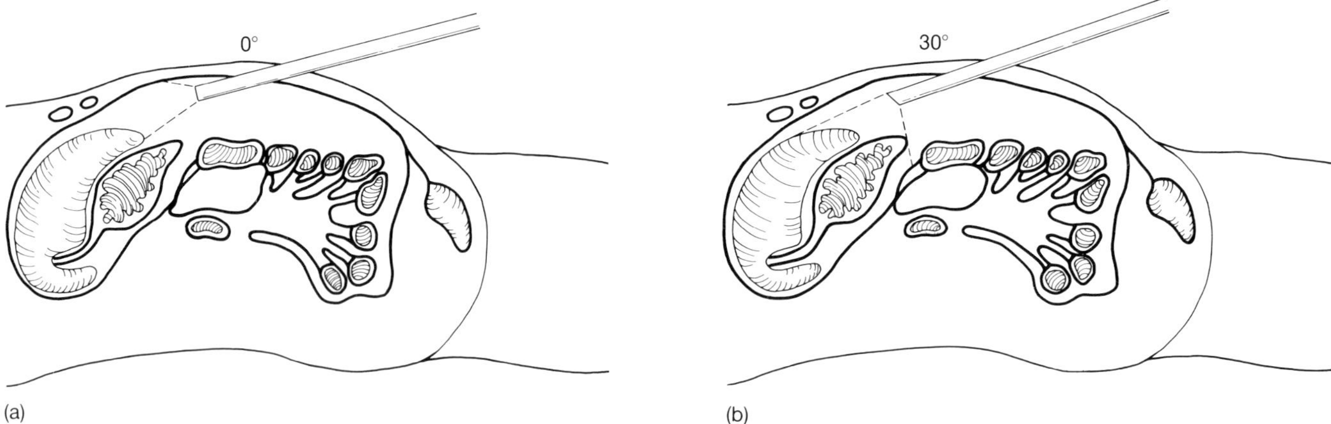

Fig. 3.9 Diagrammatic represention of the visual field of (a) 0° forward viewing and (b) 30° forward oblique telescopes.

the anaesthetist has caught up with the replacement of the blood loss.
5 Obtain the assistance of a vascular surgeon.

Laparoscopes and CCD cameras

Type and size of laparoscope

All modern laparoscopes are based on the Hopkins rod lens system. The improved models have additional lenses within the optical system to correct the peripheral barrel distortion which is inherent to the Hopkins optical system. For optimum viewing, the large 10.0 mm laparoscope is necessary. The 7.0–8.0 mm telescopes are suitable for diagnostic laparoscopy but do not provide sufficient light transmission for laparoscopic surgery. As previously described, the 5.0 mm telescope is useful for guided entry into the peritoneal cavity in difficult cases.

The viewing angle of the telescope is important and in practice two are commonly used: the 0° forward viewing and the 30° forward oblique. For the same diameter, the forward-viewing telescope transmits more light than the oblique variety and is easier to use, as the visual field is constant irrespective of the axis of rotation in which the telescope is held. However, the use of the forward oblique telescope carries considerable advantages which outweigh these limitations. It permits the surgeon to 'look down' on the operative field instead of tangentially, as pertains with the forward-viewing type (Fig. 3.9a,b). This considerably facilitates difficult dissections. Furthermore, by rotation of the axis of the telescope the operative field can be changed from looking downwards (light cable attachment pointing upwards), to looking from the right, upwards and from the left. This 360° scan of the object is invaluable in advanced laparoscopic surgery (Fig. 3.10). The forward-viewing telescope is better for obtaining on overall scan of the peritoneal cavity and its contents, as in diagnostic laparoscopy.

The ideal set of optics which the authors recommend should consist of:
1 × 5 mm 0° forward viewing—for guided entry into the peritoneal cavity

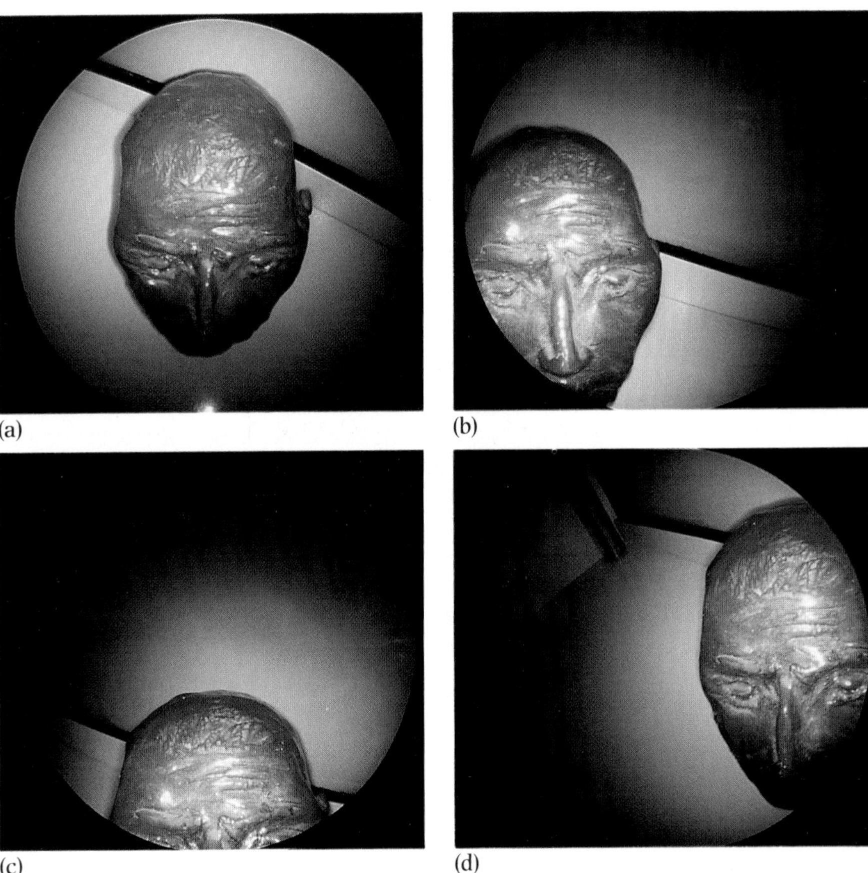

Fig. 3.10 Viewing of the operative field by rotation of the 30° forward oblique telescope. (a) Looking down, (b) from the right, (c) upwards and (d) from the left.

1 × 10 mm 0° forward viewing—initial scan of the peritoneal cavity
1 × 10 mm 30° forward oblique—for operative surgical procedures.

CCD cameras, light sources and monitors

A good CCD (charged-couple device) camera and high-resolution monitors are essential for safe laparoscopic surgery. The resolution of the camera is dependent on the size and number of chips and the number of pixels. The highest resolution and colour rendition are obtained by the three-chip cameras, but these are currently rather bulky. A high-resolution single-chip camera (16 mm), preferably with a zoom facility, gives sufficient definition and obviates the weight problem, and is currently the best buy.

Two monitors are essential: one facing the surgeon and the other the assistant. Accurate placing of the monitors diminishes eye and neck strain during long procedures. A high-intensity halide or xenon light source is required. The majority of the high-resolution camera systems incorporate control units that have an automatic light adjustment, which abolishes the 'glare spots' as the optic is moved closer to the operative field.

The Laparocamera consists of an optic which is permanently fixed to the CCD camera. There are no advantages to this system and it has a number of limitations. In the first instance, it precludes direct monocular vision through the telescope, and secondly, the surgeon cannot change the optic, e.g. from forward viewing to oblique. More recently, flexible laparoscopes which incorporate the sensing chip have been introduced. Again, there are no particular advantages to the use of these laparoscopes, although they may become useful once endoscopic 3-D television systems come on stream.

A corrected-beam splitter can be interfaced between the optic and the camera (Fig. 3.11). This allows simultaneous television and endoscopic vision and carries a number of practical advantages. There is no doubt that the resolution obtained by direct viewing through the telescope gives an incomparably sharper image than that provided by television monitoring. There are situations when the identification of structures proves difficult: a typical example is an anterior cystic artery which can be mistaken for the cystic duct. Direct monocular vision rapidly solves this problem. The other advantage of the beam splitter is in obtaining still coloured endophotographs. In this case, a sterile optical arm is used to connect the camera/flash unit to the beam splitter.

The CCD cameras can be sterilized by soaking in glutaraldehyde solution or with ethylene oxide gas. The authors prefer to cover the camera and cable with a plastic sterile sleeve, which avoids the need for chemical disinfection.

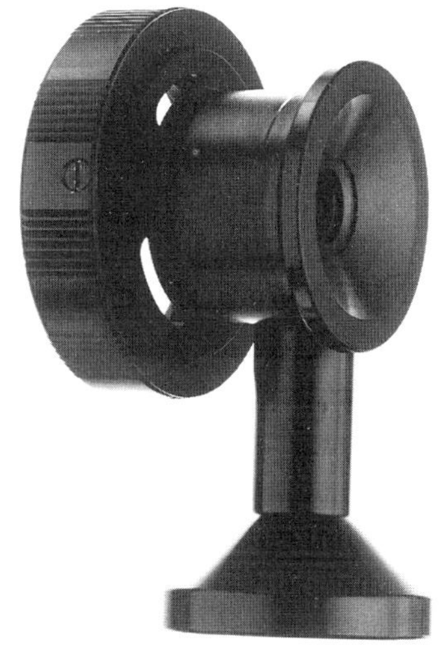

Fig. 3.11 Corrected-beam splitter which is interfaced between the telescope and the camera and allows simultaneous television and direct endoscopic viewing.

Optics warming and cleaning

Prior warming of the laparoscope is essential to establish and maintain a good view, since this prevents condensation of the warm saturated air inside the peritoneal cavity on a cold lens surface. Commercial dry-heat telescope warmers are available (Fig. 3.12). However, warming of the laparoscope is

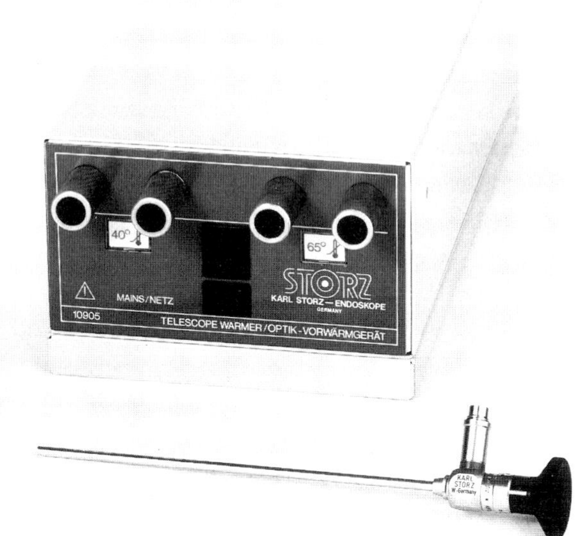

Fig. 3.12 Telescope warming device.

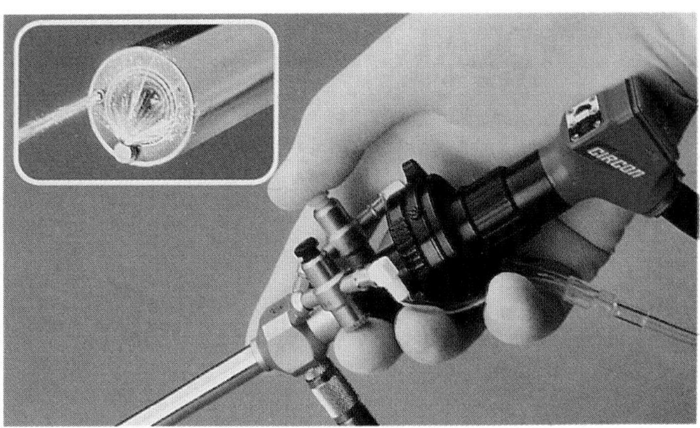

Fig. 3.13 Hydrolaparoscope system which permits irrigation of the lens and the operative field (Circon, ACMI).

best achieved by immersion of the optics in a cylinder filled with warm sterile water and kept in a waterbath set at 50°C. During operations, blood and tissue may cloud the lens and this hot sterile-water system is used to immerse and clean the optic while at the same time rewarming it. Fouling of the lens is often caused by the accumulation of loose tissue and blood clot inside the telescope cannula. This problem is remedied by withdrawal of the optic, followed by the insertion of a pledget swab mounted in a forceps to wipe the inside of the cannula. An alternative solution consists in irrigating of the cannula with warm isotonic saline contained in a large bladder syringe.

More recently, the hydrolaparoscope system has been introduced (Circon ACMI). This features an integral distal lens-wash and tissue irrigation. Both can be activated independently by fingertip control (Fig. 3.13). The lens-wash facility avoids the need to remove the telescope for cleaning, and thus permits the progress of the dissection without any interruptions. In this respect it saves considerably on the operating time.

Teamwork, assistance, cannula position and laparoscope holder

Teamwork and assistance

There is no doubt that good-quality experienced assistance greatly facilitates the conduct of difficult laparoscopic dissections. A team approach is essential. Endoscopic surgery proceeds smoothly only if the same group of people (anaesthetist, surgeons and nurses) work routinely together. Frequent changes of staff are detrimental and often delay the procedures.

Cannula positioning

An inspection of all the quadrants of the abdomen is essential to ensure that the diagnosis is correct and that the pathology is suitable. On this, a decision is made either to progress to the operative phase or to abandon it in favour of an open procedure. The siting of the accessory cannulae follows this laparoscopic inspection and must be carefully planned. The two main ones must be so placed that, within the operative field, the ends of the instruments meet at a 90° angle to each other. Great difficulties in the execution of surgical manoeuvres (dissection, ligation, suturing) will be encountered if the respective positions of the cannulae are such that the instruments when introduced are too close, or worse still, parallel to each other. The third cannula is sited primarily with a view to optimum retraction. All cannulae are inserted under direct vision through the laparoscope.

Camera operator and laparoscope holders

It is a great advantage to the surgeon to have the laparoscope held and directed correctly throughout the operation, thereby allowing both hands to be free to manipulate the instruments. Most surgeons employ a surgical trainee or nurse to support the telescope/camera assembly and rapidly change its position in response to the surgeon's needs or verbal requests, or by anticipation of the next operative manoeuvre as seen on the video monitor. This is fine so long as the assistant is experienced and dedicated to the task. In addition, this practice is very useful for training, as it engages the assistant's attention and participation, allowing procedures to be learnt in a

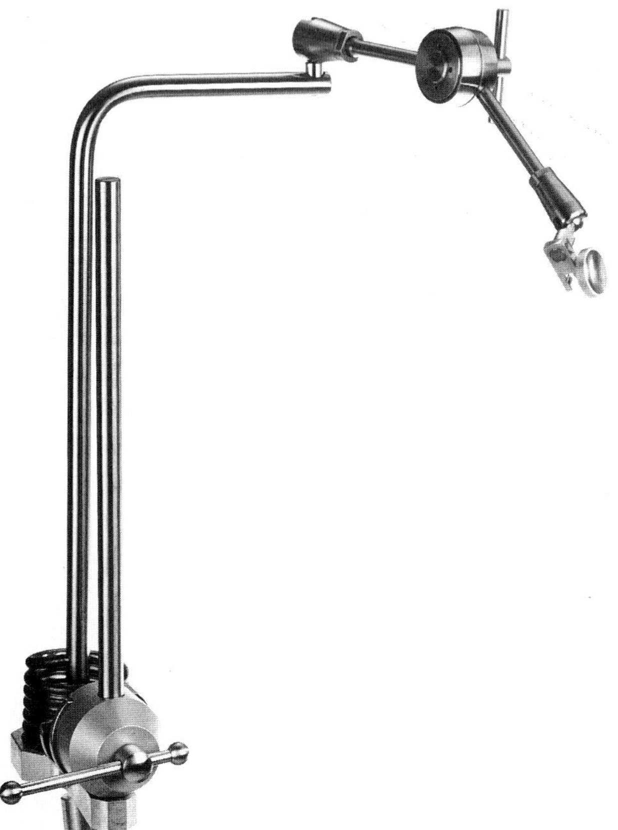

Fig. 3.14 Martin's arm laparoscope holder.

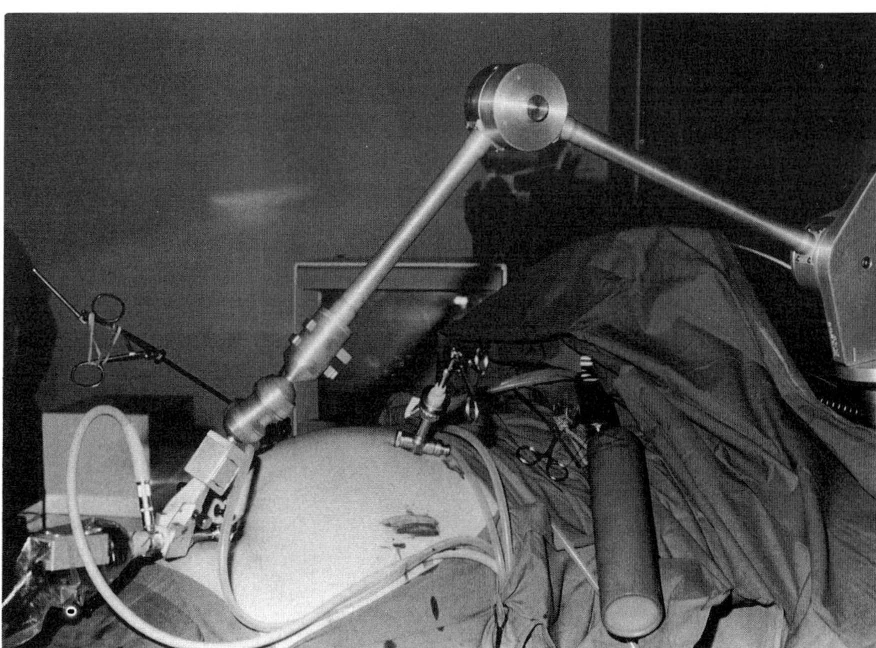

Fig. 3.15 Vacuum-lock pneumatic robotic arm—First Assistant. This allows rapid adjustment of the operative field by the surgeon and disposes with the need of a camera holder for most of the time during an operation (Leonard Medical, Philadelphia.)

systematic fashion. As the camera operator's ability to assist the surgeon in other ways, i.e. retraction, suction irrigation, etc., is restricted, a further assistant is needed to undertake these tasks. This often leads to overcrowding of the immediate operating environment, restricting elbow room and manipulations by the surgeon. This problem can be resolved to a large extent by the use of laparoscope/camera holders.

The ideal holder should permit rapid and smooth adjustment in all directions: sideways to monitor and guide instrument insertion toward the operative field; in and out to change from wide-angle to close-up viewing; and up and down to change the incident angle with the horizontal. Stainless steel metal holders such as the Martin's arm (Fig. 3.14) are based on a universal joint which controls the articulations and can be locked and unlocked by a single fixation-screw mechanism. They work reasonably well but have a limited flexibility and range. For these reasons, the authors prefer the vacuum-lock robotic arm—First Assistant (Leonard Medical, Philadelphia). This reproduces all the movements of the human upper limb and is capable of rapid fingertip-controlled adjustment by the surgeon (Fig. 3.15).

Specific organ exposure and retraction

This must be approached in the same manner as in open surgery. Apart from the limitations in depth perception imposed by the two-dimensional imaging, an excellent view of the relevant anatomy should be available. If not, adoption of the techniques described below will ensure adequate exposure. Great care must be exercised during the insertion and use of the fine-pointed instruments to avoid accidental organ injury. As one instrument is removed from the cannula, the direction of the cannula should be maintained until the replacement instrument appears in the operative field. Even so, the instrument should glide effortlessly without any hold-up and on no account must pressure be exerted. Again the importance of repositioning the optics to observe the entry of any sharp instrument through the end of the cannula towards the operative field should be stressed. This is the safest way to minimize the risk of instrumental injury to organs beyond the field of vision.

Gas leaks

An absolute requirement for the smooth progress of the operation is the maintenance of a constant pneumoperitoneum. This is achieved by using cannulae and instruments which seal properly, so avoiding gas leaks, and the use of the electronic high-flow insufflator to ensure rapid gas replacement as required. The 5.0 mm instruments can be introduced down the 11.0 mm trocar if they are initially preloaded into the appendix extractor, which acts as a reducer tube. During suction a considerable amount of CO_2 is lost and requires rapid replacement by the electronic insufflator set at maximum, otherwise deflation ensues with sagging of the anterior abdominal wall and loss of vision.

Gravity

By virtue of their various peritoneal attachments, the abdominal organs can be differentially moved by tilting the table, either head-up for upper abdominal surgery, or head-down for pelvic work. Lateral tilt of the table helps to enhance this exposure. However, care must be taken to anchor the pelvis if tilt is used, to prevent movement of the patient on the inclined surface. This is probably best achieved by the placement of a safety belt anchoring the pelvis. Apart from the obvious danger of slipping off the table, lesser degrees of displacement can easily result in pressure on vulnerable bony points and nerves.

Falciform lift

This simple technique helps to increase the exposure around the porta hepatis. An atraumatic 60.0 mm straight needle with 0 prolene is inserted percutaneously just to the left of the linea alba in the upper abdomen. Under visual control, the needle is made to enter the peritoneal cavity to the left of the falciform ligament. It is then grasped by the 5.0 mm needle-holder and passed below and to the right side of the ligament before being pushed through the peritoneum and abdominal wall. As the needle emerges through the skin it is grasped and withdrawn. When the two ends are tied the suture acts as a sling, elevating the falciform ligament. Care must be taken not to tie or pull up the sling too firmly, as the suture could cut through fat and vessels, causing a haematoma. The falciform sling also exerts tension on the round ligament and thus helps to lift the liver, thereby opening up the subhepatic pouch. The other benefit of the technique is that an accessory cannula can be inserted in the left upper gradient without the instruments becoming entangled in the falciform ligament during insertion and withdrawal.

Abdominal wall lift

A sustained CO_2 pneumoperitoneum induces cardiovascular haemodynamic changes which, though less marked than those following air insufflation [5,6], can be significant in patients with compromised cardiac function due to ischaemic heart disease. Carbon dioxide insufflation results in a rise in the central venous and systemic arterial pressures. The rise in the blood pressure is largely due to a sympathetic drive consequent on the hypercarbia, and to a lesser extent to the increased pressure on the abdominal aorta [6–8]. When the intra-abdominal pressure exceeds 20 mmHg (2.7 kPa), the CVP and blood pressure fall in association with a significant diminution of the cardiac output [9], which on average is reduced by 0.5 l/min (16% drop) during CO_2 insufflation [10]. Arrhythmias are common with CO_2 insufflation; the most frequent is bradycardia. This is due to reflex vagal stimulation from stretching of the peritoneal surface and local irritation by CO_2. Premedication with atropine can prevent this [11]. Other more serious arrhythmias include bigeminal rhythm, ventricular ectopic beats and ventricular tachycardia. However, these are mainly the result of inadequate ventilation, especially when the patient is in the Trendelenburg position [11]. Carbon dioxide insufflation is also accompanied by a rise in the arterial $p\text{CO}_2$ and a fall in the arterial pH and $p\text{O}_2$ [12]. In addition, the serum chloride level drops due to a shift of chloride ions into the red blood cells in exchange for bicarbonate ions consequent on hypercarbia. This respiratory acidosis is more marked if

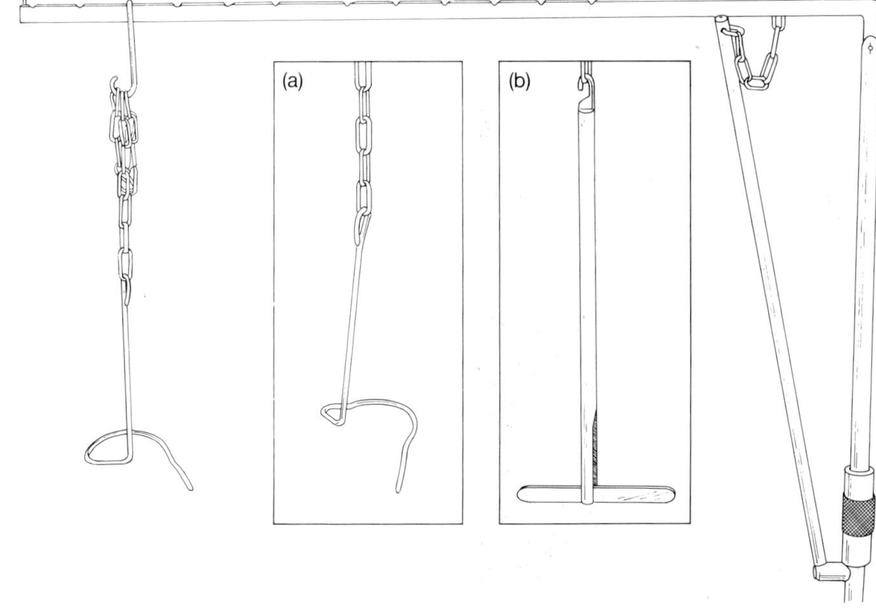

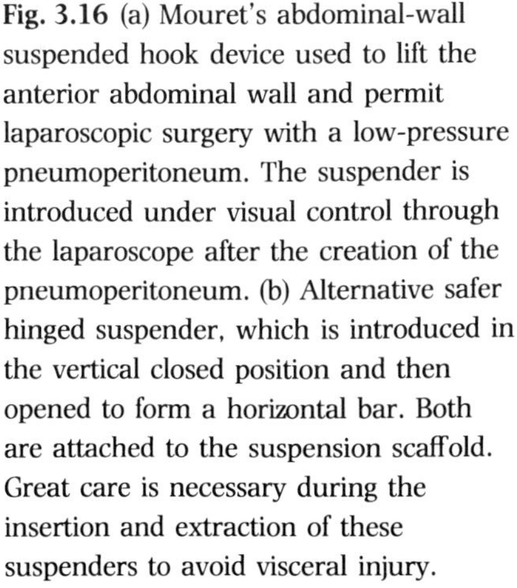
Fig. 3.16 (a) Mouret's abdominal-wall suspended hook device used to lift the anterior abdominal wall and permit laparoscopic surgery with a low-pressure pneumoperitoneum. The suspender is introduced under visual control through the laparoscope after the creation of the pneumoperitoneum. (b) Alternative safer hinged suspender, which is introduced in the vertical closed position and then opened to form a horizontal bar. Both are attached to the suspension scaffold. Great care is necessary during the insertion and extraction of these suspenders to avoid visceral injury.

during general anaesthesia the patient is allowed to breathe spontaneously, as opposed to controlled ventilation [13].

Although fit patients (ASA I and II) can cope with these changes, particularly if expert anaesthesia with controlled ventilation is administered, patients with diminished cardiac reserve are at risk. These patients should undergo laparoscopic surgery with a low-pressure pneumoperitoneum (4.0–6.0 mmHg). Adequate exposure can be obtained in this situation by the use of devices which enable the abdominal wall to be lifted up, such as the hook developed by Mouret [14], shown in Fig. 3.16a. This metal abdominal-wall suspender is inserted after the creation of the pneumoperitoneum. Both its introduction and removal have to be undertaken with great care to avoid laceration of the liver. A safer metal abdominal wall suspender is shown in Fig. 3.16b. An equally effective and safer procedure is the combined abdominal wall–round ligament lift using polyethylene tubing on a curved sharp pointed trocar. After creation of the pneumoperitoneum and introduction of the telescope, the trocar trailing the tubing is inserted high up to the left of the xiphoid process, through the abdominal wall just to the left of the falciform ligament. The trocar is passed beneath the latter and then up alongside its right side to emerge below and to the right of the xiphoid process. The trocar is then withdrawn. The sling of tubing is now placed around the abdominal wall and falciform–round ligament complex. The two external ends of the tubing are tied and the loop is lifted up by a hook and chain to the horizontal bar of the head screen (Fig. 3.17 a,b). The pneumoperitoneum is then reduced to 6.0 mmHg. An excellent working space and good exposure is obtained despite the low intra-abdominal pressure. The technique has the added advantage of lifting the medial sectors of the liver, including the quadrate lobe, as the round ligament is pulled up with the abdominal wall (Fig. 3.18).

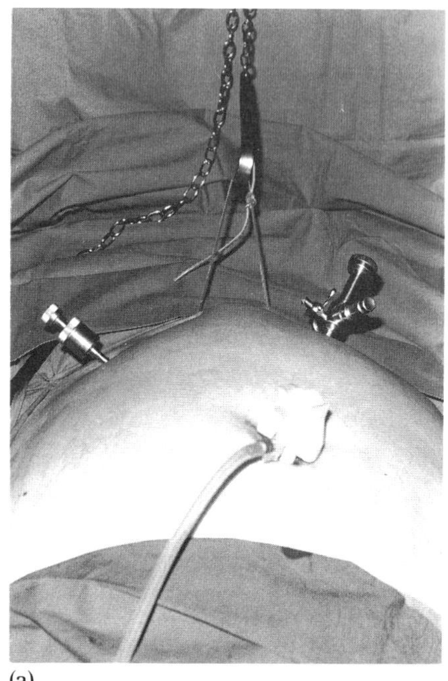

(a)

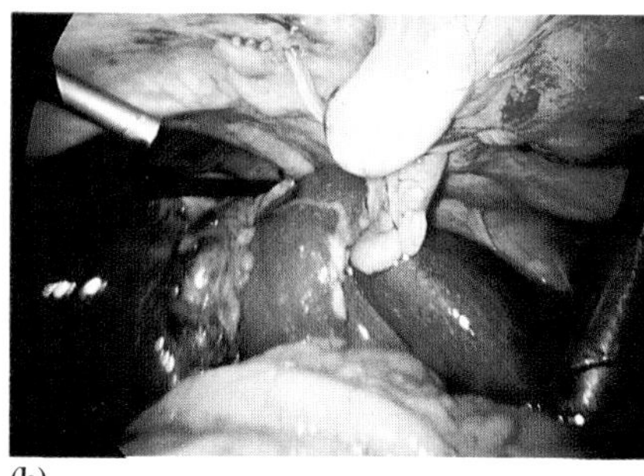

(b)

Fig. 3.17 (a) Abdominal wall–falciform lift in place. The sling is suspended by chain and hook to the horizontal bar of the head stand. (b) Internal view of tube around falciform and round ligament.

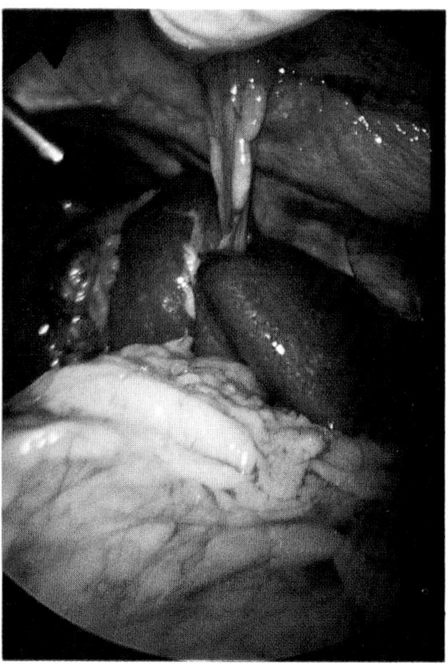

Fig. 3.18 Abdominal wall–falciform lift with intra-abdominal pressure reduced to 6.0 mmHg. In addition to providing excellent working space, the central portion of the liver is elevated by the round ligament which is pulled up with the anterior abdominal wall.

Nasogastric tube

A major factor in limiting exposure in the upper abdomen is a distended stomach. A large-bore nasogastric tube should be passed in all cases prior to induction of the pneumoperitoneum. This will also minimize the risk of penetration of the gas-filled stomach with the Veress needle, and during extubation it decreases the risk of vomiting and aspiration of gastric contents. The nasogastric tube should be removed before the patient is wheeled out of the operating theatre.

Retraction with instruments

While the techniques for retraction used in laparoscopy are different from those of open surgery, the principles of traction and counter-traction to reveal tissue planes still apply. It is surprising how adequate this can be. Much can be gained from the correct siting of the trocars and cannulae, which by optimizing the retraction that can be achieved by the instruments introduced through them, can result in an excellent view of the selected organ.

A simple probe with a smooth surface and rounded tip is useful for the manipulation of friable tissues. A variety of tissue-grasping forceps is available, ranging from ones with atraumatic tips, including bowel-holding types, to heavy and sharp traumatic claw forceps. Careful stepwise lifting of tissue, using two instruments (through separate trocars), forms the basis of manipulation.

The laparoscope itself can be used to displace organs but great care should be taken to avoid contact with the tip of the laparoscope, which may cause burns from the heat generated by the light transmitted through the fibre bundles.

Endoretraction

In biliary tract surgery this concerns the retraction of the liver to expose the cystic pedicle and the common bile duct. The simplest manoeuvre consists of grasping the fundus of the gallbladder with a traumatic forceps, which is then used to elevate and rotate the right lobe of the liver. This is effective in most instances but fails if the liver is firm and enlarged or the quadrate lobe is prominent. Under these circumstances, upward retraction of the liver medial to the cystic pedicle is necessary. This is achieved by an extra cannula placed below and to the right of the xiphoid process, through which a retracting rod or expanding retractor is inserted (Fig. 3.19). This extra retracting port is necessary for adequate exposure in cases undergoing laparoscopic exploration of the common bile duct.

A better alternative to the use of an extra retracting port is the employment of the Nathanson–Cuschieri dipping endoretractor. This fits inside an 11.0 mm cannula and has its own 8.0 mm 30° forward oblique

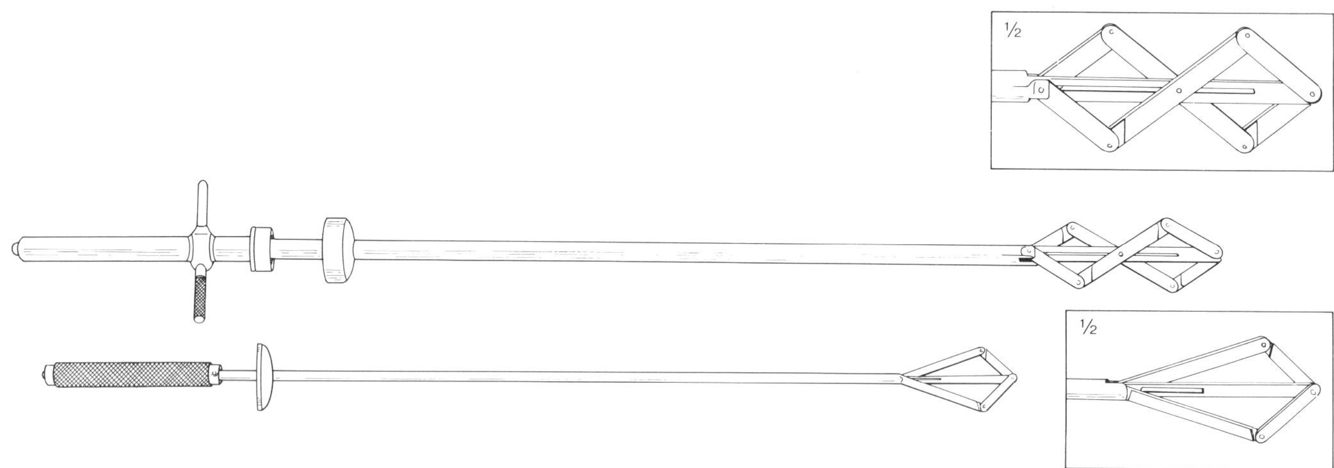

Fig. 3.19 Types of expanding retractors.

optic, which is used instead of the standard optic (Fig. 3.20 a). The endoretractor has three components: (i) a hollow telescope conduit with an inferiorly placed viewing window and a terminal hinged dipping rod which drops down to an angle of 120° (Fig. 3.20 b,c); (ii) a telescopic system to advance and withdraw the optic through the 5.0 cm viewing window; and (iii) a 30° forward oblique telescope, preferably with an integral light bundle to enhance light transmission (Storz, Tuttlingen, Germany). The liver retraction and exposure of the common bile duct obtained with this instrument is unsurpassed. It also carries the advantage of avoiding the need for the insertion of an extra port to retract the liver.

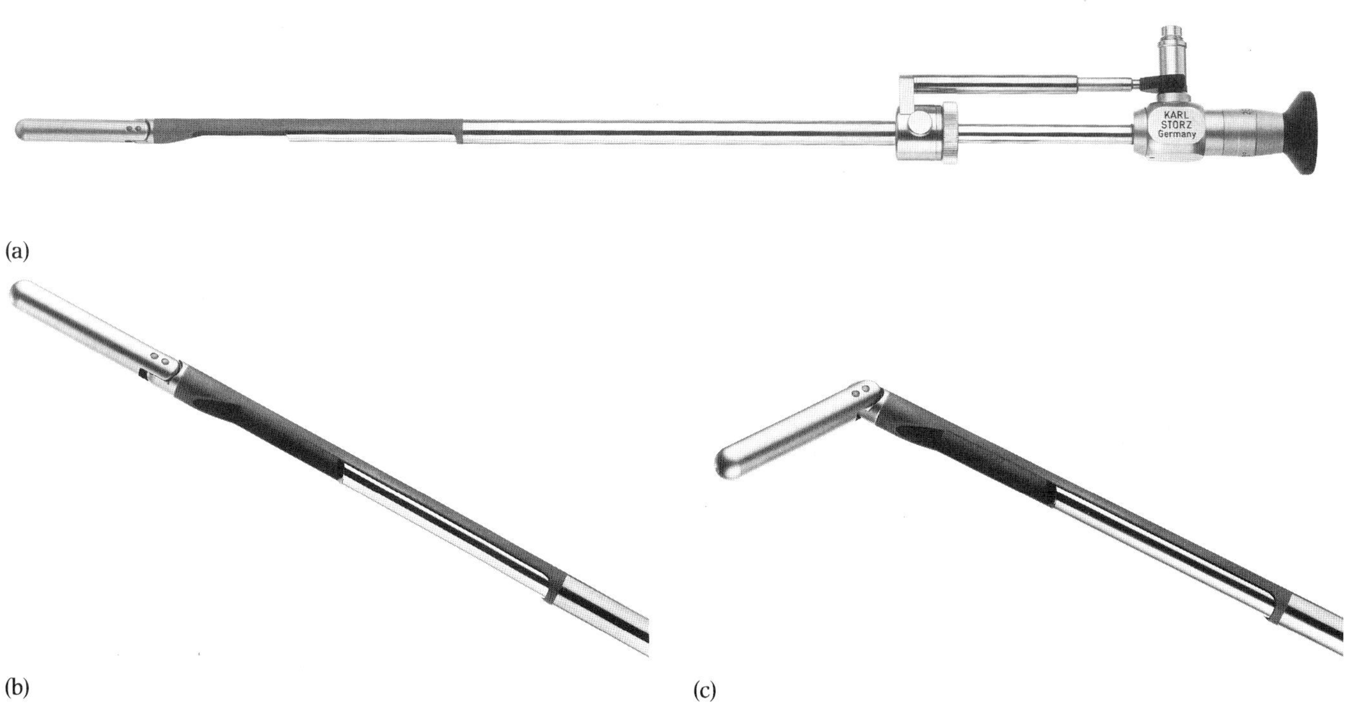

Fig. 3.20 (a) Profile of the dipping endoretractor. (b) The hinged terminal section. (c) Drops down ahead of the operative field to an angle of 120° (Karl Storz, Tuttlingen, Germany).

Tissue dissection

Blunt dissection

As in open surgery, various methods of dissection along tissue planes are used. As even minor blood loss considerably impairs vision during laparoscopic surgery, a meticulous bloodless dissection technique is essential, and paradoxically, speeds up the procedure. Blunt dissection of mature adhesions with smooth instruments is easily achieved. A 'peanut' swab mounted on a grasping forceps introduced through the 11.0 mm cannula after preloading with the appendix extractor will allow this method of dissection to be used (Fig. 3.21 a–d).

Another technique is hydrodissection with a pressurized jet of warm saline, which teases tissue planes gently apart. This hydrojet dissection can be especially useful in separating inflamed organs and has been likened to 'an extension of the surgeon's finger'. The same jet of fluid can be used to separate other tissue planes, e.g. for dissection of the pelvic side walls, in which case a small nick is made in the peritoneum and the jet of saline directed underneath the peritoneal lining to infiltrate and lift the adipose fascial planes, thereby dissecting and isolating the vessels, nerves and ureter. This allows sharp dissection (e.g. for lymph node sampling) to proceed more safely.

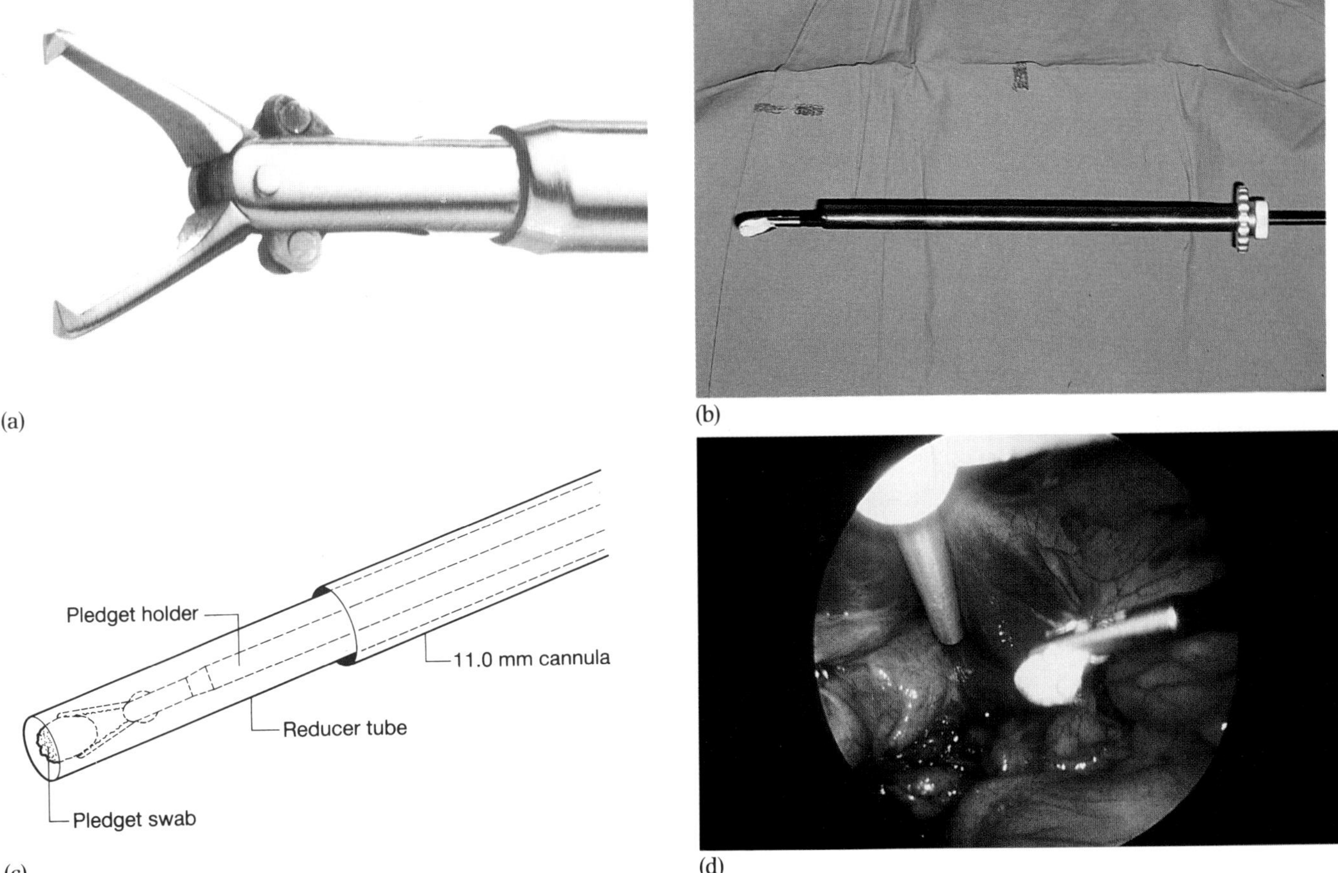

Fig. 3.21 (a) Peanut pledget holder. (b) This is inserted inside a reducer tube before the pledget is grasped. (c) For introduction and removal from the peritoneal cavity, the pledget swab is retracted inside the reducer tube. (d) Endophoto showing pledget swab dissection.

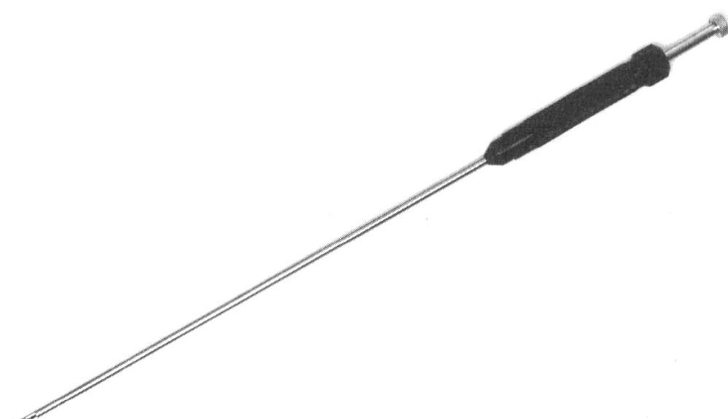

Fig. 3.22 Retractable diamond knife.

Sharp dissection

Scalpels of various shapes can be inserted down the 5.5 mm cannula. Great care is needed during their insertion and use to avoid accidental organ injury. Again, the introduction of the knives through the accessory cannulae must be conducted under visual control to minimize the risk of accidental injury to organs beyond the field of vision. The best scalpel in terms of safety and sharpness is the retractable diamond knife (Fig. 3.22), which is the only one used by the authors. The sharpness of the diamond knife and its cutting properties are unrivalled. Furthermore, the knife can be extruded or retracted inside the protecting sheath by a fingertip-controlled spring-loaded mechanism. This knife is extremely useful for laparoscopic common duct exploration and for opening bowel and gallbladder during the performance of laparoscopic cholecystojejunostomy for inoperable pancreatic cancer (Chapters 9, 10).

Scissors dissection

There has recently been significant progress in the design, size and type of scissors for laparoscopic work. In terms of their mechanical function, scissors, irrespective of type, are either single- or twin-action. The former have only one moveable blade, whereas in the twin-action variety both blades move (Fig. 3.23). A large straight blunt-nosed scissor is available for use with 11.0 mm cannula. Similar but finer scissors for use with the 5.5.mm cannula are very useful for general dissection, much as Metzenbaum or Macindoe scissors are used in open-access surgery. Sharp-tipped straight or curved microdissecting scissors allow precise work, especially when the optics are brought up close to magnify the structures being dissected.

The authors favour a two-handed scissor dissection as it mimics most closely the well-established surgical craft with which most surgeons are familiar. Hook scissors are the safest way to cut tubular structures in

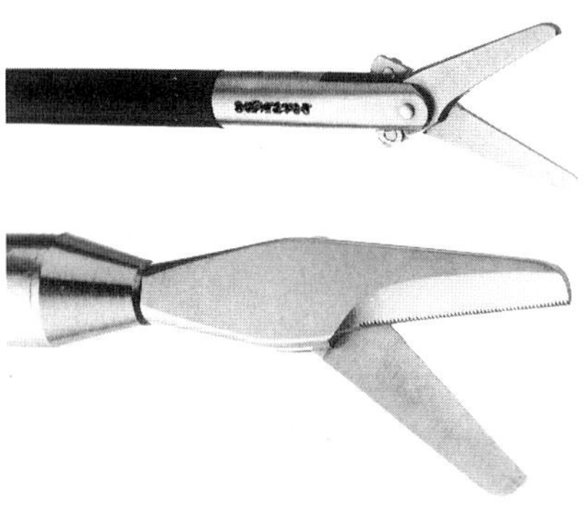

Fig. 3.23 Scissors: twin-action (top), single-action (bottom).

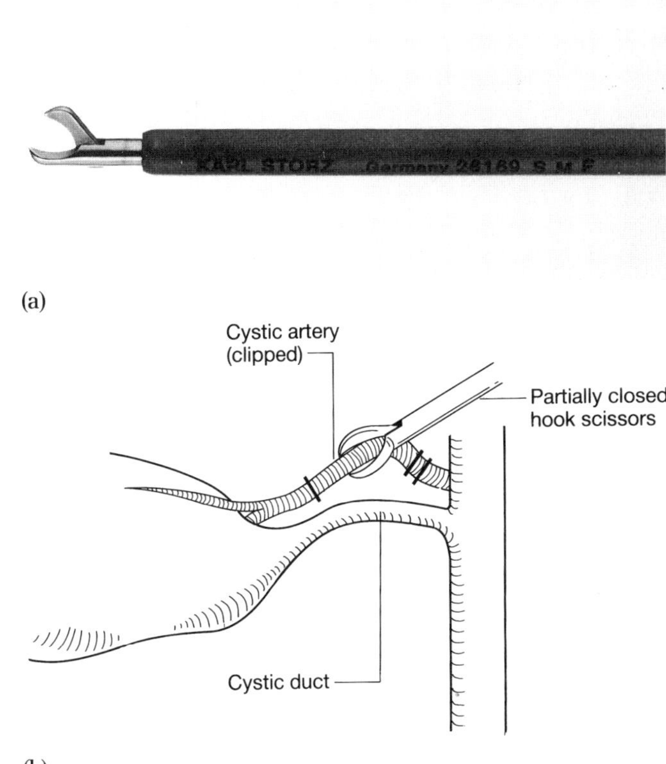

Fig. 3.24 (a) Hook scissors. (b) Partial closure of the hook jaws allows the structure to be lifted off subjacent tissues before it is cut.

confined areas such as the cystic artery and cystic duct. Partial closure of the hook jaws allows the structure to be lifted before it is cut (Fig. 3.24), ensuring restriction of the cut to the intended structure.

The use of insulated scissors will allow monopolar coagulation of small vessels as dissection proceeds, without changing instruments. However, repeated electrocoagulation (especially forced) results in blunting of the cutting edges of the scissors. An electrocoagulating current should be applied

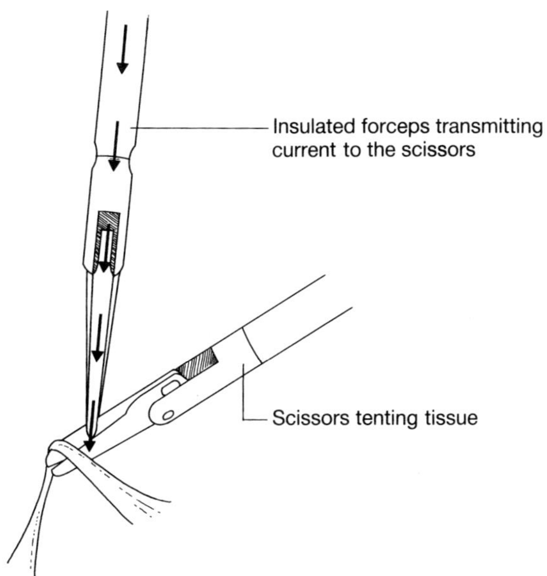

Fig. 3.25 Technique of applying soft electrocoagulation through the dissecting scissors, which does not damage the instrument and retains the sharpness of the cutting blades. If soft coagulation is used (less than 200 V), electric arcs which cause instrument damage are not generated.

to dissecting scissors only when the jaws of the instrument are closed, and the current voltage should not exceed 200 V (soft coagulation). As sparks are not generated by this current, damage and blunting of the scissor blades are considerably minimized. The best technique for applying soft coagulation through insulated scissors is illustrated in Fig. 3.25. The closed ends are used to tent the vessel away from subjacent tissue before the current is applied.

Scissors dissection necessitates a two-handed technique. The tissue is grasped by an atraumatic grasper and the correct tension applied before the scissors are used to cut peritoneal surfaces and then tease areolar tissue planes.

High-frequency electrosurgical dissection

Dissection with monopolar current requires extra care with insulation (see below). A useful instrument is the insulated electrosurgical hook knife, the hook end of which is used to dissect and lift up the desired tissue before the coagulating or cutting current is activated. A very important practical consideration is tenting of the tissue by the hook before the current is applied. This manoeuvre, by creating a constriction in the tissue, localizes the energy to the intended site and limits the spread of thermal damage (Fig. 3.26). The excessive use of high-frequency electrosurgery should be avoided, as tissue planes can be obscured by the charring effect and the heat-induced contraction of tissue obscures cleavage planes. Another problem with the electrosurgical hook knife is the accidental entanglement of the tip in omentum and other tissues, although this is less of a problem with the L-shaped as distinct from the curved device. Constant cleaning of the electrosurgical hook knife to remove charred tissue debris is essential for optimum function. As electrosurgery generates smoke, an integral suction channel activated by fingertip control is essential. Even this does not prevent smoke obscuring the visual field. When encountered, this problem is overcome by temporarily withdrawing the optic inside its cannula and opening one of the taps on the access ports for a few seconds to achieve a rapid gas exchange.

Bipolar coagulating and cutting high-frequency generators with sensor electronics incorporated in the functional hand pieces are currently being

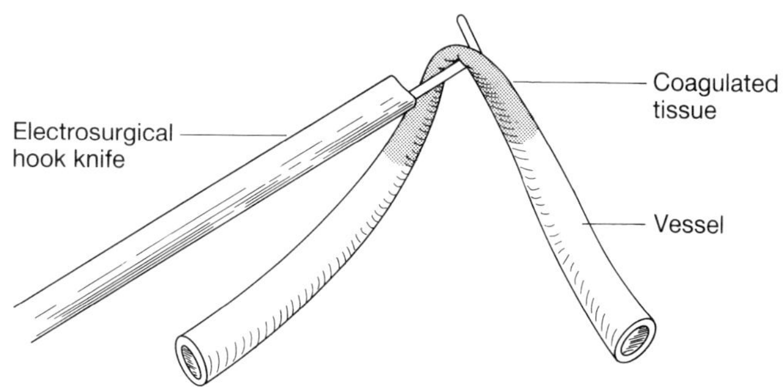

Fig. 3.26 During electrosurgical dissection the tissue is tented by the hook before the current is applied. This manoeuvre, by creating a constriction in the tissue, localizes the energy to the intended site and limits the spread of thermal damage.

evaluated, and will replace monopolar machines for laparoscopic surgery in the near future.

Laser dissection

Laser surgery is undoubtedly elegant and achieves bloodless dissection. The two most commonly used lasers in laparoscopic surgery are the Nd-YAG (1066 nm), which is invisible and therefore requires a guiding beam (usually helium–neon), and the potassium titanyl phosphate laser (KTP) which is produced by frequency-doubling Nd-YAG by a KTP crystal. This produces high-intensity green light (532 nm). Laser energy can be applied either as a non-contact beam or in the contact mode by bare fibres or special hand/terminal pieces. As the contact mode results in a greater power density when applied directly to tissues, it is more precise and requires less output from the laser device to achieve the same effect as the free laser beam. Hence it is the optimal system for laparoscopic work. The other advantage to contact laser in surgical practice (laparoscopic or otherwise) is that the delivery system maintains the tactile feedback which is so important to surgeons. By adjustment of the power output (watts), spot size and duration of exposure, coagulation, cutting and vaporization can be achieved. The recommended output for laparoscopic cholecystectomy, where the KTP laser is used to cut the cystic duct and artery and to dissect the gallbladder from the liver bed, is 15.0 W with the exposure duration set to continuous. There are two specific dangers inherent to laser dissection: past pointing and beam deflection. Past-pointing injuries are caused by the laser energy penetrating through the entire thickness of the tissue (e.g. the gallbladder) with resultant damage to the deeper structures. It may complicate laser dissection using either the free beam or the contact mode. Deflections of the free laser beam due to collision of the probe with other instruments or from hand tremors may result in injury to adjacent structures.

Despite its advantages, laser dissection is by no means necessary or indeed desirable for laparoscopic surgical procedures. Undoubtedly, there are certain disadvantages to its use. In the first instance, the current generation of machines is bulky and adds to the already crowded operating theatre. It requires additional technical staff and is far more expensive than high-frequency electrosurgery, with regard to both use and maintenance. Laser dissection is probably more time-consuming than electrosurgery [15,16] and it introduces an extra element of risk to both patient and staff. There is no evidence that it generates less smoke than high-frequency electrosurgical dissection. The long-term consequences (if any) of the effect of green high-intensity laser light on the peritoneal lining consequent on the photoactivation of haemoglobin, are unknown.

Many of the technical problems encountered with the present generation of lasers will disappear with the introduction of small hand-held diode array lasers, which are currently being developed. The incorporation of non-linear crystals into these new-generation laser systems will result in low-cost, low-maintenance portable devices with the capacity for tunability over a wide range of wavelengths.

Ultrasonic dissection

There is no doubt that for major endoscopic surgery such as thoracoscopic dissection of the oesophagus and laparoscopic colonic mobilization, the ultrasonic dissecting probe provides a more rapid and significantly less bloody dissection. Early clinical evaluation of the laparoscopic 5.0 mm ultrasonic dissecting probe for these procedures has been most encouraging. Separation of the gallbladder from the liver is also considerably expedited, especially when the organ is shrunken and fibrotic or largely intrahepatic. The authors have also found it useful for dissection of the common duct during laparoscopic supraduodenal exploration.

The harmonic scalpel works on the same principle as the ultrasonic dissector, except that the vibration frequency of the tip is much higher, in the harmonic range. This results in a cutting (as opposed to plane separating) device which generates sufficient heat by friction to gently coagulate the cut surfaces.

Peritoneal lavage and suction equipment

One of the major advances possible with laparoscopic surgery is the avoidance of bowel cooling and drying. The environment in the pneumoperitoneum is saturated with water vapour, and lavage of blood and debris is easily achieved with a suitable cannula. The instilled Ringer's lactate or saline solution should be heated to 37°C. An adequate pressure head is necessary for effective irrigation; this is achieved by the use of purpose-designed pump delivery systems such as the Aquapurator (Fig. 3.27), or foot-operated roller pumps. Failing the availability of this equipment, a bag of warm crystalloid solution is placed inside a Fenwell pressure cuff inflated to a pressure of 200–300 mmHg.

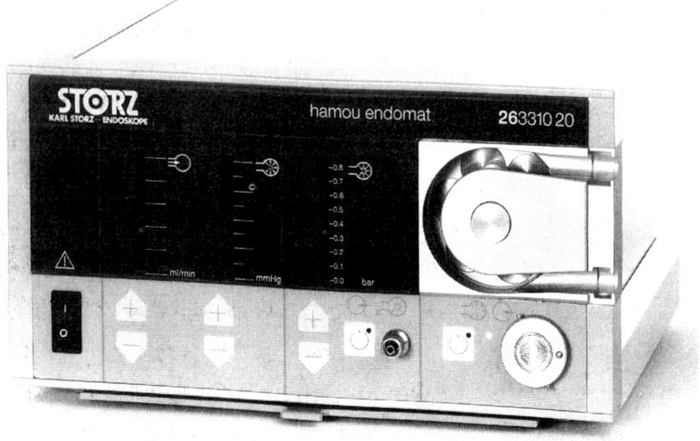

Fig. 3.27 Aquapurator for pressurized irrigation (Storz, Tuttlingen, Germany).

The same cannula is used to aspirate blood, irrigating solution, pus and escaped visceral contents using ordinary wall suction. The ideal suction/irrigation cannula has finger tip control valves (mechanical or electronic) which permit the single-handed operation of both irrigation and suction, since this frees the other hand for the retraction of tissues as necessary. If omentum or other tissues are caught in the cannula during suction, this is immediately stopped and the trapped tissue released by opening the irrigation valve.

Haemostasis

General principles

Haemostasis is essential in laparoscopic surgery. Apart from the obvious surgical principle of avoiding blood loss, extravasated blood and clots obscure the visual field both directly and by absorbing the available light. The control of bleeding is less easily achieved than in open surgery. Cut vessels often retract within surrounding fibrofatty tissue and can then be difficult to identify and pick up prior to coagulation, clipping or ligature. Thus any structure which is considered to be vascular must be coagulated or secured prior to division.

Oozing can be a problem during some dissections. There are several adjuncts which may be used in this situation. Local compression by adjacent tissues (grasped in an atraumatic forceps), or by a pledget swab is often successful. Irrigation of the field with Ringer's lactate solution is also helpful. In patients with constant ooze, blunt dissection with the suction probe and intermittent suction is the only measure which allows the dissection to proceed during the critical stages. At the end of oozy procedures, absorbable haemostatic agents (microfibrillar collagen, cellulose, etc.) may be inserted over the raw areas. It is also a wise precaution to drain these cases.

In general, vessels less than 3.0 mm in diameter can be safely coagulated. Vessels between 3.0 and 5.0 mm may be clipped or ligated, but larger vessels should be secured by ligature.

Coagulation

At present, there are three available methods of coagulating blood vessels during laparoscopic surgery: electrocoagulation, heater endocoagulation and photocoagulation. Electrocoagulation using modulated high-frequency current may be achieved by monopolar or bipolar circuits. Bipolar electrocoagulation is safer and should be used in preference to the monopolar mode in anatomically crowded regions, as it eliminates the risk of thermal damage to adjacent structures. The generator should have a capacity not exceeding 100 W and be of the isolated circuit variety. The safest monopolar electrocautery is achieved by using a voltage of less than 200 V (soft coagulation). With this setting, as electric arcs are not generated the risk of thermal

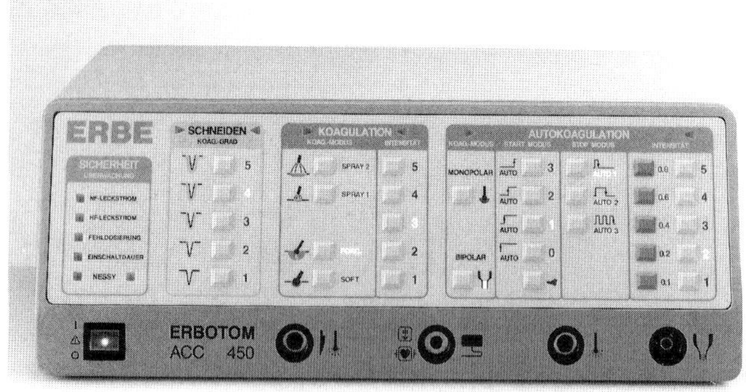

(a)

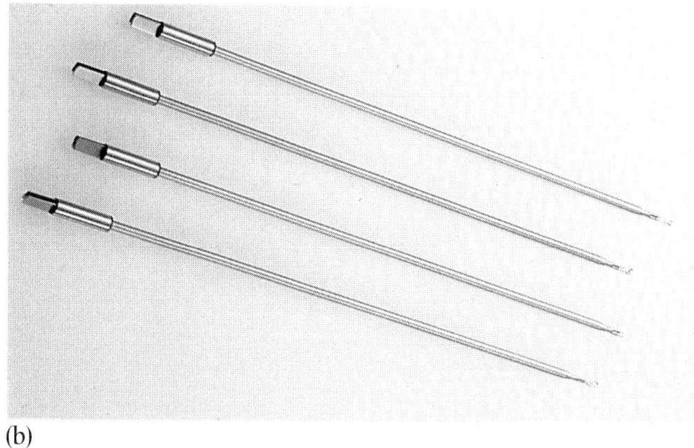
(b)

Fig. 3.28 (a) Microprocessor-controlled high-frequency generator. (b) Array of bipolar peripherals with sensor electronics which allow automatic bipolar coagulation (Erbe, Tübingen, Germany).

damage to adjacent structures is greatly reduced. In addition, damage to the instrument tips (including scissors) by the electric energy is minimized. Shorting of the non-insulated terminal segment of the instrument by contact with adjacent tissue (e.g. liver) or metal cannula must be avoided. Care must be exercised that the insulation of the instruments remains intact to prevent current leakage to the cannula. A very simple safety measure is to observe the area of coagulation very carefully. If local effects are not produced as the machine is activated, electrocoagulation should be stopped immediately and all connections and insulation checked.

In monopolar electrosurgery, the return current travels from the site of delivery through the arteries (e.g. hepatic), down the aorta and iliac vessels to exit at the site of the applied ground pad. This path may be altered by several factors, including the pooling of significant amounts of the isotonic saline used for irrigation. This errant return current may cause distant visceral injury. For this reason, electrosurgery should not be applied unless the area is reasonably dry of irrigating fluid and blood. As a further precaution, the use of Ringer's lactate as an irrigating solution is better than isotonic saline because it is less conductive. In this respect the safest is glycine solution, although there are unproven concerns regarding the possibility of increased adhesion formation with this solution.

Automatic bipolar electrocoagulation employs probes which contain sensor electronics and a microprocessor-controlled generator (Fig. 3.28). When programmed, the system initiates and stops the coagulation process when the optimal vessel occlusion has been achieved. The surgeon simply applies the bipolar probe to the vessel, which is coagulated with the right amount of energy commensurate with its thickness. This is a new and perhaps safer method of electrocoagulation, but more information is needed to document its advantages over conventional electrocoagulation.

Another method favoured by gynaecologists is the Semm endocoagulator. This is in effect a sealed heater probe which electronically maintains its tip at a temperature adjustable between 100 and 120°C. The tip rapidly cools when not activated, and no current passes through the patient. The instrument is autoclavable. The disadvantage of the endocoagulator is its relatively slow action. Photocoagulation is best achieved by the KTP laser in the contact mode.

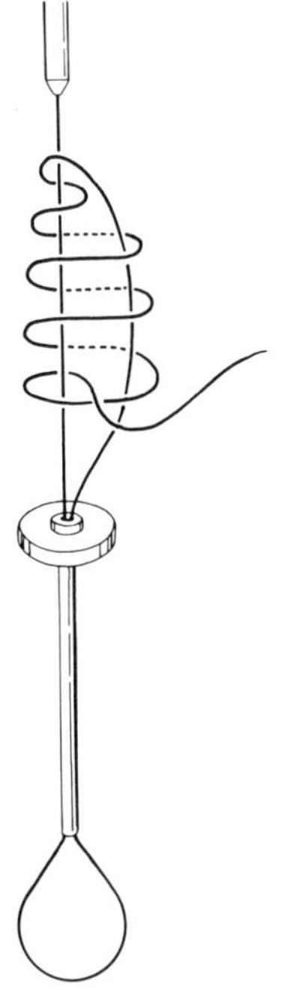

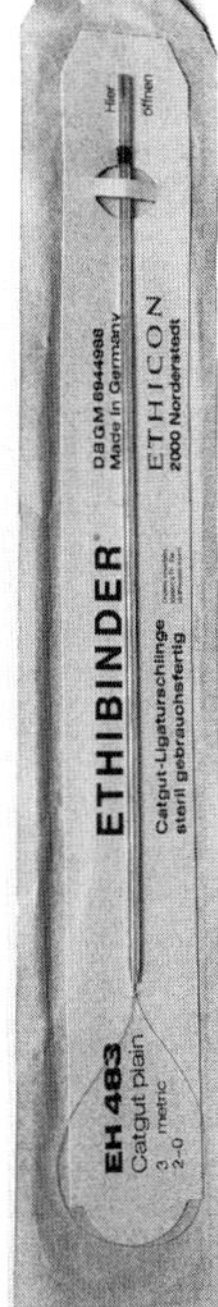

(b)

Fig. 3.29 (a) Diagrammatic representation of the Roeder slip-knot. (b) Ethicon preformed catgut endoloop based on the Roeder knot. The equivalent USSC product is the Surgitie.

Clips

Non-absorbable metal clips (stainless steel, titanium) are available in various sizes. Clip appliers are available in two sizes (for clips 6 and 9 mm in length). As in open surgery, selection of the appropriate size clip for the pedicle in question is important. Care must be taken during their application and a second clip should be used on the proximal end of arteries. The clip applicator must be carefully examined before use to ensure that it can be inserted with an airtight seal through the cannulae in use. Disposable preloaded clip applicators with automatic delivery of the clip to the jaws (Endoclip USSC, Ethicon Corporation) are useful for long procedures and have certain advantages. These instruments allow rapid precise repeated clipping without the need of withdrawal of the instrument for loading, thereby speeding the procedure considerably. They are, however, costly and are not essential for routine cholecystectomy.

The current limitation of all clip appliers (disposable and non-disposable) relates to the fixed-size clip that each instrument can apply. This entails the use of different clip applicators for small, medium and large clips, and is an important practical consideration because clip security after application is dependent on using the appropriate size of the clip in relation to the occluded vessel. The risk of slippage is especially high if the clip is too small and does not project beyond the whole width of the vessel, or is not applied at right-angles to its long axis. Furthermore, accidental brushing or traction can result in the slippage of clips. Metal clips, especially stainless steel, interfere with both computed tomography and magnetic resonance imaging, although this is less of a problem with the modern titanium varieties.

Absorbable polydioxanone (Ethicon Corporation) clips provide an attractive alternative to metal ones, and applicators designed to allow their laparoscopic use are available. Again, clip selection to match the size of the pedicle is important. If the clip applied is too small the locking mechanism will not operate. On the other hand, a clip which is too large will not anchor securely and tend to slip off the pedicle. Absorption of these clips takes about 6 months.

Ligatures

The adaptation of knotting techniques to laparoscopic surgery was started in the mid 1970s by Semm and his coworkers [17,18].

Preformed endoloops

The first techniques adopted was the use of the endoloop of gut (Ethicon) based on the slipknot first described by Roeder for use during tonsillectomy (Fig. 3.29 a,b). The item is packaged with the long tail of this endoloop threaded through a push-rod. The endoloop is loaded into the suture applicator and this is then introduced down a 5.5 mm cannula (Fig. 3.30). The equivalent Surgitie (USSC) is packaged with a disposable suture applicator. After the loop is placed around the pedicle or tissue to be ligated, the knot is tightened by the push-rod under visual control until it is locked firmly in place. Catgut is the preferred material for this ligating technique, as it resists reverse slipping better than any other suture material. In addition, as hydration of the catgut occurs *in vivo*, the material swells, thus increasing the security of the knot. This property of swelling by hydration is also shared (to a lesser extent) by silk. The catgut Roeder knot can be safely used for the ligation of vessels up to 3.0 mm diameter. This assertion is backed up by studies the authors have performed (see below) and the experience of its use in Kiel with gynaecological operations performed since 1977. For large vessels the Kiel surgeons advocate the application of three loops for added safety. A chromic catgut endoloop preloaded in a suture applicator should be available on the scrub nurse's table for rapid introduction into the abdomen and application in the event of unexpected bleeding. The alternative course of action in this eventuality is the application of a metal clip to the bleeding vessel. Preformed endoloops with PDS (Ethicon) or Polysorb (USSC) which employ modified slip knots are now available, and are preferable to catgut for securing larger arteries.

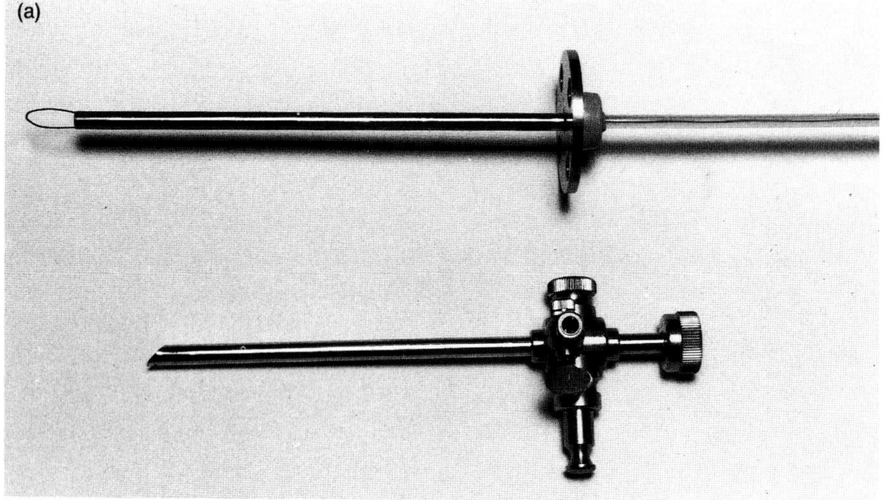

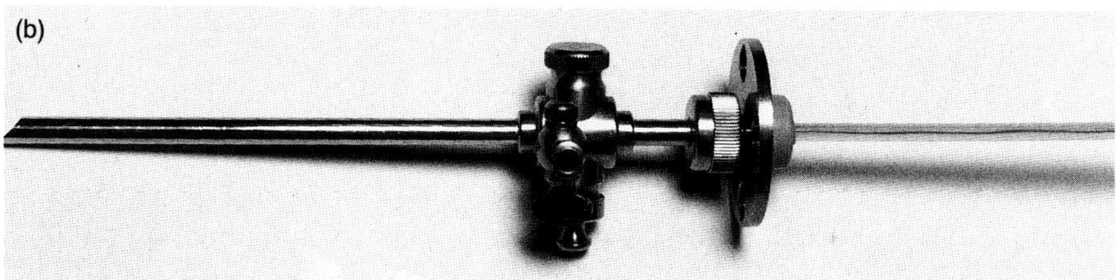

Fig. 3.30 The endoloop preloaded in the suture applicator is passed down the 5.5 mm cannula.

Ligature of blood vessels in continuity using external slip knots

As in open surgery, the safest technique is to ligate the vessel in continuity before it is divided. This cannot be achieved by the preformed endoloop. There are a variety of external slip knots; two are especially useful: the Roeder knot for catgut and the Tayside knot for all other materials.

Roeder knot. For this purpose a catgut suture is threaded through the push-rod which is loaded inside a suture applicator. The steps of this important technique are illustrated in Fig. 3.31 a–i. Two needle-holders are needed to execute this procedure. A 3.0 mm one (which allows room for the suture lying alongside it within the suture applicator), is used to grasp the end of the suture (leaving the push-rod outside) and is inserted together with the suture applicator down a 5.5 mm cannula. The end of the suture is advanced by the needle-holder around the desired pedicle and grasped momentarily by the 5.0 mm needle-holder (inserted via another cannula) before it is transferred back to the 3.0 mm holder and then withdrawn to the exterior through the suture applicator. To prevent damage to the tissue by serration from the suture during the withdrawal process, the 5.0 mm needle-holder is inserted inside the loop to take the tension and friction off the vessel. Once the end of the suture emerges from the cannula the assistant seals the suture applicator by finger occlusion to prevent gas leakage, while the Roeder knot is tied and trimmed before it is laid down to the desired site by the push-rod under visual control. Once locked in place the suture is cut with hook scissors.

The authors have been interested in the safety of the Roeder knot and so have conducted experiments to investigate the tension experienced by vessel ligatures, and the tension at which reverse slipping of the Roeder knots occurs. Table 3.1 shows data concerning the tension exerted on a ligature during the *ex-vivo* perfusion of blood vessels.

We then tested the safety of the Roeder knot by cutting the loop and distracting the two cut ends to determine the load required to induce reversed slipping. Catgut sutures stored in alcohol were opened and allowed to dry for 10 minutes before knotting. Dry-packaged sterile catgut is available commercially, designed for laparoscopic ligating. It is preferable to the usual alcohol-packaged variety because its stiffness decreases twisting and tangling as the knot is laid down. In our experiments the knot hydration which occurs *in vivo* was simulated by soaking knots in sheep amniotic fluid. The findings of this study are shown in Table 3.2. Dry catgut gave the best performance and the safety of this knot improved sixfold after hydration, due to swelling of the material.

The measured tension of a small artery was thus found to be only a few grams and the calculated tension by the cystic duct (assuming a diameter of 5.0 mm which ties down to 2.0 mm and a maximum biliary pressure of 30.0 cmH_2O) is approximately 1.1 g wt. These data serve to indicate the high safety margin of the Roeder knot using dry chromic catgut.

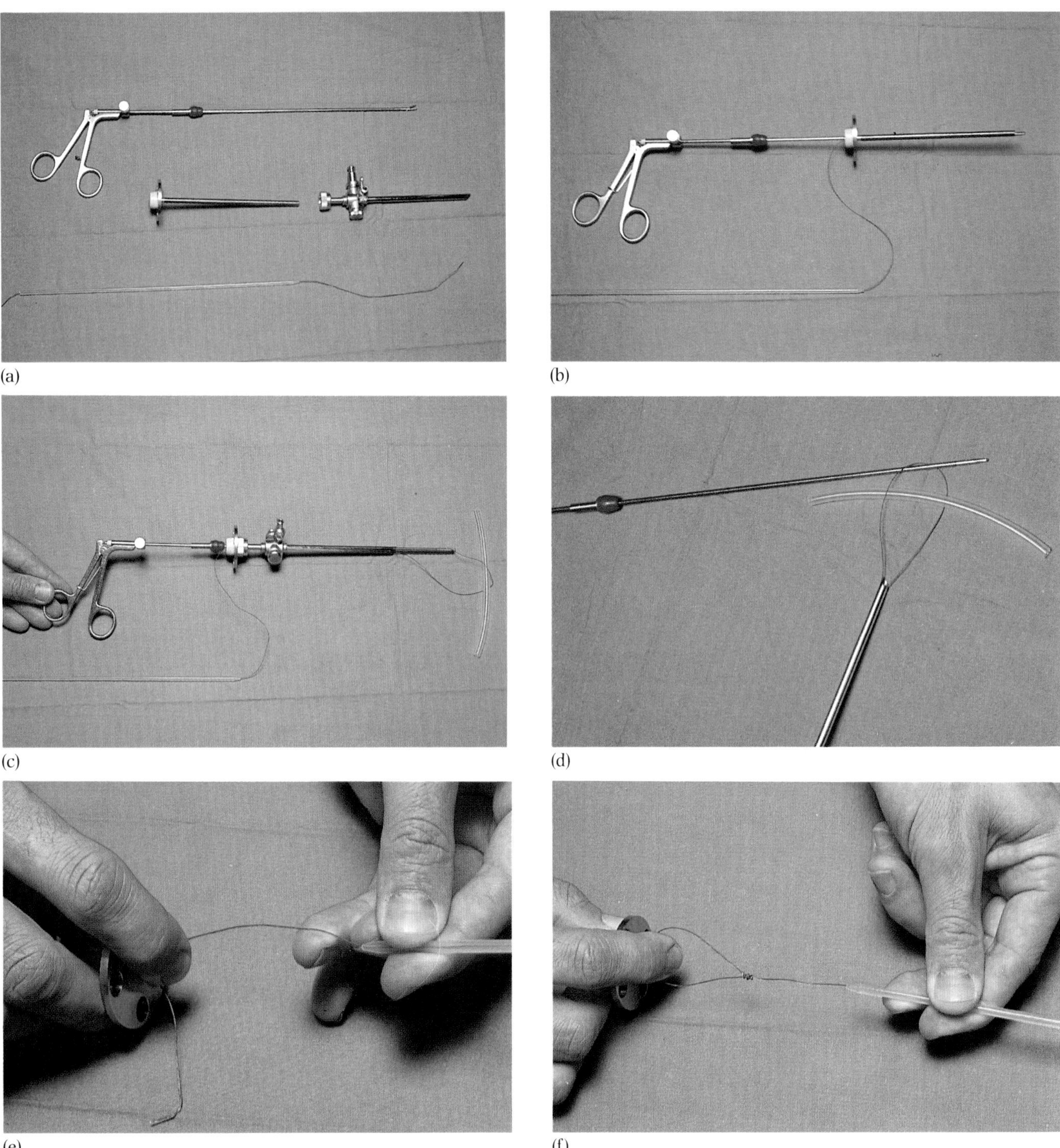

(a) (b) (c) (d) (e) (f)

Fig. 3.31 Photographic demonstration of the steps involved in ligating tubular structures using the Roeder slip knot with catgut. (a) The instruments needed are an accessory 5.5 mm cannula, a suture applicator, a push-rod containing the suture, a 3.0 mm needle-holder, hook scissors (not shown) and a grasping forceps. (b) Step 1: loading of suture applicator with 3.0 mm needle-holder grasping the suture. (c) Step 2: insertion of the loaded suture applicator into the trocar and placement of the suture around the 'structure'. (d) Step 3: withdrawal of the suture through the suture applicator with grasping forceps, preventing serration of the structure. (e) Step 4: assistant's finger sealing the suture applicator. (f) Step 5: completed Roeder knot. (g) Step 6: knot engaged into the suture applicator. (h) Step 7: Roeder knot slipped down by the push-rod with counter-traction on the tail of the suture. (i) Step 8: final locking of the knot.

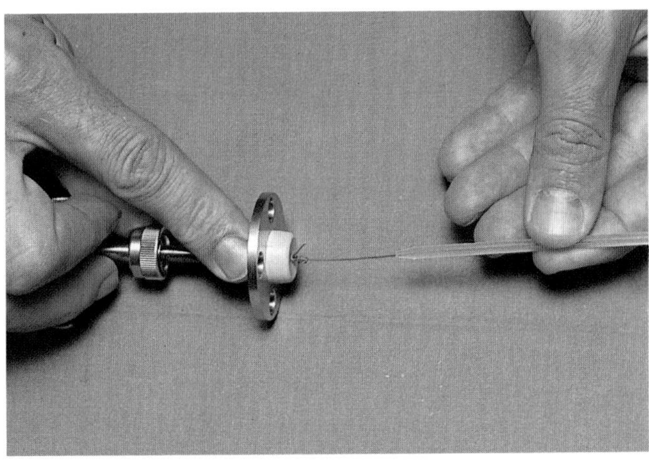

(g)

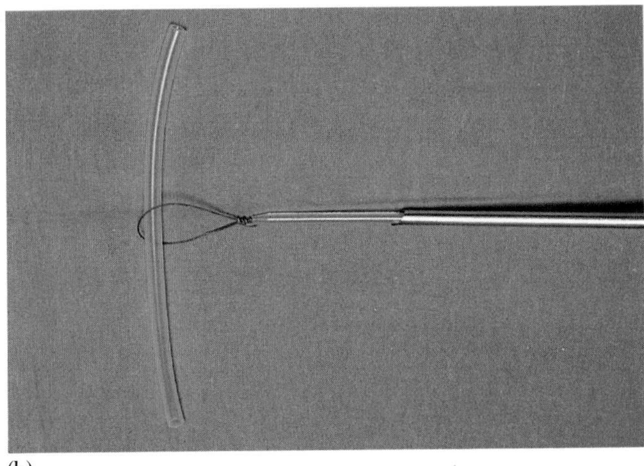

(h)

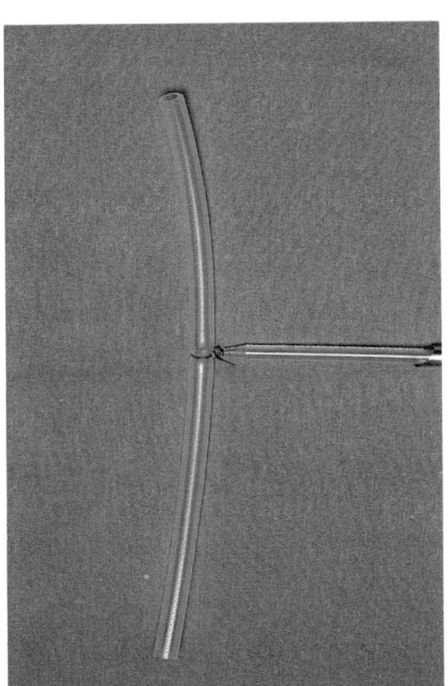

(i)

Fig. 3.31 *(continued)*

Tayside knot. This is the safest external slip knot, which can be used with any material (braided or monofilament, absorbable or non-absorbable). Laboratory studies with the tensiometer have shown that this knot resists a slipping force of 4.0 kg, which is equivalent to that of a surgeon's knot. It is outlined in Fig. 3.32 and is the knot the authors use for large vessels such as the azygos vein in oesophageal dissections, and the inferior mesenteric artery in colonic resections. Apart from its absolute security, the knot is quicker and easier to tie than the Roeder slip knot. The Tayside knot is pushed down and locked in place with a plastic push-rod in the same fashion as the Roeder knot.

External surgeon's knot. The two ends of the ligature are exteriorized inside a suture applicator or reducer tube. While the assistant puts a finger between

Table 3.1 Comparison of observed and derived* values for tension on ligatures on blood vessels perfused at 200 cmH_2O pressure (147 mmHg)

Vessel diam. (mm)	Radius at ligated site (mm)	Ligature tension (g)	
		Observed	Derived*
Veins			
2.6	0.40	2.3	1.4
3.7	0.40	4.0	2.0
6.0	0.75	10.6	6.0
8.0	0.70	14.0	7.5
9.4	0.80	18.0	10.0
Arteries			
4.4	0.90	9.6	5.3
4.5	0.75	8.3	5.0
6.2	0.90	17.6	7.5
9.0	2.15	55.0	26.0

Values for observed ligature tension were the mean of three readings.
*The derived tension was obtained with the formula $T = 3/2\ pr\delta$, where p = pressure within vessel, r = radius of vessel and δ = radius of vessel at point of ligation.

Table 3.2 Roeder knots: tension required for reversed slipping

Suture type	Tension (g, median & range)	
	Immediate	After hydrating (48 h)
00/Chromic	1125 (750–1575)	1100 (750–1400)
0/Chromic	1125 (225–2700)	1700 (1500–1875)
0/Plain gut	2000 (650–2450)	1800 (1575–2000)
1/Chromic	1400 (700–3050)	1650 (1150–1950)
1/Dry plain gut	475 (275–550)	3175 (2150–4000)
00/Polyglactin	300 (150–800)	325 (225–575)

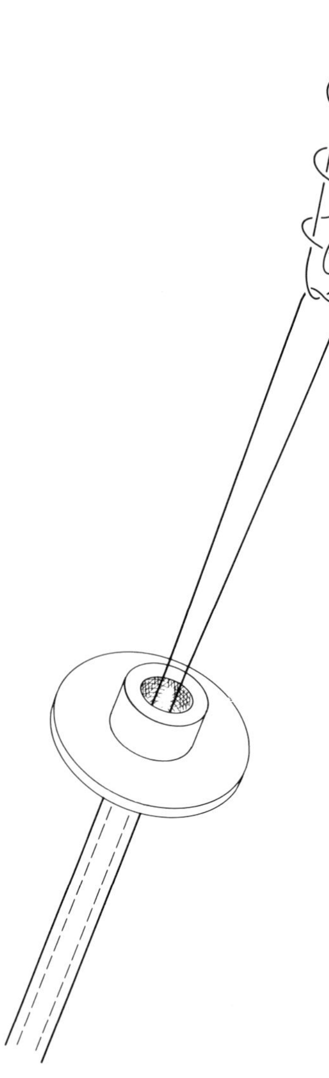

Fig. 3.32 Tayside external slip knot which works with any material and resists a reverse slipping force of 4.0 kg.

the two strands on top of the suture applicator to prevent gas leaks, the first component of the surgeon's knot (a double hitch) is fashioned. The hitch is then slid into place by means of a knot-pusher (Fig. 3.33). The second and third components of the knot are also fashioned externally, pushed down and locked in place with the knot-pusher. In practice there are several disadvantages to this type of knotting in laparoscopic surgery: the technique

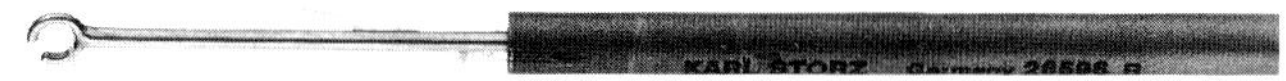

Fig. 3.33 Knot-pusher used to slide the first double hitch of an external surgeon's knot. This technique has considerable disadvantages.

is slow, some materials do not slide easily after the creation of the first double hitch, and the grip on the vessels by this may loosen while the second hitch is slid down, resulting in a knot which does not securely compress the vessel.

Internal knotting

This is used in relation to suturing and is executed with two needle-holders. There are two types of knot which can be executed: the standard microsurgical knot and the tumbled square knot. Internal knotting requires practice to be performed smoothly and quickly, and this is best achieved by use of the practice bench with foam or resected specimens. Mechanical devices for internal knotting such as the Endotyer (Solos Endoscopy) are cumbersome, require several instrument insertions and are an inferior substitute for manual internal knotting.

Another alternative system to internal knotting is the application of compressible silver beads or small polydioxanone clips to the suture at the desired points. These are undoubtedly quick and can facilitate continuous suturing, but carry the intrinsic disadvantage of suture damage at the point of compression, with the risk of subsequent breakage.

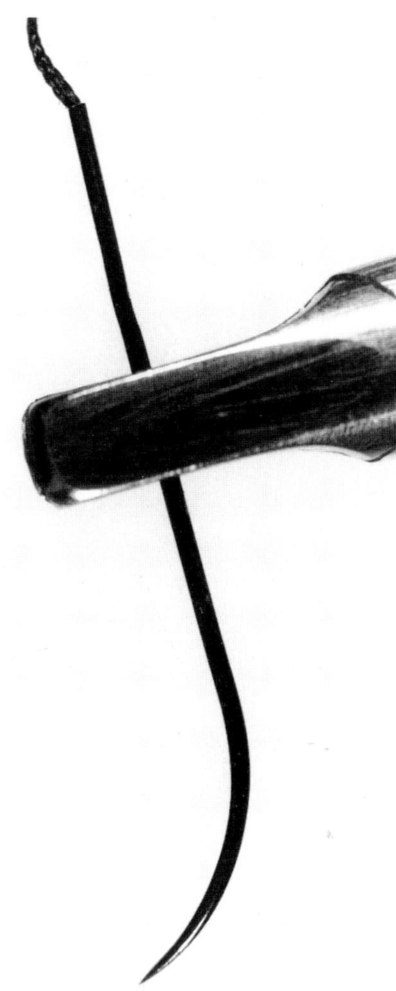

Fig. 3.34 Dundee endoski needle for laparoscopic suturing.

Tissue approximation

The preformed catgut endoloop or Surgitie combined with push-rod can also be used for tissue approximation. The loop is fed into the peritoneum, an instrument placed within the loop grasps the tissue to tent it up, the loop is tightened around it and the tail is cut. This technique is suitable for dealing with fresh perforations, for securing the base of the appendix during appendectomy, etc. Again, the advantages of this technique are convenience and speed.

Laparoscopic suturing

The sutures must be atraumatic. Although straight and half-circle needles can be used, the best needle shape is the endoski (Fig. 3.34). This considerably facilitates both continuous and interrupted suturing [19,20]. The atraumatic suture is introduced into the peritoneal cavity inside a suture applicator or reducer tube. The problem of needle swivel has been overcome to some extent by improved needle-holder design. Once inside the peritoneum, the active 5.0 mm needle-holder is used to grasp the needle and the tissue is sutured by passing the needle through the tissue to the 3.0 mm needle-holder and then regrasping it with the 5.0 mm needle-holder. The techniques of laparoscopic suturing are described in Chapter 10.

Maintenance, care and sterilization of equipment

The more commonly used laparoscopic instruments are shown in Fig. 3.35.

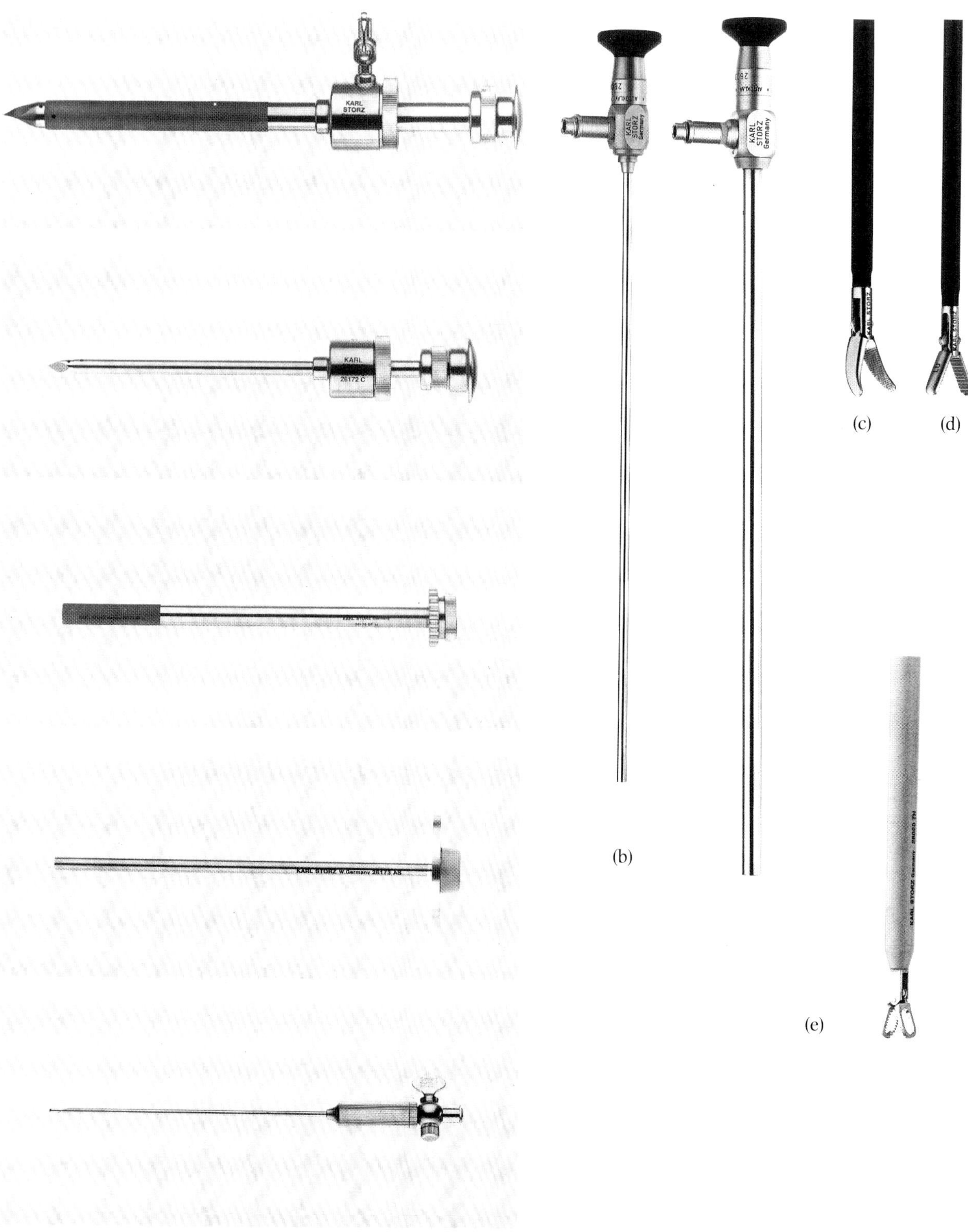

(a) (b) (c) (d) (e)

Fig. 3.35 Commonly used laparoscopic instruments. (a) Top to bottom: flap-valve 11.0 mm trocar and 5.5 mm trocar, reducer tube, suture applicator, Veress needle. (b) 10.0 and 5.0 mm telescopes. (c) Curved grasping forceps. (d) Atraumatic grasping forceps: round-ended. (e) Heavy-duty traumatic grasping forceps. (f) Clip applicators: (left) non-disposable for metal clips, (right) non-disposable for absorbable clips (g) Berci dissecting spatula (insulated) and electrosurgical hook knife (insulated). (h) Suction/irrigation cannula. (i) Cholangiographic cannula.

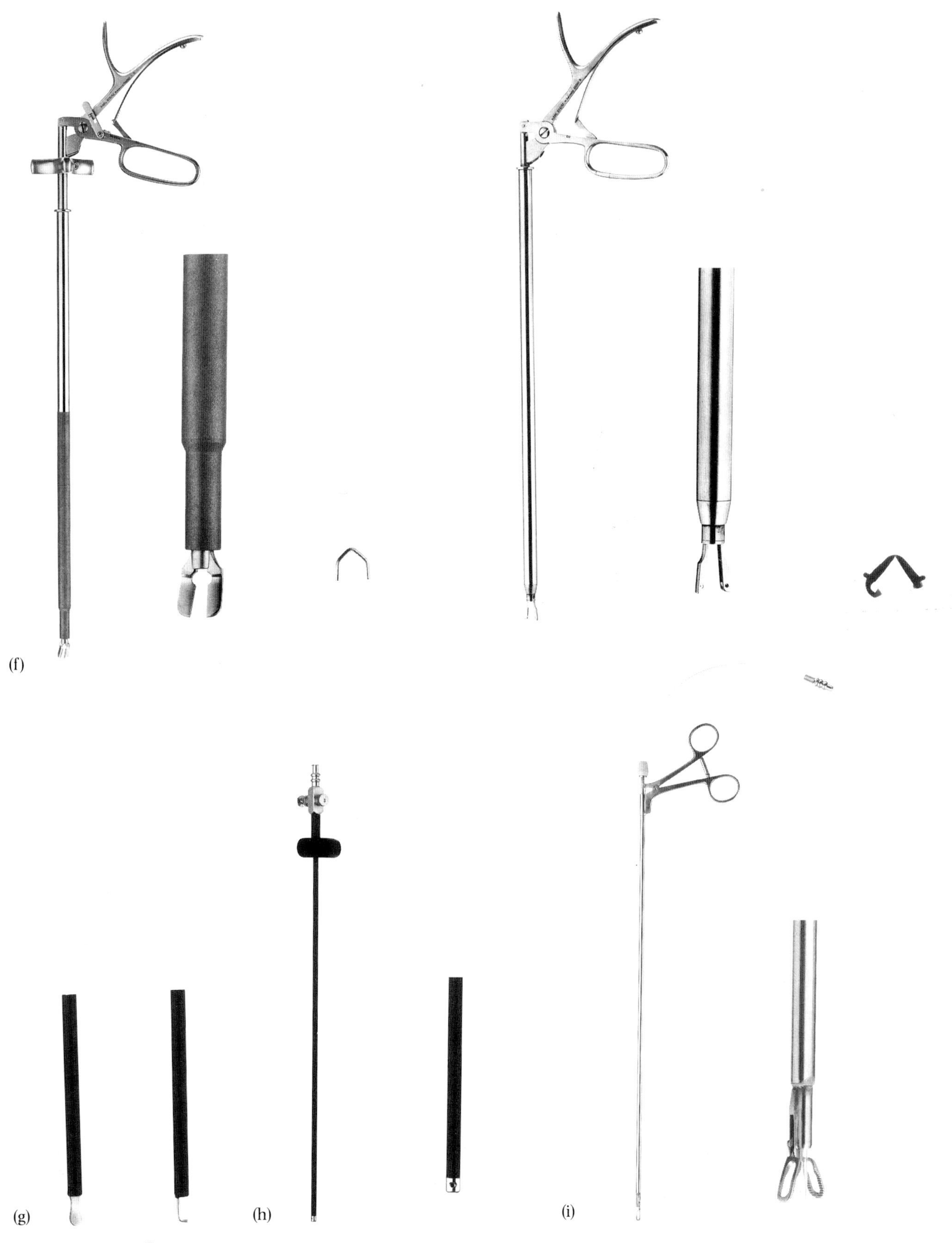

Fig. 3.35 *(continued)*

These are delicate and should be handled with care to avoid damage. The success of laparoscopic procedures is to a large measure dependent on the availability of all the instruments which may be required (to cover any eventuality) in working order. Ideally the cleaning, maintenance and packaging should be designated to one person. These instruments will inevitably be damaged or lost if they are processed through the central sterile supply unit together with the large instruments used in open-access surgery.

There are three options for sterilization: gas sterilization in ethylene oxide, steam autoclaving and chemical sterilization. The ethylene oxide method is undoubtedly the best and least harmful to the instruments, including the optics. The entire set is packaged in one tray before sterilization. Its disadvantage is the delay, which can amount to several days before the instruments can be used.

Steam autoclaving is often recommended by some manufacturers. Although this is a perfectly feasible option for metal instruments, it is not ideal for the optics as these may sustain damage during the process, particularly if the cooling period is not carefully controlled, and this does happen in busy departments. In the authors' experience, telescopes of the rod-lens system deteriorate if subjected to repeated steam autoclaving, even if this is conducted with care.

Chemical sterilization by soaking in glutaraldehyde is useful, particularly when the set is to be used on two consecutive cases, and for quick sterilization of specific items such as the camera and any dropped instruments, but meticulous rinsing is essential. Before instruments are subjected to chemical sterilization, they have to be cleaned meticulously. This applies in particular to instruments which cannot be dismantled, where congealed blood may remain around joints and in between the push-pull rod and the outer sheath, the dead space of which normally measures only 2–3 ml.

Disposable and reusable instruments

With the exception of the optics, almost all laparoscopic instruments are now available as disposable items from several well-established and many newer companies. There are obvious advantages inherent to disposable products. The instrument when used is guaranteed to be in its peak functional state, and therefore the risk of malfunction is considerably diminished. This is undoubtedly an important consideration, especially when it applies to complex instrumentation such as disposable cartridge staplers and preloaded clip appliers. However, when it is extended to the more common instruments there are practical disadvantages which must be borne in mind. The first of these is the increasing cost, which is directly proportional to the number of disposable items used per case. The disposable instruments create additional problems for the hospital by increasing the administrative task of ordering, inventory and storage. On a more practical level, an adequate stock of disposable equipment to cover all the contingencies is essential for a successful practice and to ensure the uninterrupted progress of laparoscopic operations. There is also the risk, human nature being what it is, that disposable equipment will be cleaned, sterilized and reused a number of times. This is a dangerous practice, as the ability of these disposable items to be cleaned is limited, and their functional performance deteriorates rapidly. They are only safe and reliable if used once only. The ecological consequences inherent to the disposal of the plastic material are real and will assume increasing importance, particularly in Europe.

For the common instruments such as graspers, scissors, hooks etc., a good reusable instrument is much cheaper in the long run, even if additional manpower and time are needed for maintenance, cleaning and sterilization. The way ahead amid this controversy is the development of semidisposable instruments, where the functional part is disposable but the rest of the instrument is reusable.

References

1 Sigel B, Golub RM, Lauric A *et al.* Technique of ultrasonic detection and mapping of abdominal wall adhesions. *Surg Endosc* 1991; **5**: 161–165.

2 Ravintharan T, Shimi S, Banting S, Hassan AK, Sinclair D J, McCullough AS, Cuschieri A. Prospective blind evaluation of the ultrasound visceral slide technique in the location of adhesions in patients undergoing laparoscopic cholecystectomy. *Surg Endosc* (in press).

3 Cuschieri A. Tissue approximation. In: Berci G (ed), *Problems in General Surgery*. JB Lippincott, Philadelphia, 1991; pp. 365–377.

4 Hasson HM. Modified instrument and method for laparoscopy. *Am J Obstet Gynecol* 1971; **110**: 886–887.

5 Booker WM, Johnson A. Pneumoperitoneum: physiological effects. *Anaesth Analg* 1944; **2**: 23–26.

6 Elwood BJ, Piltz GF, Potter BP. Electrocardiographic observations on pneumoperitoneum. *Am Heart J* 1940; **19**: 206–208.

7 Gordon NLM, Smith I, Shwapp GH. Cardiac arrhythmias during laparoscopy. *Br Med J* 1972; **1**: 625.

8 Scott DB, Julian DG. Observations on cardiac arrhythmias during laparoscopy. *Br Med J* 1972; **1**: 411–413.

9 Motew M, Ivancovitch A, Bieniac J *et al.* Cardiovascular effects and acid–base and blood gases during laparoscopy. *Am J Obstet Gynecol* 1973; **115**: 1002–1012.

10 Lenz RJ, Thomas TA, Wilkins DG. Cardiovascular changes during laparoscopy. *Anaesthesia* 1976; **31**: 4–12.

11 Carmichael DE. Laparoscopy: cardiac considerations. *Fert Steril* 1970; **22**: 69–70.

12 El-Miawi MF, Wahbi O, El-Bagouri IS *et al.* Physiologic changes during CO_2 and N_2O pneumoperitoneum in diagnostic laparoscopy. *J Repro Med* 1981; **26**: 338–346.

13 Hodgson C, McClelland N, Newton JR. Some effects of the peritoneal insufflation of carbon dioxide at laparoscopy. *Anaesthesia* 1970; **25**: 382–390.

14 Mouret P. Le pneumopéritoine en suspension. *Endomag* 1991; **2**: 2–4.

15 Voyles CR, Petro AB, Meena AL, Haick AJ, Koury AM. A practical approach to laparoscopic cholecystectomy. *Am J Surg* 1991; **161**: 365–370.

16 Hunter JG. Laser or electrocautery for laparoscopic cholecystectomy? *Am J Surg* 1991; **161**: 345–349.

17 Semm K. Tissue-puncher and loop ligation. New aids for surgical–therapeutic pelviscopy (laparoscopy) = endoscopic intra-abdominal surgery. *Endoscopy* 1978; **10**: 119–124.

18 Semm K, Mettler. Technical progress in pelvic surgery via operative laparoscopy. *Am J Obstet Gynecol* 1980; **138**: 121–127.
19 Nathanson LK, Nathanson PDK, Cuschieri A. Safety of vessel ligation in laparoscopic surgery. *Endoscopy* 1991; **23**: 206–209.
20 Shimi S, Banting S, Cuschieri A. Laparoscopy for advanced pancreatic cancer: bilio-enteric anastomosis for advanced disease. *Br J Surg* 1992; (in press).

4 : Technique of laparoscopic cholecystectomy

Anaesthesia

The patient is premedicated with temazepam (20–30 mg) 2 hours prior to induction and receives a small dose of intravenous midazolam (4.0 mg) on arrival in the anaesthetic room. Induction is carried out with thiopentone (5.0 mg/kg) and neuromuscular blockade is established using alcuronium (0.2 mg/kg), or vercuronium (0.1 mg/kg) in patients with hypertension. All patients are intubated with a cuffed endotracheal tube and ventilated mechanically. Nitrous oxide (66%), oxygen and enflurane are used to maintain anaesthesia, with increments of alcuronium and fentanyl (0.04–0.08 mg/h) as required.

Monitoring during anaesthesia includes ECG, blood pressure (Dinamap), oxygen saturation (Datascope Accusat), end-tidal CO_2 (Datex Multicap) and urine output. End-tidal CO_2 is maintained at 30 mmHg. Fluids are replaced using Hartmann's solution (250 ml/h). An intravenous injection of a cephalosporin such as cephuroxime (1.0–1.5 g) is administered at the start of the operation.

At the end of the procedure, neuromuscular blockade is reversed with neostigmine and atropine. Oxygen is administered for the first 3 hours after operation and morphine is used for postoperative analgesia as required.

Position of the patient, layout, skin preparation and draping

Laparoscopic cholecystectomy can be performed with the patient either in the modified lithotomy or the supine position.

Modified lithotomy position

This is favoured by European surgeons, particularly the French. The patient is positioned supine on the operating table (with the distal section removed) such that the lower limbs are suspended on Lloyd Davies stirrups in an abducted position with the knees slightly flexed (Fig. 4.1a). This allows the surgeon to operate sitting down facing the patient's abdomen. The table is tilted 20° head up (reverse Trendelenburg position). A diathermy pad is placed underneath the buttocks and connected to the high-frequency electrosurgical generator, which must be of the isolated-circuit variety. The advantage of the modified lithotomy approach, apart from the sitting position which is an important consideration in lengthy procedures, is that the surgeon can steady his wrist movements by resting his elbows on the patient's abdomen.

The assistant stands on the patient's left and the scrub nurse on the opposite side. The insufflator, suction/irrigation system, telescope heater, electrocautery unit and xenon light source are positioned on the right of the

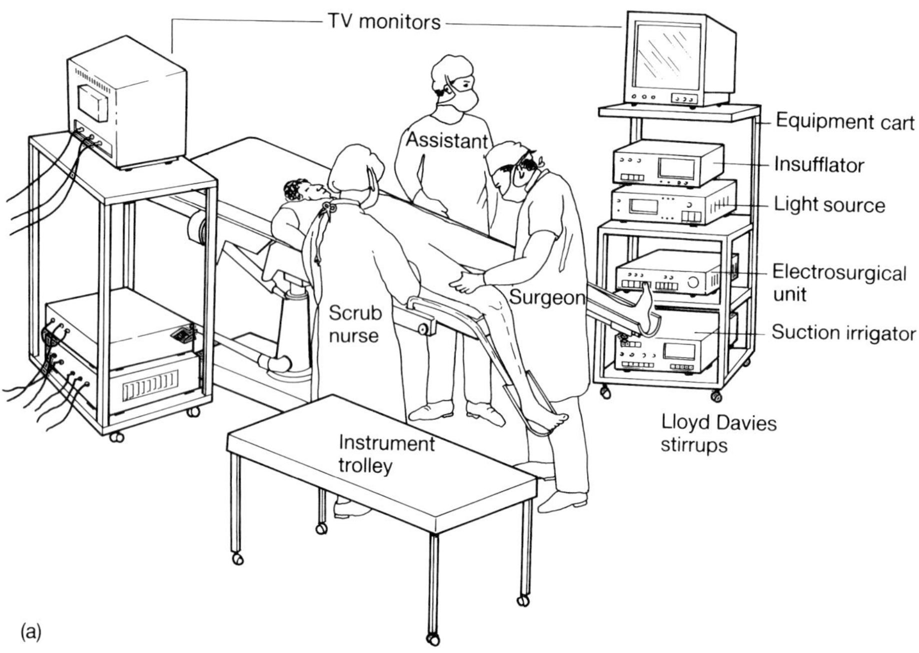

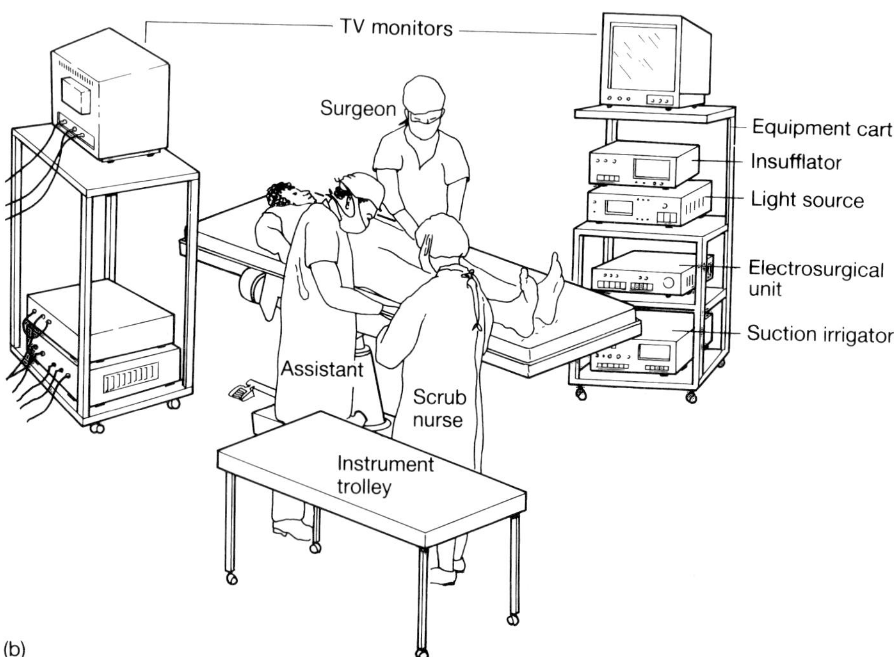

Fig. 4.1 Layout of patient, staff and equipment. (a) Modified lithotomy position. (b) Supine position.

surgeon. The instrument trolley is placed on the left of the surgeon between him or her and the scrub nurse. The TV monitor (linked to the endovideo camera) is placed on the right side of the patient so that the assistant and scrub nurse can clearly visualize the progress of the operation (Fig. 4.1a). If the operating theatre is dedicated to laparoscopic surgery, the TV monitor is best ceiling-mounted with a pivot arrangement to enable adjustment of the viewing angle to suit the needs of the team.

Supine position

This is popular in North America and the UK. The patient is placed in the ordinary supine position, with the table tilted 20° reverse Trendelenburg with the surgeon on the left and the assistant on the right of the patient. The best layout in this situation is shown in Fig. 4.1b. This is now the authors' preferred position because it allows greater manoeuvrability and is less likely to result in compression trauma to the patient's calf veins. The supine position necessitates the availability of two television monitors, one facing the surgeon and the other facing the assistant (Fig. 4.1b).

Nasogastric intubation and bladder catheterization

It is the authors' custom to insert a nasogastric tube to ensure complete gastric deflation during the procedure, since a distended stomach and duodenal cap can obscure the operative field. As a safety precaution, the urinary bladder is catheterized prior to the insertion of the Veress needle and the creation of a pneumoperitoneum. If the latter is not adopted as a routine measure, it is important that the suprapubic region is percussed for dullness to exclude a distended urinary bladder before the Veress needle is inserted. Both the nasogastric tube and the bladder catheter are removed at the end of the operation.

Skin preparation and draping

The skin of the abdomen from the level of the nipple line to the pubic region is prepared with chlorhexidine soap followed by chlorhexidine–alcohol antiseptic solution (or a suitable alternative depending on the surgeon's preference). If the patient is in the modified lithotomy position, drapes with integral leggings and a central cutout should be used. The central cutout is positioned to expose the entire upper abdomen, including the costal margins. The edges of the drapes are sutured temporarily to the skin. This practice is better than the use of skin clips, especially if cholangiography is contemplated. Some surgeons prefer to use disposable drapes. Standard towelling as for open cholecystectomy is used for the supine position.

Pneumoperitoneum, insertion of main trocar/cannula and diagnostic laparoscopy

Pneumoperitoneum

The technique and measures that ensure the safe creation of a pneumoperitoneum are outlined in Chapter 3. Special precautions are necessary in patients with an abdomen scarred due to previous surgery, and in some of these patients a decision may be taken to proceed with open laparoscopy.

Main trocar/cannula

This should have an external diameter of 11.0 mm and is used for the introduction of the video-laparoscope. Its use together with a 10.5 mm reducer results in an adequate space between the telescope and the inner surface of the cannula, thereby ensuring free gas flow and maintenance of the pneumoperitoneum during the course of the operation. Some prefer to use a disposable sheathed cannula to minimize the risk of visceral injury during this step of the operation. This is not, however, a substitute for good technique as visceral and vascular injuries can be sustained by the sheathed cannula due to the phenomenon of sheath drag [1]. If a non-disposable cannula is used, this should be of the flap-valve (trap-door) variety, as compared to the trumpet valve type this permits unrestricted movement of the telescope. The available trocars are either conical or pyramidal, with sharp cutting edges. The latter type results in a more controlled direct 'cut-penetration' of the abdominal parieties, but is unsuitable for entry by the 'Z' technique as the cutting edges lacerate the muscle fibres and associated arterioles instead of separating them, with the risk of significant abdominal wall bleeding. The non-disposable metal trocars are hollow and have a hole near to the pointed tip. This provides an important safety feature during insertion (see below).

Insertion of main trocar/cannula

The optimal site for insertion is the immediate subumbilical region. The skin incision used for the insertion of the Veress needle is extended in a vertical or transverse direction to 1.5 cm and deepened until the hiss of escaping gas is heard. In large or obese individuals with a long stretch between the umbilicus and the right costal margin, siting of the laparoscopic cannula is at a higher level on either side of the umbilicus.

The trocar/cannula is held in the right hand with the butt firmly pressed against the palm, and the index finger alongside the long axis of the shaft some 2.5 cm away from the tip (Fig. 4.2).

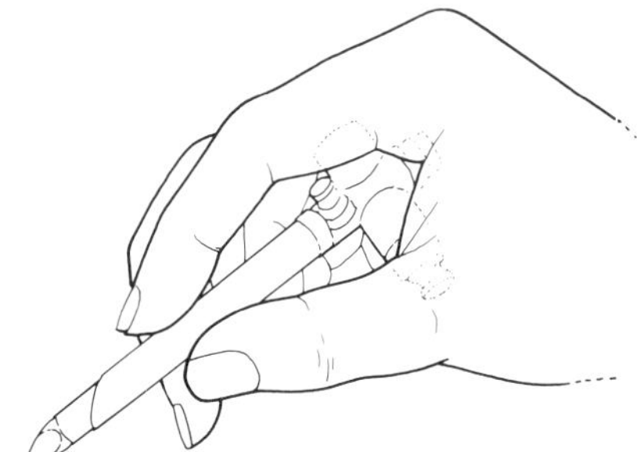

Fig. 4.2 Safe technique for introducing the main trocar/cannula. Pressure is exerted from the wrist and not from the shoulder. The index finger acts as a safety stop in case of sudden give. The periumbilical region is lifted by the left hand.

The periumbilical region is pulled firmly up by the left hand so that the abdominal wall is tented upwards and the trocar/cannula is introduced through the subumbilical incision parallel to the axis of the aorta, pointing to the centre of the pelvis. Alternatively, two strong Littlewood's forceps or towel clips are applied to the edges of the skin wound and the abdominal wall is pulled up by traction exerted on the forceps by the assistant. Pressure from the wrist accompanied by to-and-fro rotational movement is used to 'ream' the trocar/cannula through the parieties. Pressure against the palm of the hand prevents riding of the trocar inside the cannula as it encounters the resistance provided by the abdominal wall. The tip of the index finger against the long shaft of the assembly acts as a safety stop in case of sudden give. With the disposable sheathed cannula, a click is heard due to snapping of the sheath over the trocar point as soon as the peritoneal lining is breached. By contrast, with the non-disposable type, the perforation near the tip of the trocar leads to a sudden escape of gas, with a resultant audible hiss, as soon as complete penetration of the abdominal wall is achieved. Irrespective of type of system used, the trocar is withdrawn before the cannula is advanced further. The gas line is then connected to the side port of the cannula and the tap opened to maintain insufflation of the peritoneal cavity.

Laparoscopic inspection

The previously heated 10.0 mm laparoscope is attached to the endo camera (sterile or inside a transparent plastic sterile sleeve). After activation of the high-intensity light source, the light cable is attached to the telescope. The latter is then introduced down the cannula under vision. If blood clot or tissue debris is seen (usually near the terminal segment of the cannula), the telescope is withdrawn and the cannula is cleaned (see Chapter 3) before reinsertion of the laparoscope.

The initial laparoscopic inspection is one of the most crucial steps of the entire procedure. It has three objectives:

1 The detection of inadvertent injuries caused during insufflation and insertion of the main trocar/cannula.
2 The exclusion of additional unsuspected intra-abdominal pathology.
3 The assessment of the feasibility of laparoscopic cholecystectomy.

Detection and management of laparoscopic injuries

With care and attention to detail, laparoscopic injuries are rare and usually minor. The commonest problem is entanglement of the Veress needle in the omentum, with insufflation of the peritoneal fat causing bubble formation which, if extensive, may obscure the field of vision. This usually clears rapidly.

Minor oozing from the stab wounds in the abdomen is common and almost invariably stops spontaneously. Arterial bleeding may occasionally be encountered from epiperitoneal and muscular vessels close to the posterior rectus sheath. This problem is more common with the pyramidal trocars, particularly when the indirect 'Z' technique of cannula introduction is used, or when the trocar/cannula is inserted to the right or left of the midline. It requires immediate attention to avoid extensive haematoma formation within the rectus sheath. To achieve control, a secondary accessory 5.0 mm cannula is inserted in the right upper quadrant. The easiest technique consists of the use of the suture holder which is loaded with a 2/0 ligature and introduced under vision to one side of the bleeding area. The ligature is then disengaged and the suture holder withdrawn and inserted on the other side of the bleeding area. The internal end of the ligature is loaded in the suture holder, which is then exteriorized. The two external ends of the ligature are then pulled and tied over a gauze swab. An alternative technique consists in introducing a 2/0 non-absorbable suture on a 60 mm (hand) cutting needle to the left of the bleeding point. The needle is grasped internally with a needle-holder, pulled into the peritoneal cavity and then brought out to the right of the bleeding area. The two ends of the suture are then pulled tight and tied over a small gauze roll. Minor bleeding points in the omentum may require electrocoagulation. Needle-stab wounds to the viscera and solid organs are inspected closely for leakage.

More extensive injuries and active arterial bleeding from large vessels are dealt with by immediate laparotomy (see Chapter 3).

Exclusion of additional unsuspected pathology

A systematic inspection of the contents of the four quadrants and the pelvis is undertaken. This is equivalent to the exploratory laparotomy in routine biliary surgery. Common disorders of a benign nature, for example colonic diverticular disease, pelvic adnexal disease in the female etc., are noted but do not preclude the performance of laparoscopic cholecystectomy. More serious findings, particularly if considered to be neoplastic in nature, may necessitate conversion to open laparotomy or postponement of the surgical treatment pending further investigations and preparation of the patient.

Assessment of the feasibility of laparoscopic cholecystectomy

This is an assessment of the technical difficulty and safety of gallbladder excision via the laparoscopic route. To a large extent the decision is influenced by the experience of the surgeon in laparoscopic surgery. The situations which may be encountered are:

Easy cases. The patient is thin and the intraperitoneal fat is minimal. The gallbladder is floppy and non-adherent. When the gallbladder is lifted and retracted upwards by a grasping forceps, the cystic pedicle (fold of peritoneum covering the cystic artery, duct and lymph node) is readily identified as a smooth triangular fold between Hartmann's pouch and the common duct (Fig. 4.3). These patients are undoubtedly better served by laparoscopic than open cholecystectomy. Such cases should be done initially, before the surgeon has acquired the experience to tackle more difficult cases.

Feasible but difficult cases. These include obese patients in whom the cystic pedicle is fat-laden. A gallbladder containing a large stone load is difficult to grasp, and this causes problems with retraction and exposure. The gallbladder may be distended due to the cholecystitis, or because of a stone impacted in the neck or Hartmann's pouch. Difficulties may also be encountered due to adhesions from previous surgery. Provided the surgeon is experienced and

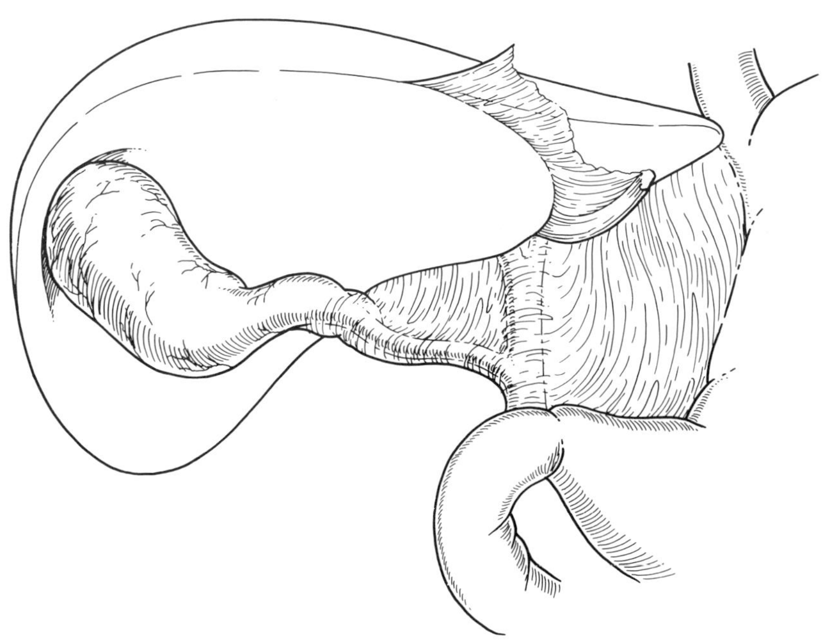

Fig. 4.3 Anatomy of the cystic pedicle.

is prepared to proceed slowly, these patients can undergo laparoscopic cholecystectomy with safety and a good outcome. Special measures are needed in these difficult cases, and these are dealt with in Chapter 5. In any event the operation takes longer.

Cases of uncertain feasibility—trial dissection. This group includes patients with dense adhesions, those in whom the cystic pedicle cannot be visualized, in situs inversus, and in patients with contracted fibrotic organs where the neck or Hartmann's pouch appears to be adherent to the common bile duct. In all these situations a careful trial dissection is commenced. The feasibility or otherwise of the procedure becomes apparent as the dissection proceeds. In adopting this approach, common sense should prevail and trial dissection should not be equated with a long hazardous procedure. If the surgeon cannot for any reason clearly identify and expose the structures of the cystic pedicle in the triangle of Calot in reasonable time, further laparoscopic endeavour should be desisted and the case converted to open surgery. Ideally length of cystic duct not less than 1.0 cm is needed for a safe laparoscopic cholecystectomy.

Unsuitable cases. These include patients with the following findings: severe acute cholecystitis with gangrenous patches or gross inflammatory phlegmon obscuring the structures of the porta hepatis; chronically inflamed gallbladder with the neck being adherent to the common bile duct indicative of a Mirizzi syndrome; and cirrhosis with established portal hypertension and large high-pressure varices surrounding the gallbladder and cystic pedicle. In patients with severe acute cholecystitis, which precludes safe dissection, a laparoscopic cholecystostomy (see Chapter 8) may be performed, with interval cholecystectomy at a later date. The cholecystostomy is carried out by aspiration of the gallbladder fluid contents through healthy fundus, followed by the insertion of a self-retaining balloon catheter.

It is foolhardy to attempt laparoscopic cholecystectomy in patients in whom the gallbladder neck/Hartmann's pouch is densely adherent to the common bile duct, since the risk of damage to the bile duct is considerable and in the author's opinion, unacceptable. These patients are best served by open cholecystectomy. Even in experienced hands, some 5% of patients with symptomatic gallstone disease are found to be unsuitable for laparoscopic cholecystectomy because of these findings on the initial inspection. In these patients the procedure is simply converted to the open operation at the same sitting. This is one of the reasons why laparoscopic cholecystectomy should only be attempted by fully trained biliary surgeons. The decision to convert to open surgery reflects good surgical judgment, and simply indicates that for the particular patient, open cholecystectomy is the appropriate treatment. Elective conversion must not in this context be equated with surgical failure; it results in a much better clinical outcome than persistence with the laparoscopic approach in the presence of technical difficulties, which often result in iatrogenic injury with enforced conversion and enhanced morbidity.

Insertion of accessory cannulae

These 5.0 mm cannulae are required for the insertion/withdrawal of the various laparoscopic instruments. They may either be disposable or non-disposable. The latter should have a flap valve in preference to a trumpet valve, as the latter requires to be depressed before instruments can be moved inside the cannula. This is an important practical consideration, as jamming of instruments inside the cannula not only slows down the procedure but carries the risk of stab injuries as a result of the increased force needed to advance the instrument. The sudden give may result in overshoot trauma to the surrounding organs. Another frequent occurrence which is encountered with both disposable and non-disposable cannulae is dislocation of the access

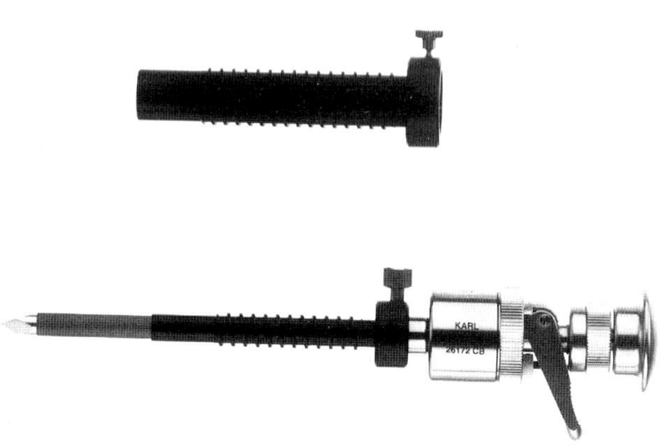

Fig. 4.4 Non-disposable trocar/cannula with screw relief to minimize the problem of inadvertent cannula dislocation during instrument manipulation.

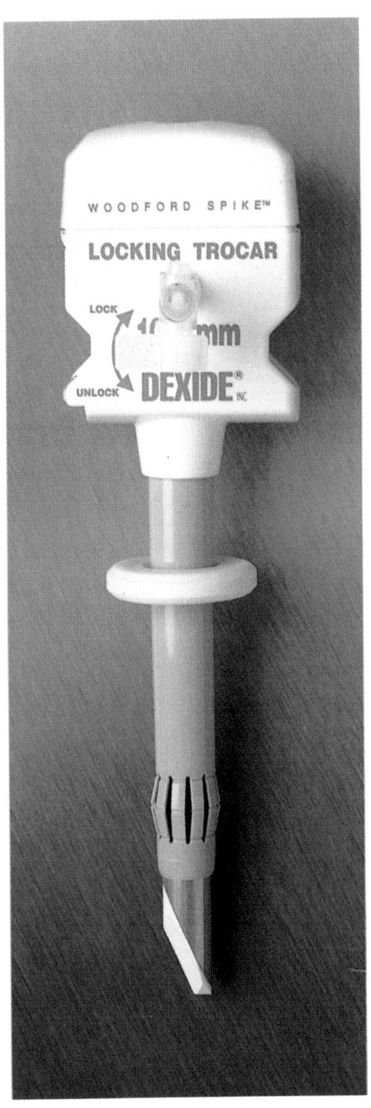

Fig. 4.5 Locking trocar cannula (Dexide Inc., Texas). Other makes incorporate a balloon near the tip to prevent dislocation during instrument manipulation (Marlow Surgical Technologies, Willoughby).

cannula during instrument manipulation, due either to valve sticking or congealed blood between the instrument shaft and the inside of the cannula. In relation to non-disposable systems, cannulae with an external spiral screw relief minimize this problem (Fig. 4.4). Cannula fixation outer screws serve the same function with disposable cannulae. This problem has led to the design of new disposable cannulae which either incorporate an internal inflatable balloon or have a retractable flange (operated through a sliding mechanism) which locks once the cannula is inserted (Fig. 4.5). All non-disposable cannulae require careful maintenance for optimum function.

Number and position of accessory cannulae

In the majority of patients three accessory cannulae are needed. The location of these depends on the technique used to expose the triangle of Calot. Irrespective of the approach used, all the accessory cannulae are inserted under vision. In practice the North American technique is easier provided the right lobe of the liver is soft and floppy. In the presence of a thick heavy right left lobe, the French exposure gives more adequate access and, for this reason, is safer.

French approach

In the French technique popularized by Dubois and Perissat [2–6], the liver is retracted upwards by a medially placed retractor (Fig. 4.6). The cannula sites for this technique (Fig. 4.7) are 10.0 mm upper left paramedian (for electrosurgical hook knife, scissors, etc.), 5.0 mm upper medial subcostal (for retraction, suction/irrigation), 5.0 mm lower right hypochondrial just lateral to the linea semilunaris (for grasping forceps).

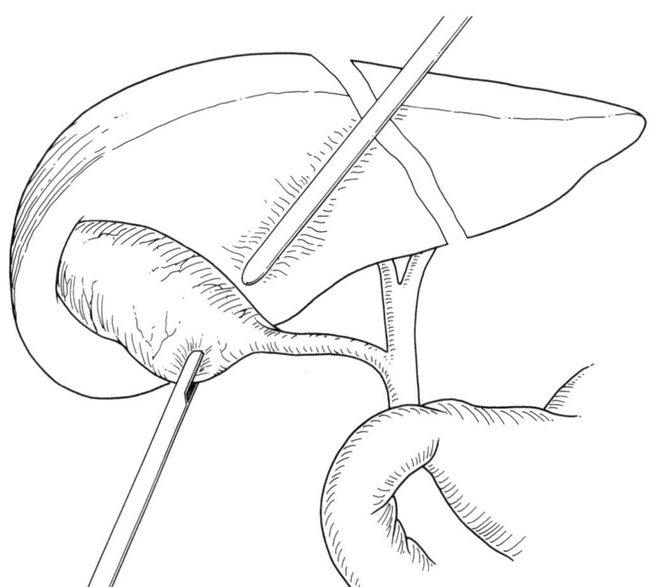

Fig. 4.6 French technique for exposure of the triangle of Calot.

North American approach

The exposure of the cystic pedicle is achieved by grasping the gallbladder fundus which is then lifted together with the right lobe, and rotated backwards (Fig. 4.8) [6,7]. The following placements are used with this technique (Fig. 4.9): 10.0 mm left upper paramedian (or just to the right of the midline, avoiding the falciform ligament), 5.0 mm right upper midclavicular and 5.0 mm right lower axillary. In some patients (obese, unexpected complications requiring additional instrumentation) a fourth cannula may be needed. This is positioned where needed, depending on the exigencies of the case.

The left upper paramedian cannula is placed about 1.0 cm lateral to the linea alba and 3.0 cm below the left costal margin [8]. Some surgeons prefer to insert this cannula just to the right of the falciform ligament to obviate any entanglement in this structure. However, this position may result in crowding of the instruments in the subhepatic pouch. The problem of entanglement with the falciform ligament when the cannula is inserted to its left is easily solved by advancing the tip of the cannula beyond the free margin of this ligament. Alternatively, in suitable cases the cannula may be passed through an avascular window in the falciform ligament. In obese patients with a heavy fat-laden falciform ligament, the use of the falciform sling (Chapter 3) imparts a number of advantages which include elevation of the liver through the round ligament. The right upper cannula, often referred as the midclavicular, is best sited by reference to the gallbladder fundus using the finger-depression technique for precise localization. It must enter the parieties just below the liver edge, at the junction of the fundus with the body of the gallbladder. Usually, but not always, this corresponds to a point 2.5 cm below the right costal margin in the

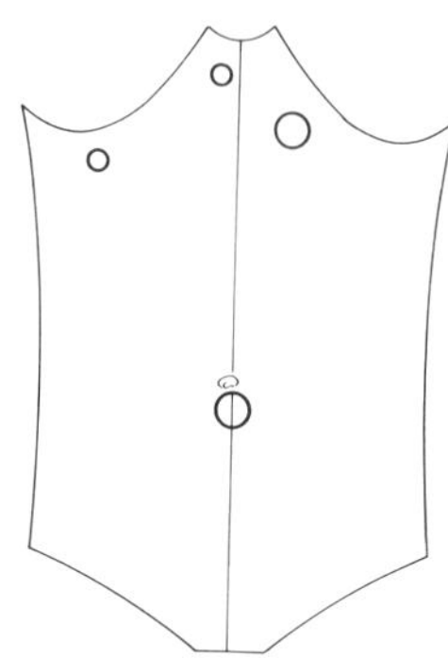

Fig. 4.7 Sites of insertion of the trocar/cannulae for the French approach.

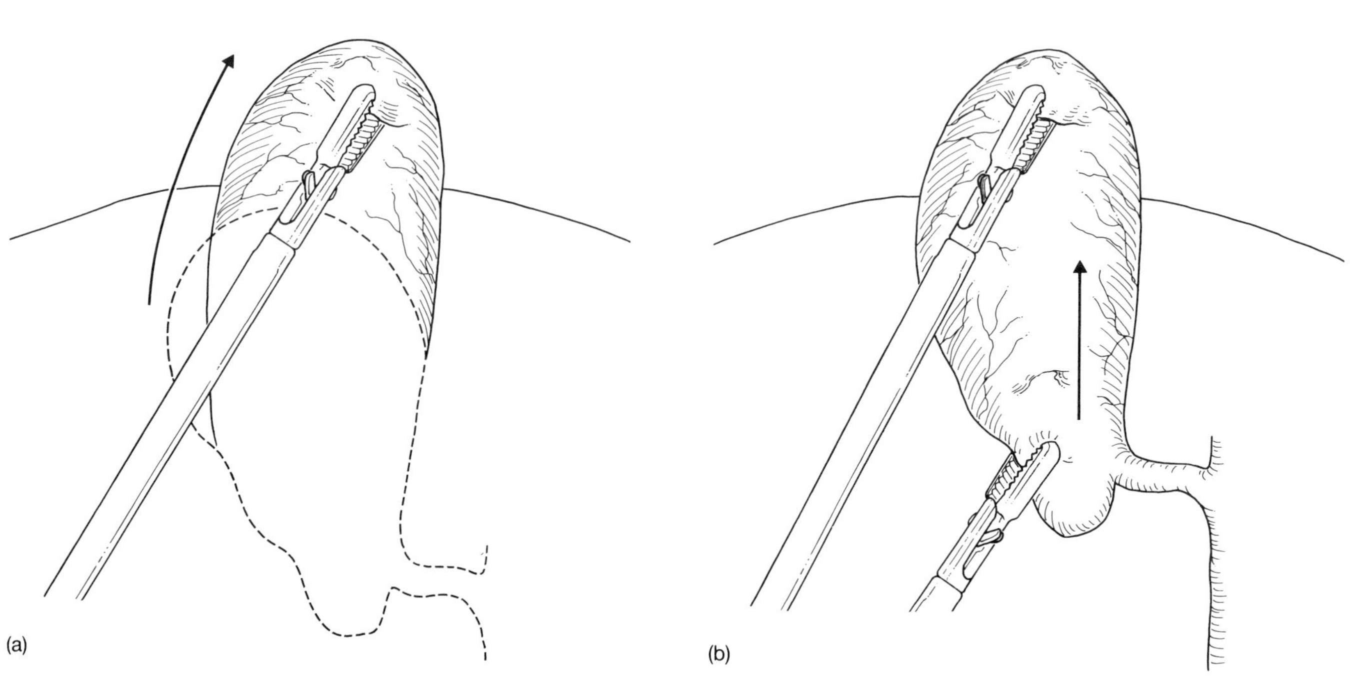

Fig. 4.8 North American technique for exposure of the triangle of Calot.

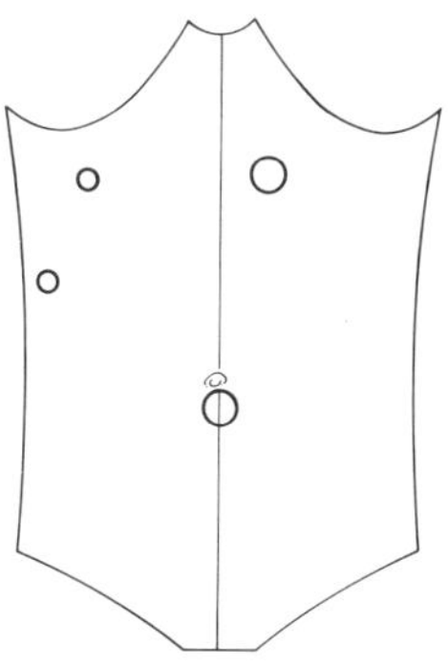

Fig. 4.9 Sites of insertion of the trocar/cannulae for the North American approach.

midclavicular line. The right lower cannula is more laterally situated along the anterior axillary some 4.0 cm below the costal margin. This cannula just skims the hepatic flexure and must be introduced with great care to avoid colonic injury.

With either approach, French or American, it is important to stress that the prescribed positions need to be adjusted in accordance with the build of the patient, and in particular, with the anatomy of the liver. Thus in patients with ptotic livers where the margins of the organ are below the costal margins, appropriate adjustments to the level of the cannulae must be made. The governing principle is to avoid any of the superior cannulae being sited above the inferior margin of the liver.

Exposure of the subhepatic region and cystic pedicle

French technique

A rod retractor or sucker is inserted through the upper medial right subcostal cannula and used to elevate the quadrate lobe. With an atraumatic grasper, introduced through the lower right hypochondrial cannula, the neck of the gallbladder is grasped and pulled anteriorly and downwards to display the cystic pedicle and the contents of the triangle of Calot (Fig. 4.10).

North American technique

A special gallbladder-holding forceps is introduced through the right lower anterior axillary cannula and used to grasp the gallbladder fundus, which is lifted in a lateral direction and rolled backwards to expose the subhepatic pouch. A second atraumatic grasper inserted through the right midclavicular

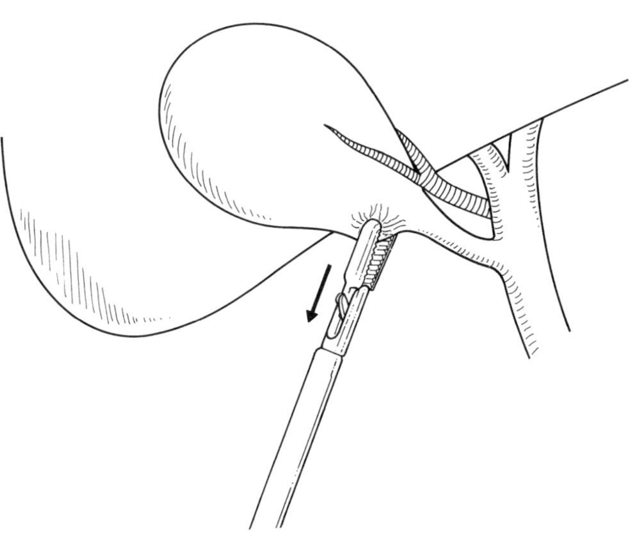

Fig. 4.10 In the French technique, the neck of the gallbladder is grasped and pulled anteriorly and downwards to display the cystic pedicle.

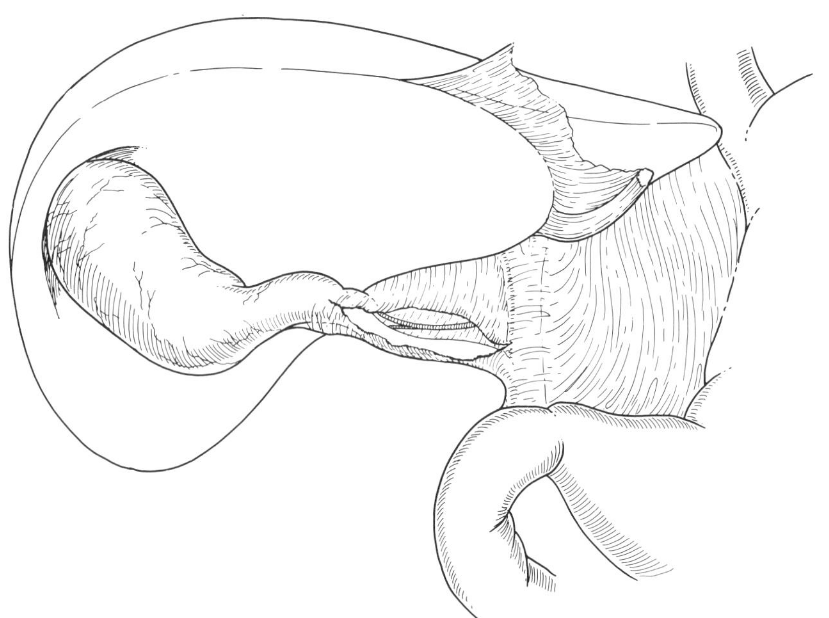

Fig. 4.11 Scissors dissection of the cystic pedicle. The neck of the gallbladder is pulled downwards to enable division of the superior leaf of the cystic pedicle, from its free edge across the triangle of Calot to the medial aspect of the gallbladder as far as the liver.

cannula is applied to the neck, which is lifted upwards and anteriorly (Fig. 4.11). Although capture and retraction of the floppy non-inflamed gallbladder presents no problems, this may be difficult in patients with a contracted fibrotic organ, or if the gallbladder is distended or tightly packed with stones. Aspiration of the gallbladder, by reducing the distension, will enable a better grasp to be obtained.

With either technique the view is at times obscured by a distended stomach and duodenal bulb. This problem is easily resolved by replacing the standard nasogastric tube with a Salem sump one. When kept on a continuous low suction, this results in complete collapse of the stomach and duodenal bulb throughout the procedure.

Inspection of the cystic pedicle

When exposure of the subhepatic pouch is achieved, the cystic pedicle is inspected by advancing the telescope to obtain a closer view. In thin patients, this appears as a triangular fold between the neck of the gallbladder and the common bile duct, which is often readily identified, especially if a forward oblique viewing telescope is used. The cystic pedicle outlines the margins of the triangle of Calot and contains between its superior and inferior leaves the cystic duct (usually anteriorly), the cystic artery (above and behind the duct) and the cystic lymph node, which is closely applied to the neck of the gallbladder between the duct and the artery. The prominent anterior free edge of the cystic pedicle is formed as the peritoneum folds over the cystic duct. Dissection will prove difficult if the cystic pedicle is foreshortened to less than 1.5 cm. A thorough appreciation of the anatomy of the cystic pedicle is crucial to the safe dissection of the cystic duct and artery.

Dissection of the cystic pedicle

Dissection of the cystic duct

The dissection of the cystic pedicle can be performed with scissors, electrosurgical hook knife, or by teasing with fine-pointed atraumatic graspers. In practice a combination of these techniques is often employed. Irrespective of the technique used, the first step consists in the division or teasing of the superior leaf of the cystic pedicle.

The *blunt teasing technique* consists in stripping the peritoneal lining covering the cystic duct and artery in a medial direction towards the common duct against counter-traction, by a grasping forceps on the neck of the gallbladder. Oozing is controlled by soft coagulation and the area is irrigated to maintain a clear view of the anatomy.

With the *scissors technique* favoured by one of the authors (AC), the gallbladder is held retracted by an atraumatic grasper applied to the neck. The dissection starts by pulling the neck of the gallbladder downwards to enable division of the superior leaf of the cystic pedicle, from its free edge across the triangle of Calot to the medial aspect of the gallbladder as far as the liver (Fig. 4.12). The dissection is kept superficial, dividing only the peritoneal covering and teasing it from the underlying structures. When complete, the cystic duct becomes obvious. The dissection is continued close to the duct, mobilizing its posterior aspect from the cystic artery. At this stage the curved dissecting grasper is very useful for opening the window between the two structures (Fig. 4.13). After this instrument is introduced in the closed position along the plane of the cleft, its jaws are gently opened to commence the separation. This procedure has to be repeated several times until sufficient posterior mobilization has been achieved. Alternatively, the

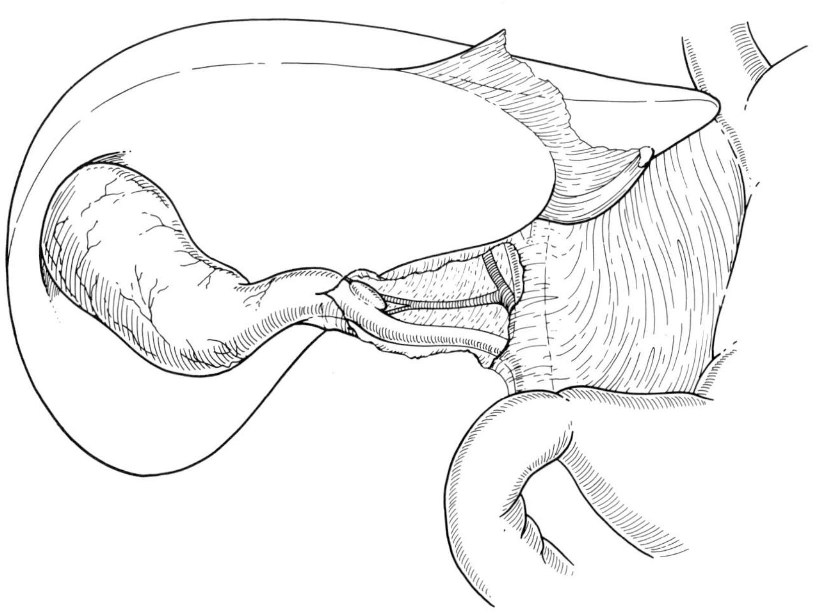

Fig. 4.12 The dissection of the superior leaf is kept superficial, dividing only the peritoneum to expose the underlying structures.

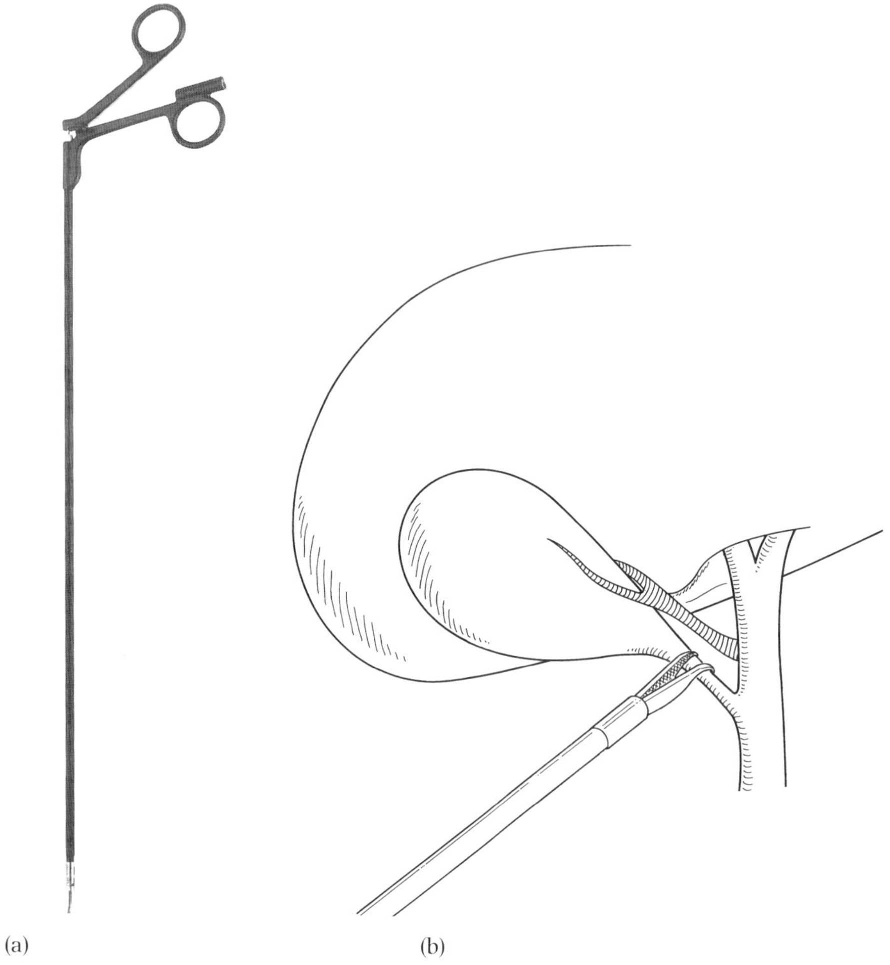

Fig. 4.13 (a) Curved dissecting grasper. (b) It is used to separate the cystic duct from the artery. This window is enlarged until the inferior peritoneal leaf is reached.

variable-curvature superelastic dissector [8] can be used, particularly in difficult cases (Fig. 4.14 a–g). There is a fairly constant branch of the cystic artery which traverses this window to supply the gallbladder neck. If identified, this is coagulated before division by the scissors. If oozing is sufficient to obscure the view at this stage, the area is irrigated and minor bleeding coagulated. It is essential to maintain a clear view throughout the dissection. The anterior fold of the cystic pedicle is then lifted upwards to expose the inferior leaf. This is divided with scissors, again keeping close to the duct and proceeding medially towards the liver. When this is completed, a gap becomes visible between the cystic duct in front and artery behind. This is opened further by grasping and lifting the cystic duct anteriorly. A few fibrous attachments on either side of the gap are divided. Finally, the cystic duct is cleared of any residual peritoneal covering on its anterior surface. In most patients with a functioning gallbladder, it is possible to isolate a 1.5–2.0 cm segment of the cystic duct (Fig. 4.15). It is much safer to gain length by extending the dissection towards the gallbladder neck rather than medially.

The *electrosurgical hook dissection* is favoured by French surgeons. The instrument consists of a hollow insulated probe with a hook (J or L-shaped) at

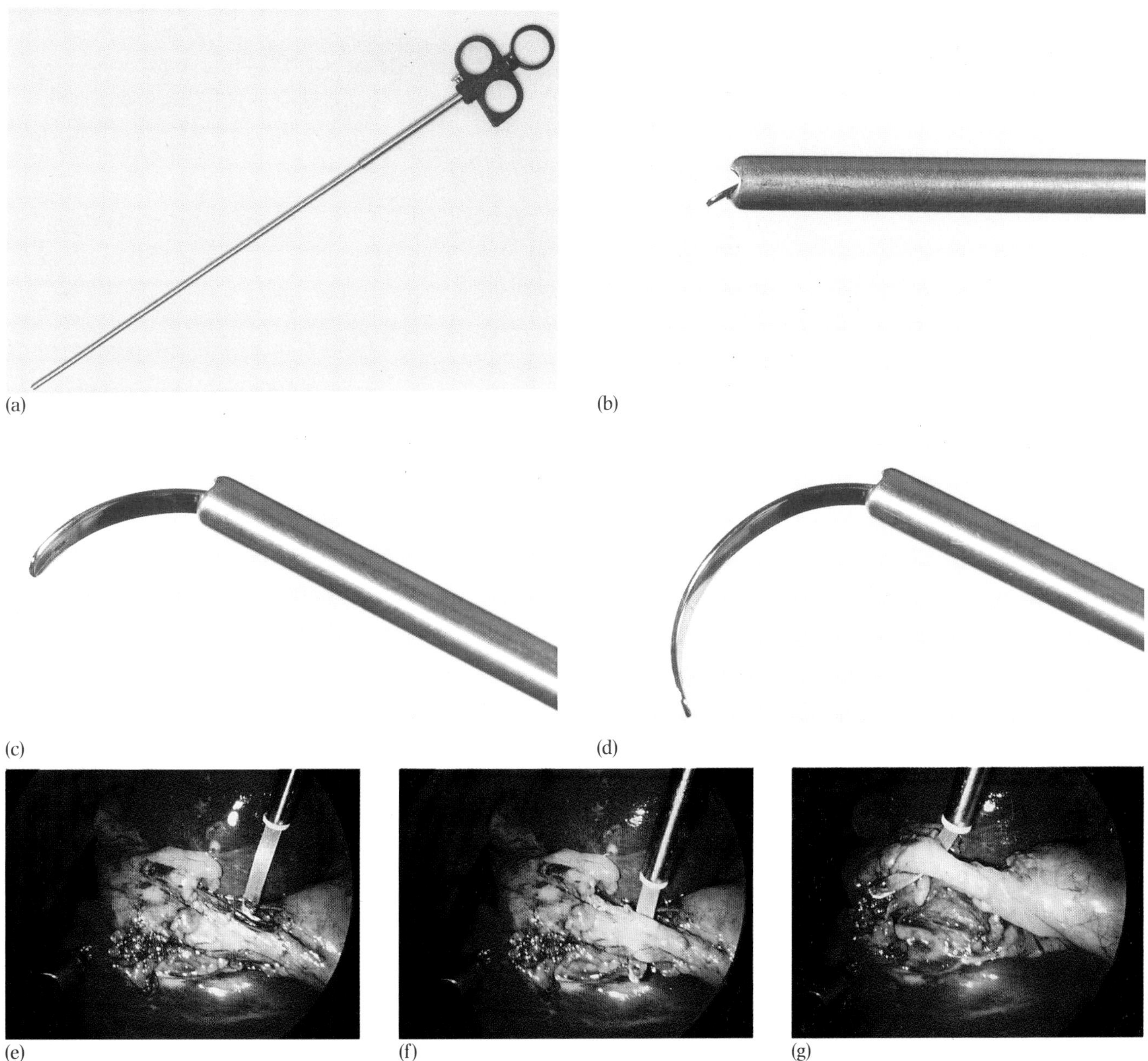

Fig. 4.14 (a–d) Shape-memory variable-curvature dissector. (e–g) Mobilization of adherent cystic duct with shape-memory dissector.

the functional end. The other extremity connects to the diathermy leads and also incorporates a suction/irrigation port, which is controlled by a trumpet valve at the external end to release smoke and permit irrigation (Fig. 4.16). Disposable types with exchangeable tips of various shapes are also available (Valley Lab). The suction capability is essential, as electrosurgical dissection generates a considerable amount of smoke which requires periodic aspiration.

The technique entails lifting the peritoneum of the cystic pedicle with the hook from the underlying structures and then applying blended high-frequency current to cut the lifted peritoneal covering (Fig. 4.17). Tenting of the tissue is essential before activating the current, for three reasons: (i) it limits the electrosurgical burn to the tissue constricted by the hook; (ii) the

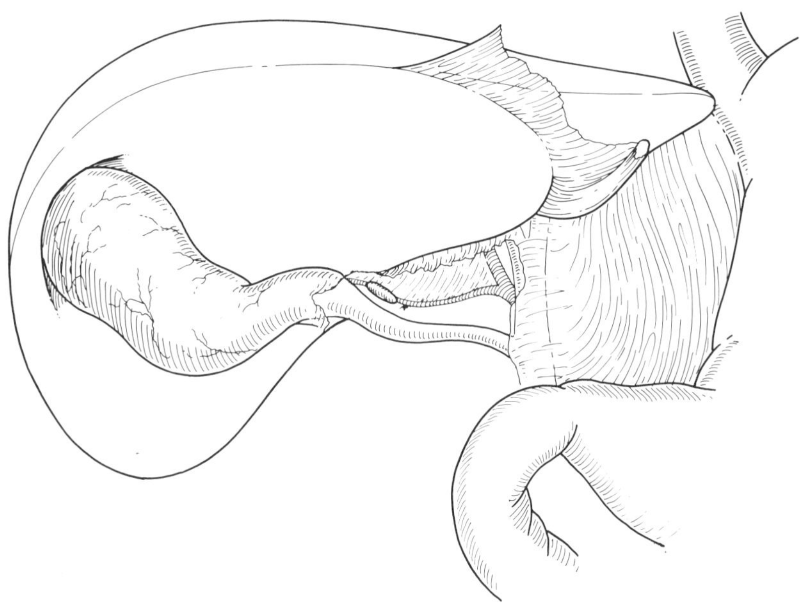

Fig. 4.15 The completed mobilization of the cystic duct. The artery has not been completely dissected.

cut is facilitated by the tension on the tissue; and (iii) the gap between the tissue and the underlying structures increases the safety margin against inadvertent thermal injury. The dissection starts on the superior leaf of the cystic pedicle and proceeds laterally towards the neck of the gallbladder, and then curves upward to the liver (Fig. 4.18). The gap between the cystic duct and the artery is identified. The heel of the hook is then inserted into this space and pushed medially before it is elevated to pick up the intervening tissue (Fig. 4.19) which is then cut by blender current. The inferior peritoneum of the cystic pedicle is divided using the same technique, keeping close to the neck of the gallbladder. Eventually, it should be possible to put the hook around the mobilized cystic duct and slide it up and down to separate

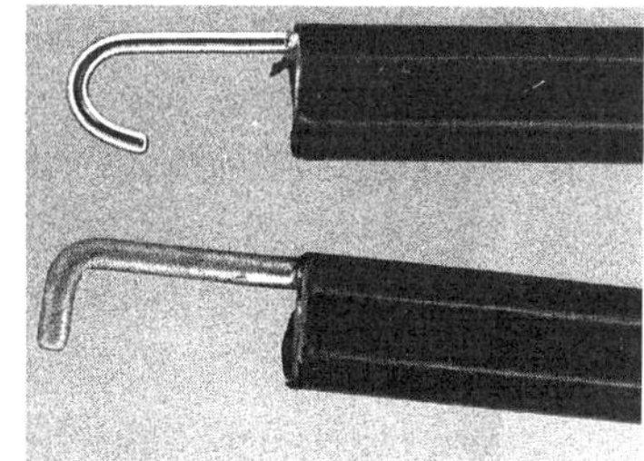

Fig. 4.16 Electrosurgical hook knives: curved and L-shaped. The latter is much less likely to get entangled and allows more precise dissection.

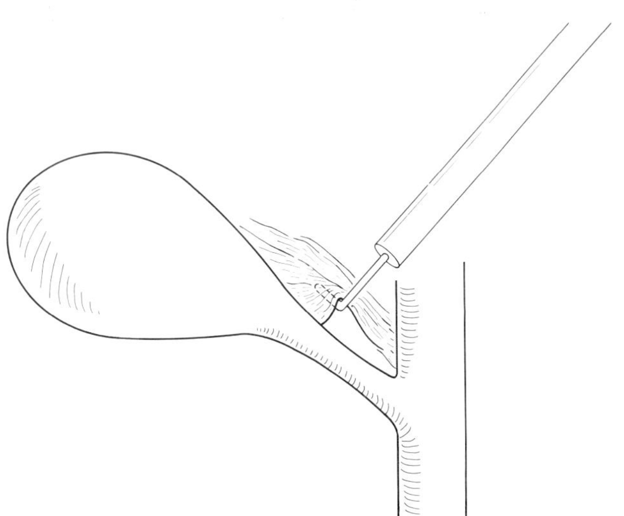

Fig. 4.17 The technique of electrosurgical dissection entails lifting the peritoneum of the cystic pedicle with the hook from the underlying structures and then applying blended high-frequency current to cut the lifted peritoneal covering.

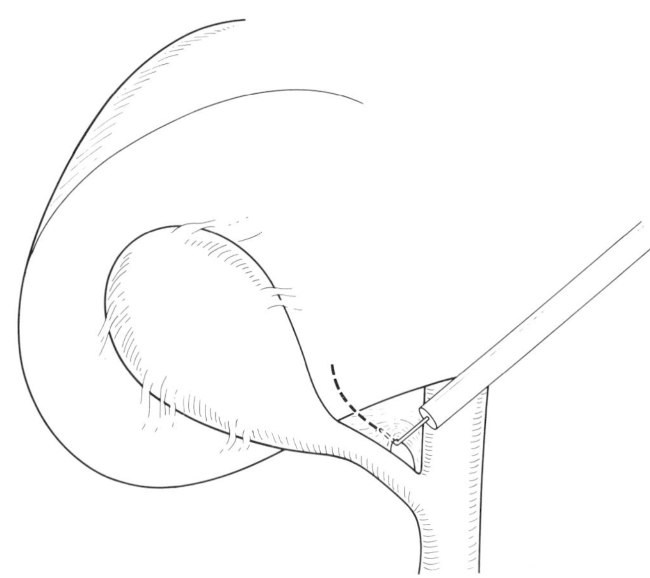

Fig. 4.18 Electrosurgical dissection. This starts on the superior leaf of the cystic pedicle and proceeds laterally towards the neck of the gallbladder and then curves upwards to the liver.

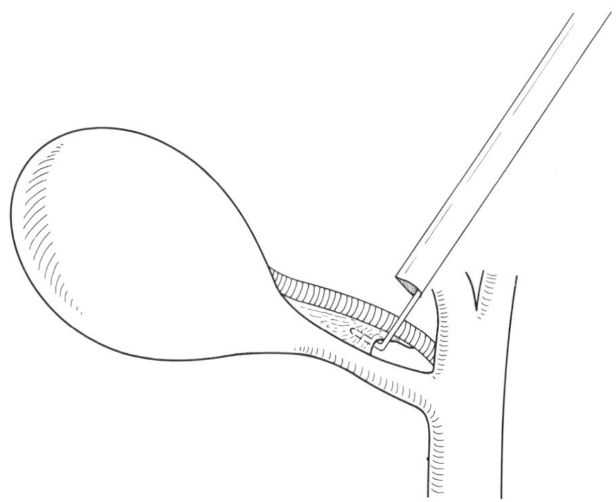

Fig. 4.19 The heel of the hook is inserted into the space between the cystic duct and the cystic artery and pushed medially before it is elevated to pick up the intervening tissue which is then cut by blender current.

any residual loose fibrous attachments (Fig. 4.20). The main disadvantage of the electrosurgical dissection is the excess smoke generation. This requires repeated suction and therefore intermittent partial loss of the pneumoperitoneum. In addition, it causes considerable charring and some contraction of tissue planes.

Identification of mobilized structure as cystic duct

In the majority of patients there is no problem: the duct is clearly continuous with the neck of the gallbladder. However, an anomalous anterior cystic artery may be mistaken for the cystic duct (Fig. 4.21) and as the cystic

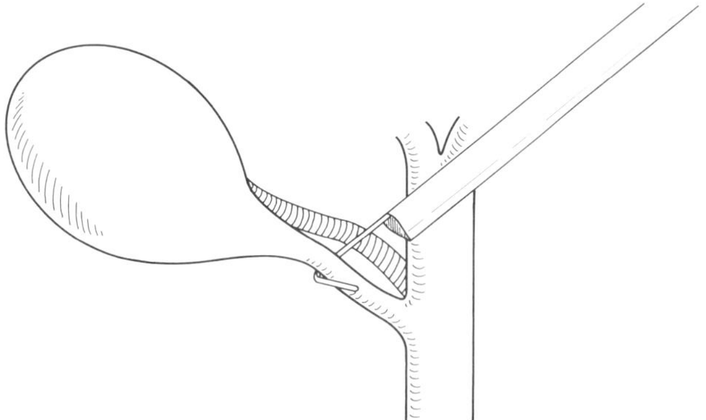

Fig. 4.20 The hook is then inserted around the mobilized cystic duct and slid alongside it to separate any residual loose fibrous attachments.

pedicle is under tension as a result of retraction of the gallbladder, pulsations may not be detected. Whenever this suspicion is raised, the telescope is advanced closer to the structure and the retraction on the gallbladder is relaxed. This simple manoeuvre, by restoring obvious pulsations, helps to identify the cystic artery in most instances. If uncertainty remains, the camera should be detached from the telescope and direct endoscopic visualization used to identify the anatomy.

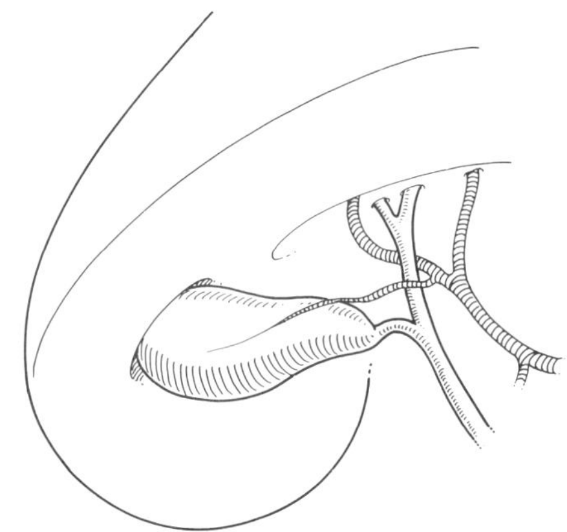

Fig. 4.21 Anterior cystic artery, which can be mistaken for the cystic duct. Release of traction on the gallbladder will restore pulsations and help to identify its true nature.

Dissection of the cystic artery

There are two options. The first consists of dissection of the artery immediately after mobilization of the cystic duct. Alternatively, the dissection of the artery is postponed until the cholangiogram has been done and the cystic duct has been ligated and divided. The correct decision depends on the anatomical findings in the individual case. If the artery is well displayed and in the normal position (Fig. 4.22), it is sensible to proceed with the dissection

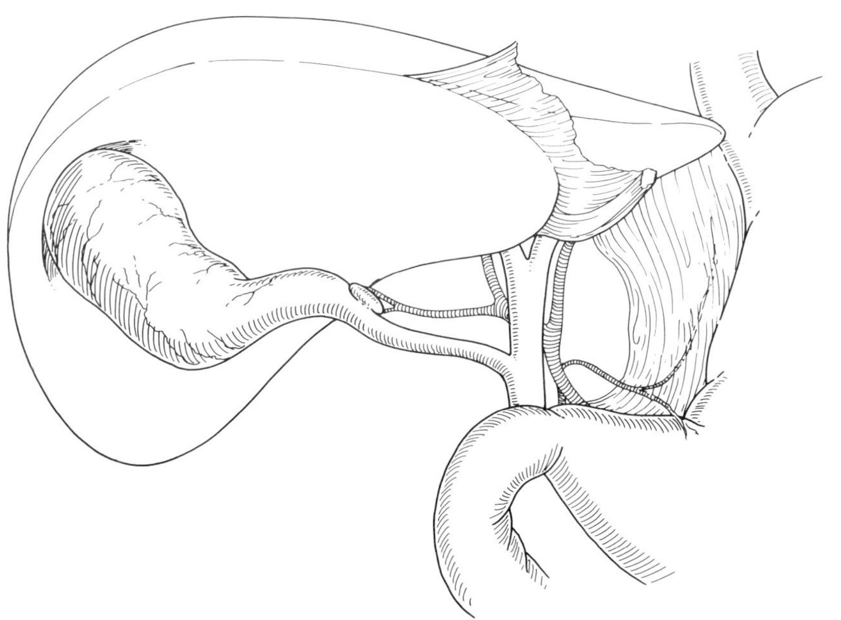

Fig. 4.22 Normal anatomy of the cystic artery in the triangle of Calot. There is a fairly constant branch which supplies the neck of the gallbladder. If identified, this is electrocoagulated and divided.

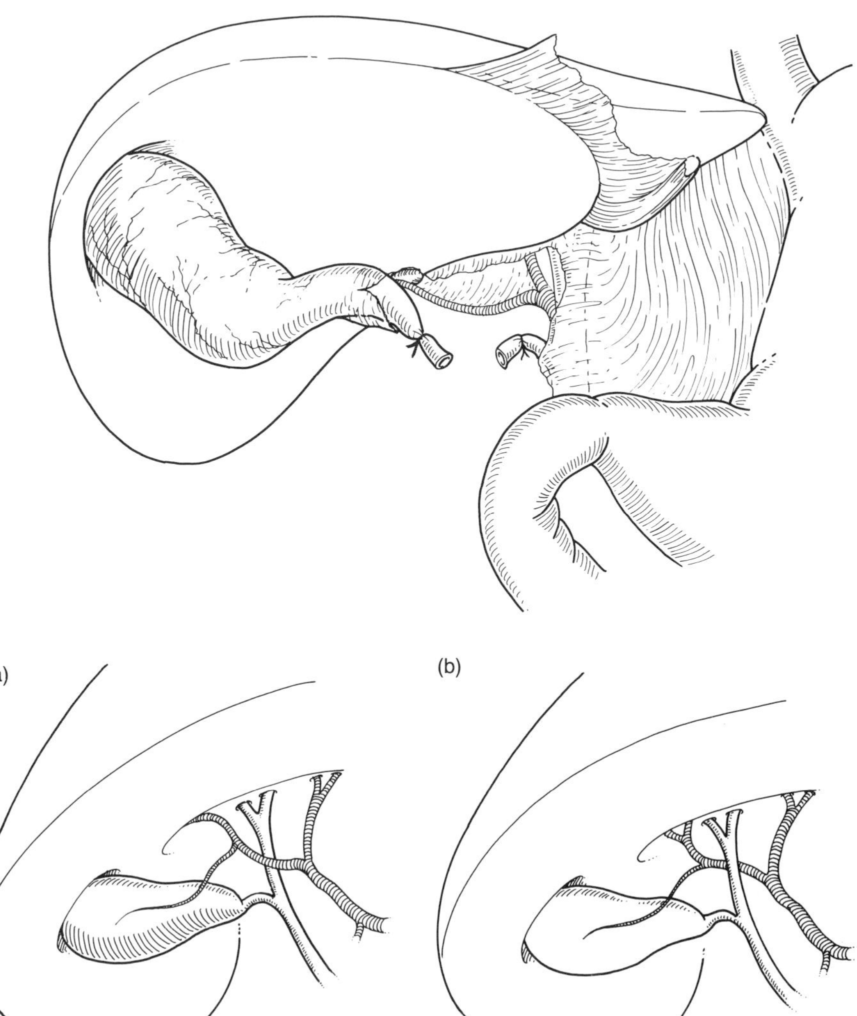

Fig. 4.23 The division of the cystic duct opens the triangle of Calot and exposes the cystic artery, especially if this is located high up in the cystic pedicle.

Fig. 4.24 Two common types of looped right hepatic artery. In (a) the right hepatic loops in front of the bile duct with the cystic branch arising from the summit of the loop. This results in a rather short cystic artery. (b) The right hepatic artery loops in the triangle of Calot behind the common hepatic duct and can easily be mistaken for the cystic artery. When suspected, the arterial anatomy must be displayed and the cystic artery clipped and divided early, without compromising the integrity of the right hepatic artery.

and mobilize the artery, which is then secured and divided before the duct. On the other hand, if the artery is not well displayed, division of the cystic duct opens the triangle of Calot and considerably enhances exposure of the artery (Fig. 4.23). The dissection of this needs to be meticulous, keeping close to the vessel. The surgeon must be constantly on the lookout for a looped right hepatic artery, which can easily be mistaken for the cystic artery (Fig. 4.24 a,b). Other important anomalies include early division of the cystic artery (Fig. 4.25) and aberrant origin of the right hepatic from the superior mesenteric artery (Fig. 4.26). A good length of the artery at least 1.0 cm should be mobilized if possible. Again, it is safer to gain the desired length by extending the dissection laterally towards the gallbladder neck. If the field is obscured by oozing, the dissection is halted to allow pressurized irrigation/suction, followed by electrocoagulation of the bleeding points. The fully mobilized artery is double-clipped proximally (Fig. 4.27). Although it is an end artery, its distal end should also be clipped before division by hook scissors at a safe distance from the proximal double-clipped end.

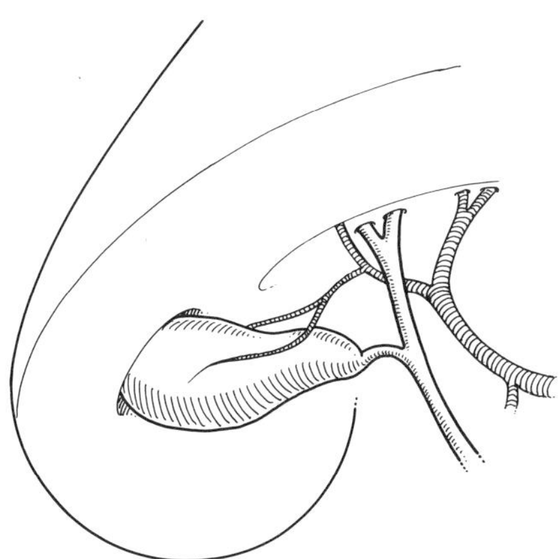

Fig. 4.25 Early division of the cystic artery in the triangle of Calot. Both branches require to be clipped separately.

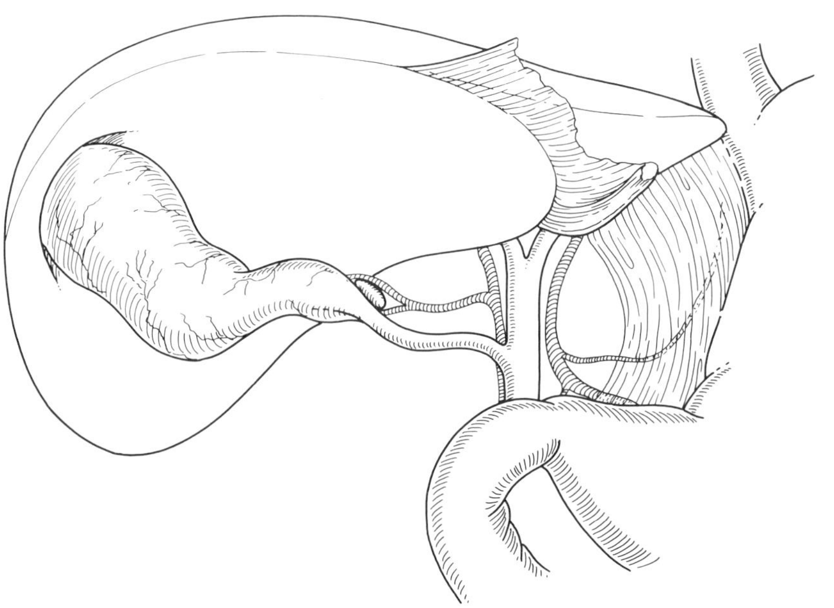

Fig. 4.26 Aberrant origin of the right hepatic from the superior mesenteric artery. Although easily identified, this may be adherent to the posterior aspect of the cystic duct at its entry into the bile duct. In this situation it is best to leave a large medial cuff of cystic duct. The cystic artery arising from an aberrant right hepatic artery is often short and bifurcates early.

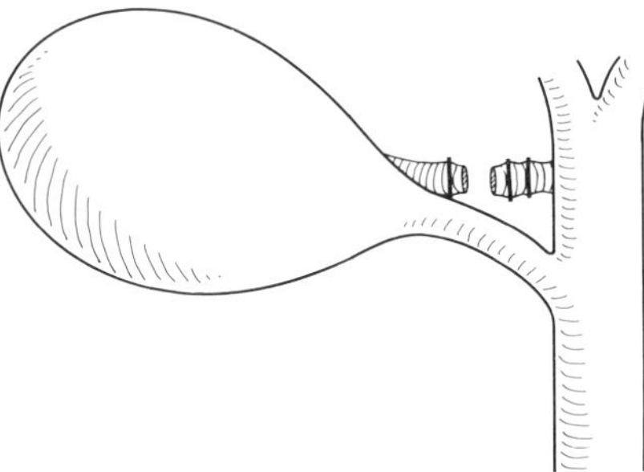

Fig. 4.27 Clipping and division of the cystic artery. For added security, the proximal end is double-clipped. Accurate demonstration of the anatomy is crucial before any structure is divided. This applies especially to clipping and division of the cystic artery.

Ligature/clipping and division of cystic duct and cholangiography

As in routine biliary surgery, cholangiography is highly desirable not only for the detection of unsuspected ductal calculi but, more importantly, to identify anomalies of the biliary tract and, in particular, where the cystic duct can be clipped or ligated medially with safety. This is the most important reason for peroperative cholangiography during laparoscopic cholecystectomy, as the cystic–common duct junction is not often clearly outlined. Partial or total clipping of the common hepatic duct (which is tented during the procedure) probably accounts for the majority of ductal injuries and postoperative bile leaks. Cholangiography provides the surgeon with a 'road map' which is specific to each patient, and must for this reason be regarded as an important adjunct for the prevention of iatrogenic bile-duct injuries. However, many surgeons do not perform peroperative cholangiography routinely but only when the preoperative work-up (LFTs, ultrasound or infusion intravenous cholangiography) suggests the presence of ductal stones.

Laparoscopic cholangiography can be performed either by injecting contrast medium into the gallbladder (cholecystocholangiogram) or into the cystic duct (see Chapter 6). In most instances, a cystic-duct cholangiogram is performed. The gallbladder end of the cystic duct is double-clipped but the medial end is left patent. The cannulation of the cystic duct is considerably simplified by the use of the cholangiography cannula. This instrument consists of a forceps with a hollow tube and terminal basket-type jaws at the distal end. It acts as a carrier for the cholangiography catheter (Cook ureteric catheter with terminal hole, 4–5 Fr). This is connected via a three-way tap to saline and contrast-filled syringes (20 ml), and is inserted inside the cholangiography instrument. The combination is then introduced into the peritoneal cavity through the right upper midclavicular accessory cannula. With the jaws of the instrument open, the catheter is pushed in until about 3.0 cm

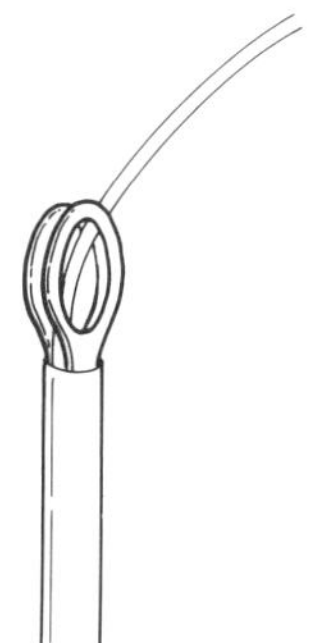

Fig. 4.28 The catheter projecting beyond the cannula is grasped at an angle to facilitate insertion.

project beyond the jaws of the instrument. A cut is made on the anterior wall of the cystic duct by fine-pointed curved microscissors, and deepened until the lumen is entered. The cholangiography cannula is then manipulated to enable the projecting part of the catheter to be threaded through the cystic duct into the common bile duct (Fig. 4.28). This step is greatly facilitated by maintaining a steady injection of saline through the catheter to lift up the mucosal folds of the cystic duct as the catheter is fed into the ductal system. Once an adequate length is in place, the cholangiography cannula is tilted medially and its jaws are closed over the cystic duct and catheter (Fig. 4.29 a,b). Contrast is injected slowly during image intensification to record the early phases of duct filling. On completion of the cholangiogram, the jaws are released and the cholangiography instrument containing the catheter is withdrawn.

There are three techniques for securing the medial end of the cystic duct: it can be ligated in continuity [9,10], clipped (metal or polydioxanone), or secured by an endoloop (Surgitie or Ethibinder).

Medial ligature in continuity. The technique of Roeder external slip-knotting is described in Chapter 3. Dry 00 chromic catgut is used (1.5 m length). This is available commercially already mounted in a push-rod. Alternatively, the alcohol-packaged material of suitable length is wiped clear of alcohol and left exposed on the sterile trolley to dry for at least 10 minutes. Ideally, this should be done by the scrub nurse at the start of the procedure to ensure that the catgut is completely dry when needed, as this material slip-knots much better when dry. The dry catgut is threaded through the push-rod and the end projecting behind the butt of the rod is knotted. The end of the catgut projecting beyond the bevelled tip of the push-rod is grasped in a 3.0 mm needle-holder and inserted inside a suture applicator through the left upper paramedian cannula. The end of the ligature is passed around the back of the cystic duct from above. It is then grasped by the 5.0 mm needle-holder (inserted through the right midclavicular cannula) below the duct and transferred back to the 3.0 mm needle, which is then used to externalize the ligature. In order to prevent the ligature serrating the duct, closed forceps are inserted inside the loop to take up the tension (Fig. 4.30). Once the end of the ligature is exteriorized, the nurse puts her index finger over the hole of the applicator while the Roeder knot is fashioned. The suture applicator is then withdrawn a few centimeters and the Roeder knot tightened in proper alignment and excess catgut beyond the knot trimmed. The assistant or the surgeon then slips the knot inside the abdomen through the suture applicator with the push-rod against controlled traction on the knotted end of the ligature beyond the butt end of the push-rod. This exercise can be performed either single-handed or by pushing the rod with the left hand and applying traction on the catgut with the right. The laying down (knot slipping) process is closely watched by the surgeon to avoid and undo any twisting. The resulting 'hangman's noose' is placed by the push-rod a few millimetres medial to the opening of the cystic duct before it

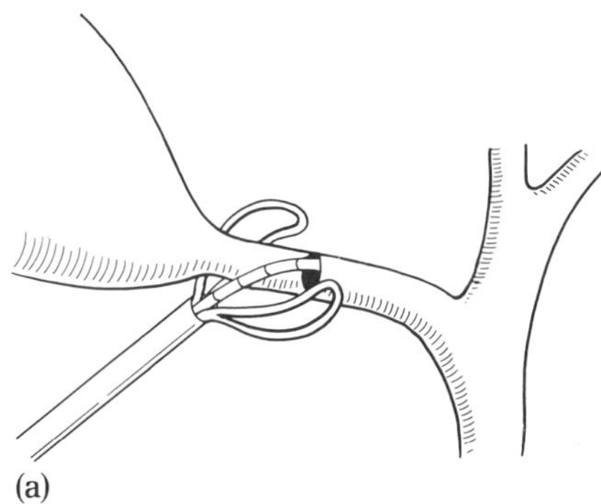

(a)

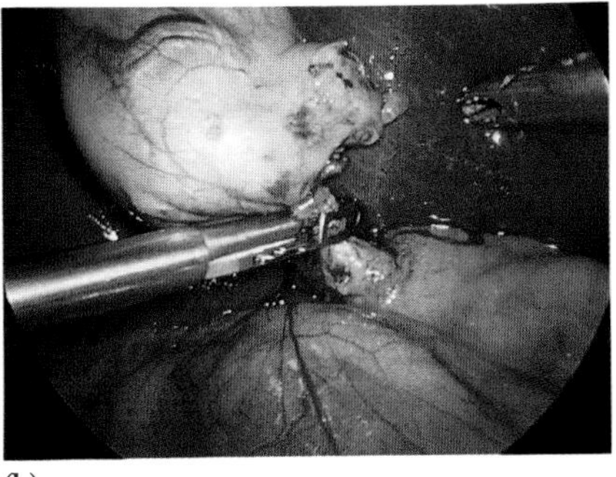

(b)

Fig. 4.29 (a) The basket jaws are closed on the cystic duct, holding the catheter in place and preventing leakage during contrast injection. (b) Endophotograph of cholangiography catheter being held by the grasping jaws of the cholangiography cannula.

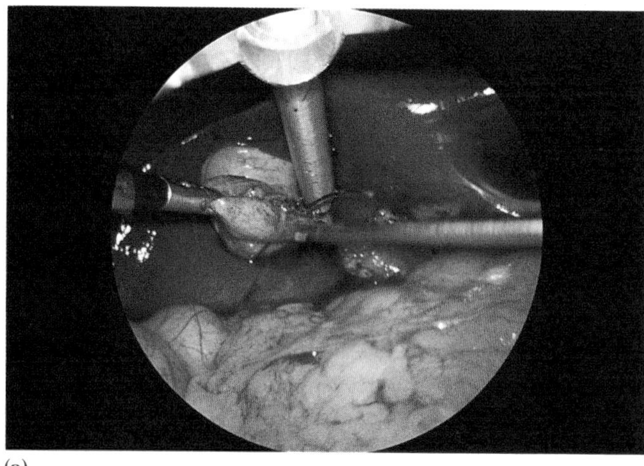

(a)

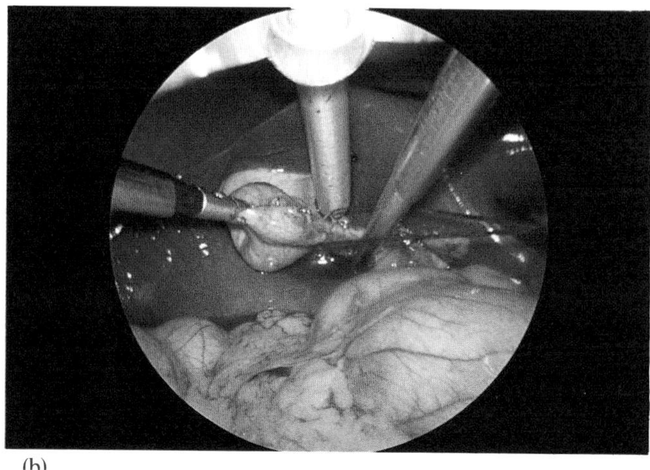

(b)

Fig. 4.30 Ligature of the cystic duct in continuity. (a) Dry catgut is passed around the cystic duct and then (b) exteriorized.

is locked tightly in the desired place. The push-rod is then withdrawn a few centimetres and the knot and its position on the duct are inspected (Fig. 4.31). If considered satisfactory, the duct is then cut by claw scissors (Fig. 4.32) and the excess suture, push-rod and suture applicator are removed.

Medial clipping of the cystic duct. Most commonly metal (titanium) clips are used (Fig. 4.33), although absorbable polydioxanone (Absolok, Ethicon) are better (Fig. 4.34) and do not carry the risk of stone formation. Either type of clip requires specific applicators. Some surgeons practise double clipping of the duct for added safety. Whatever instrument is used, it is important to apply the clips at right-angles to the long axis of the duct. Furthermore, the appropriate size of clip for the diameter of the cystic duct must be chosen, otherwise the hold achieved will not be secure. Although clipping of the

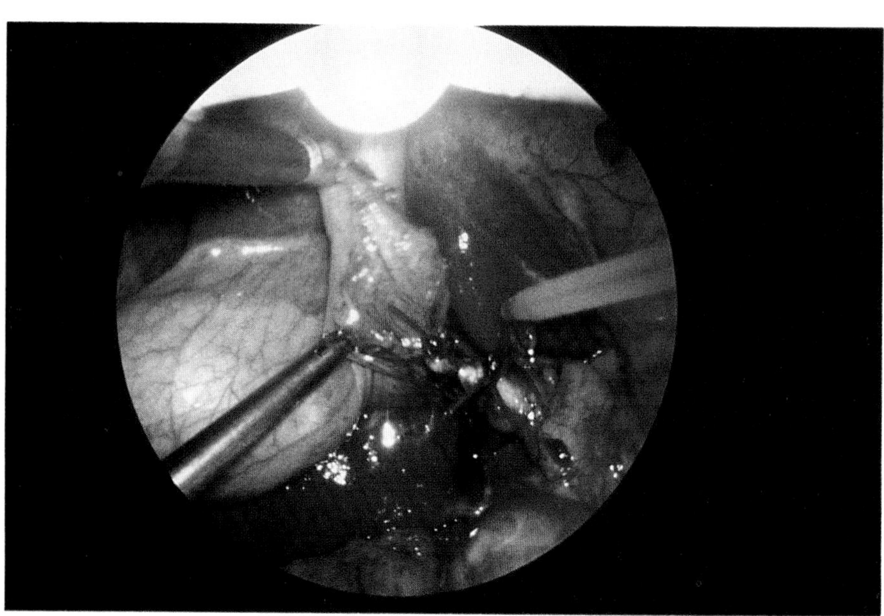

Fig. 4.31 Complete medial and lateral ligatures of the cystic duct prior to division.

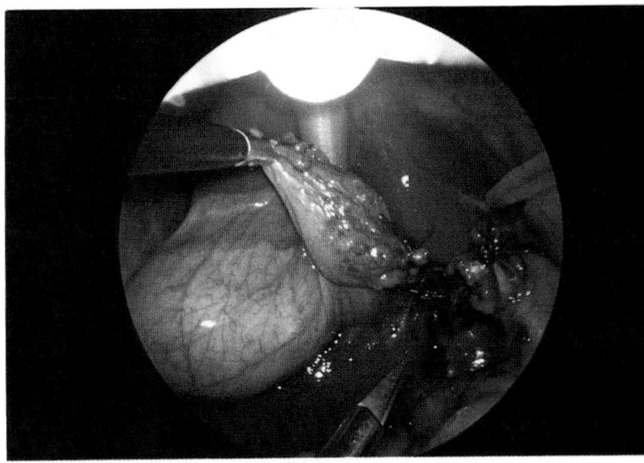

Fig. 4.32 Completed division of the cystic duct.

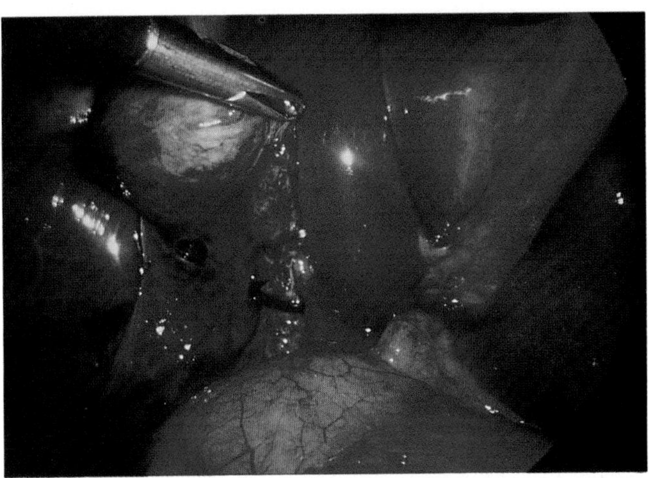

Fig. 4.33 Double proximal clipping of the cystic duct (titanium, PDS).

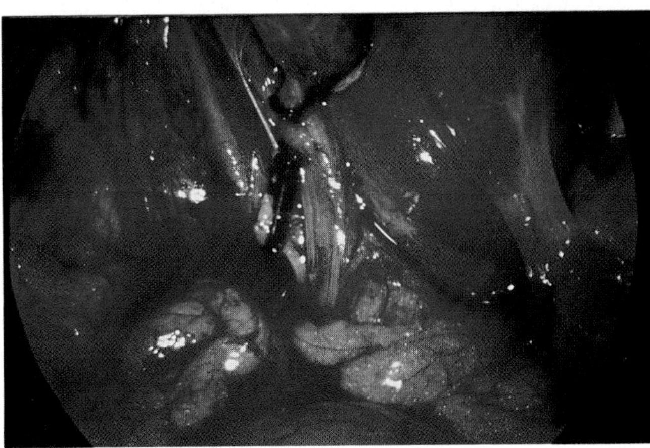

Fig. 4.34 Medial end of cystic duct secured by absorbable Absolock clip.

cystic duct is the most popular method of securing this structure, it has certain disadvantages. In the first instance, clipping requires more duct length than ligature in continuity. Unless clips are applied at right-angles to the axis of the duct, they are prone to slip. Metal clips may become incorporated in the bile duct and form calculi.

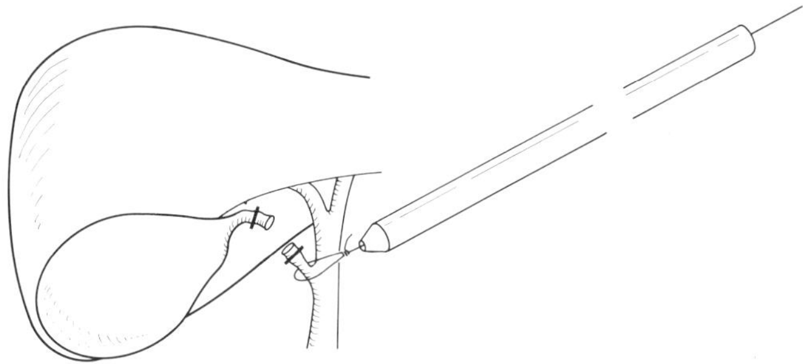

Fig. 4.35 Application of endoloop proximal to medial clip. This is less satisfactory than ligation in continuity.

Ligature by endoloop. After clipping and division of the cystic duct, some surgeons apply an endoloop just medial to the proximal clip (Fig. 4.35). This obviates the disadvantages of clipping but is an inferior substitute to ligature in continuity before division of the duct.

Irrespective of the technique used to secure it, the cystic duct is cut with hook scissors and this step completes the dissection of the cystic pedicle. The gallbladder is now detached from the structures of the porta hepatis.

Mobilization of the detached gallbladder from the liver bed

This step is relatively straightforward in patients with non-inflamed functioning gallbladder, but can be difficult in the presence of a contracted, adherent or partially buried organ. Care must be taken to keep the plane of dissection in the loose fibrous layer which separates the gallbladder from the subjacent hepatic parenchyma. If the dissection is carried too close to the liver considerable oozing is encountered, apart from the real risk of damage to the hepatic parenchyma, with significant bleeding and postoperative bile leakage. The separation of the gallbladder from the liver can be carried out with electrosurgery, scissors or laser dissection. The Berci spatula is especially useful for electrosurgical dissection of the gallbladder. The dissection starts at the gallbladder neck and should proceed along a definite plan towards the fundus: first along the anterior and posterior margins of the organ, and then between the undersurface of the gallbladder and the fibrous plate covering the hepatic parenchyma (Fig. 4.36).

The gallbladder is held on the stretch by two grasping forceps, one on the fundus and the other on the detached neck. The serosal lining on either side is divided by scissors or electrocautery hookknife 0.5 cm from the liver margin. The scissors are inserted closed underneath the cut serosa and the jaws opened to create a plane, lifting the peritoneum from the organ (Fig. 4.37). Any obvious serosal vessels are coagulated before the peritoneum is divided. This process is continued until the fundus is reached. Thereafter with the gallbladder lifted upwards and held on the stretch in this position, the central fibrovascular attachments between the inferior surface of the gallbladder and the liver are divided, with coagulation of any bleeding points. This leaves the apical fundal attachment to the superior margin of the liver.

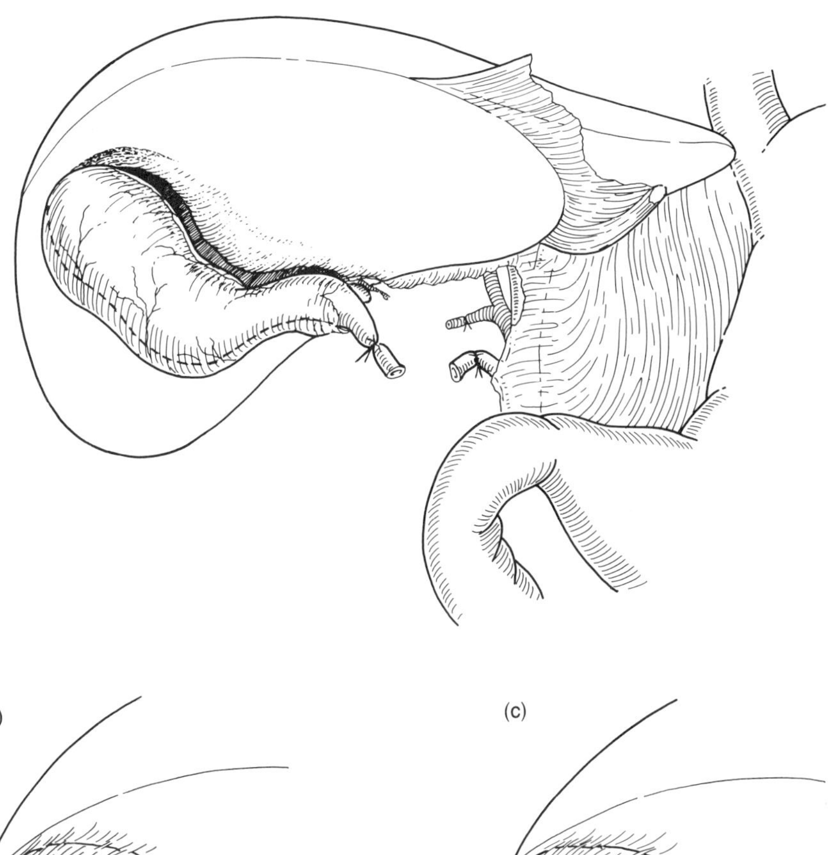

Fig. 4.36 Diagrammatic representation of the technique used for the mobilization of the gallbladder from the liver. The lines of dissection proceed along the margins of the gallbladder and subsequently between the organ and the fibrous plate covering the liver substance.

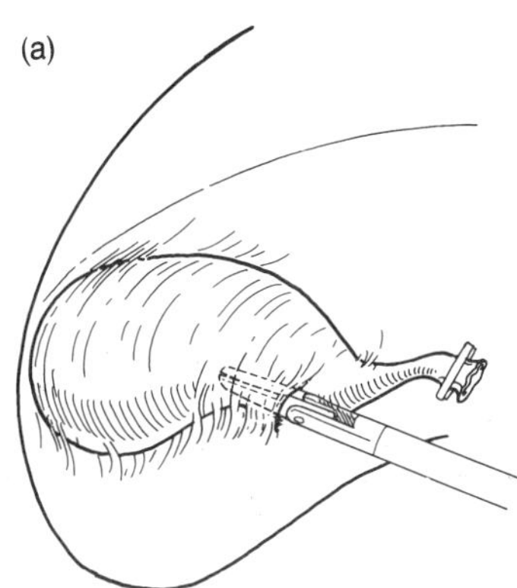

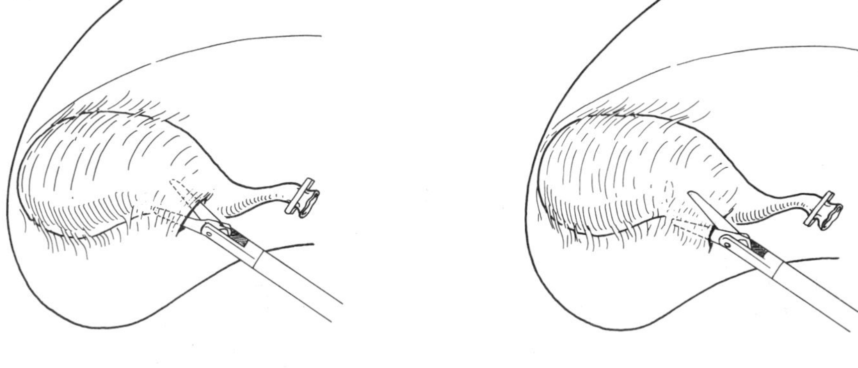

Fig. 4.37 Scissors dissection along the anterior margin of the gallbladder. (a) A small superficial cut has been made in the serosa. The blunt-nosed scissors are introduced closed in the plane between the gallbladder and the serosa. (b) The scissors are then opened to dissect the plane. (c) The undermined serosal covering is then cut.

The detachment of the fundus can prove difficult unless the position of the gallbladder is reversed. This is achieved as follows: a grasper is placed on the fibrous tissue layer on the edge of the right lobe just above the fundus, and used to elevate the liver as the gallbladder is allowed to hang down. It is steadied in this position by a grasper with traction in a downward direction (Fig. 4.38). This manoeuvre results in excellent display of the fundal attachments, which can then be divided with the electrosurgical hook knife or scissors.

In floppy gallbladders with loose attachments to the hepatic parenchyma, separation is quickly achieved by pledget swab dissection after the peritoneal margins have been divided (Fig. 4.39 a,b). Another useful technique is to hold the gallbladder on the stretch and use the argon beam spray coagulation system. This results in a very quick, safe and bloodless separation of the gallbladder from the liver parenchyma.

Once separation of the gallbladder is complete, the fundus is grasped by the assistant until the organ is extracted (see below).

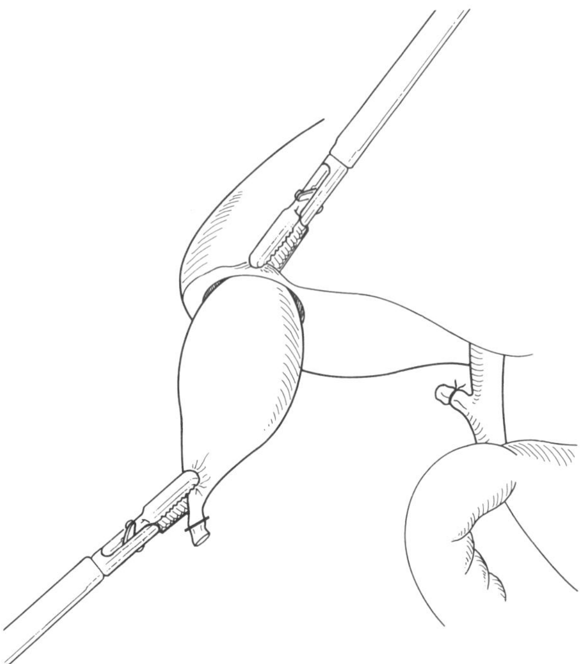

Fig. 4.38 The detachment of the fundus. A grasper is placed on the fibrous tissue layer on the edge of the right lobe just above the fundus, and used to elevate the liver as the gallbladder is allowed to hang down. It is steadied in this position by a grasper with traction in a downward direction.

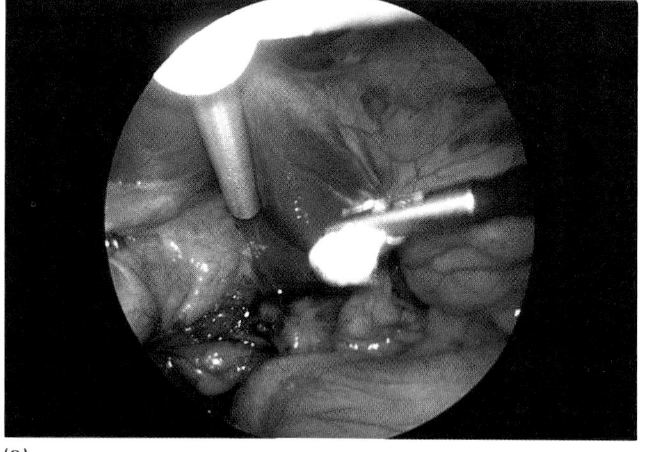

(a)

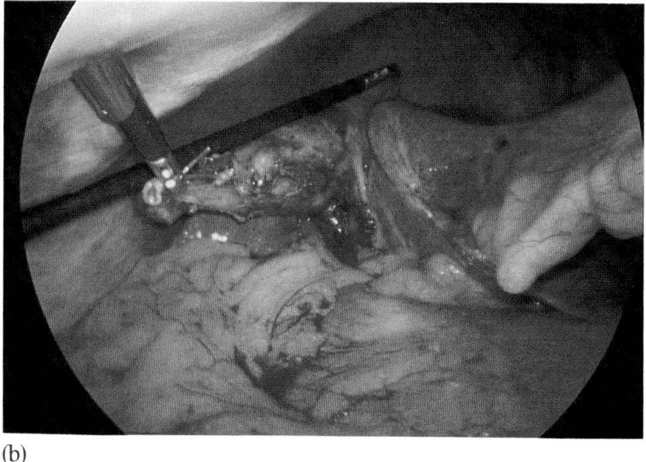

(b)

Fig. 4.39 (a) Start of pledget swab mobilization of the gallbladder. (b) Complete pledget swab separation of the gallbladder.

Extraction of the gallbladder

The gallbladder may be extracted through the left upper paramedian or the umbilical incision. If the latter site is chosen, the telescope/camera assembly are removed from the umbilical cannula and reinserted through the left upper paramedian port. If the organ is floppy and contains a small stone load, this step does not pose any problems. However, special measures are needed if the gallbladder is bulky, with a big stone load (Fig. 4.40).

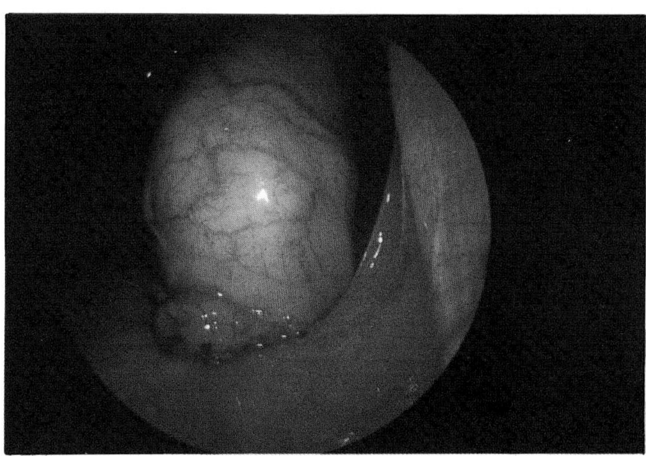

Fig. 4.40 Bulky gallbladder inside the abdominal wall.

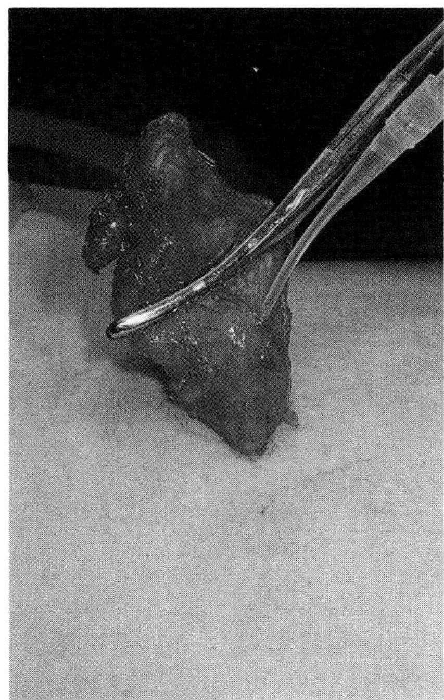

Fig. 4.41 Removal of gallbladder through subumbilical incision. After the exteriorized neck is cross-clamped, bile is aspirated to collapse the organ prior to its delivery.

Delivery of gallbladder with small stone load

A heavy self-holding grasper, such as the Semm alligator forceps, is introduced through the cannula and used to grasp the gallbladder neck. As the assistant releases the grasp on the fundus, the gallbladder is withdrawn towards the extracting cannula. Once the neck of the organ enters the cannula, this is withdrawn *en masse* with the forceps and the attached gallbladder such that the organ slides through the abdominal wall as steady traction is applied. As soon as the neck is externalized, the alligator forceps is replaced with an artery forceps applied across the whole width of the neck. If the intraperitoneal portion of the gallbladder is seen to be distended with bile, aspiration through a small cannula or suction device is performed (Fig. 4.41).

Delivery of a bulky gallbladder with a large stone load

The initial step is similar to the above. As steady traction is maintained on the gallbladder forceps, the cannula is removed over it to expose the exteriorized neck of the gallbladder, whereupon the holding forceps is replaced by a strong clamp applied across the neck of the organ. Forcible traction must be desisted at this stage as the gallbladder fundus containing the stones is trapped in the abdominal cavity by the parieties (Fig. 4.42). The manoeuvres possible are:

Manual evacuation of the gallbladder contents. The exteriorized neck is opened, the bile aspirated and a Dejardins or Randall's forceps introduced into the gallbladder lumen to crush and extract the stones (Fig. 4.43). This process must be performed under visual control. The disadvantages include risk of perforation of the fundus of the gallbladder, stone spillage, and wound contamination.

Dilatation of the wound around the gallbladder during its extraction. This is considerably facilitated by the use of the gallbladder-extracting speculum.

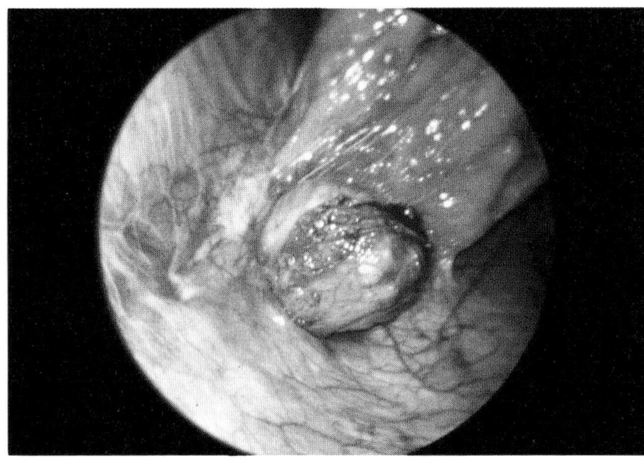

Fig. 4.42 Gallbladder with large stone load after aspiration of bile through the exteriorized neck.

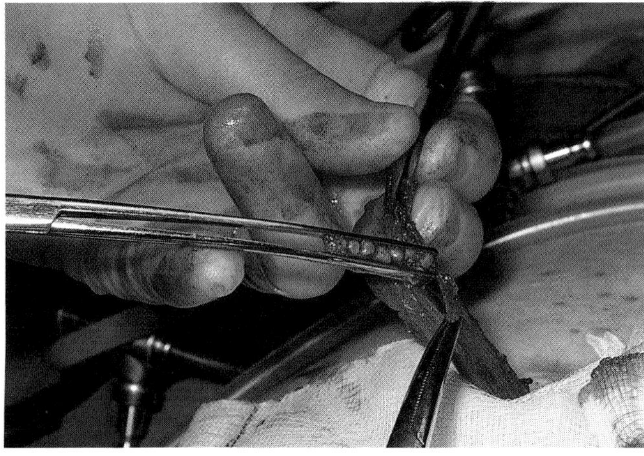

Fig. 4.43 Manual evacuation of stones. This is best performed with a Dejardins or Randall's forceps.

The instrument is placed around the cannula and its blades are inserted by rotation just beyond the peritoneal lining. Meanwhile, the gallbladder neck is grasped by a 5 mm traumatic forceps inserted through a reducer tube. After the neck of the gallbladder has been brought inside the reducer tube, the two are eased inside the cannula and then withdrawn *en masse* through the abdominal wall, until the gallbladder fundus abuts on the parietal peritoneum. At this stage the speculum blades are opened and pushed further in to grasp the widest part of the gallbladder. Steady traction is then maintained to deliver the organ (Fig. 4.44). Once the gallbladder is caught by the blades of the speculum, traction on the speculum with to and fro rotation results in delivery of the bulky organ. This procedure, although accompanied by some loss of pneumoperitoneum, is both safe and effective.

Lithotripsy. This can be achieved through the exteriorized neck by use of ultrasonic lithotripsy as practised by Perissat [6] or by the LaparoLith™ (Baxter Health Care Corporation, California). The latter is an electromechanical device which rotates a metal impeller inside a fixed protective cage (Fig. 4.45). When activated inside a dissected partially exteriorized gallbladder, the rotating impeller creates a fluid vortex which lifts the gallstones

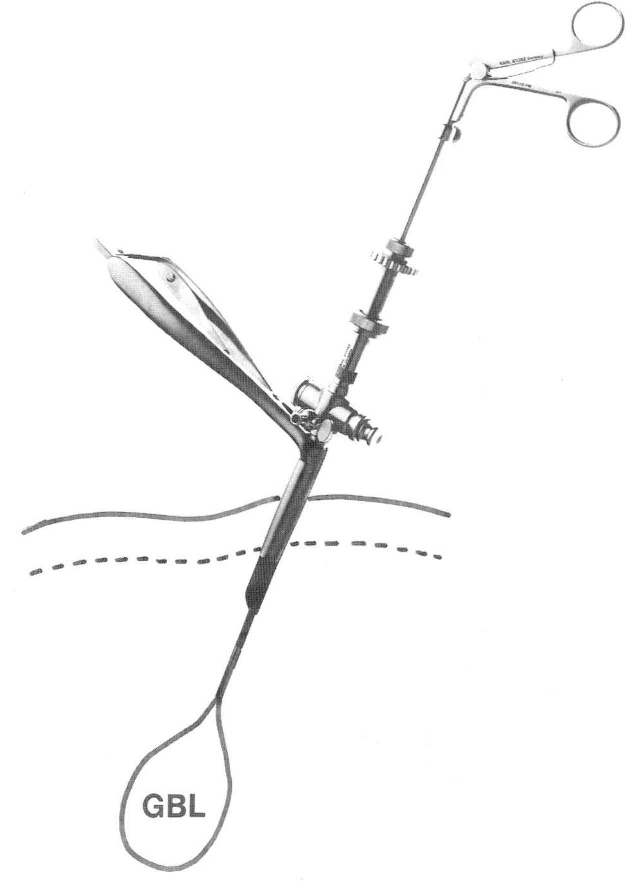

Fig. 4.44 Principle of use of gallbladder-extracting speculum. The gallbladder neck is withdrawn inside the reducer tube and the two inside the cannula, which is then eased outside the abdominal wall. The speculum blades are then pushed further in and opened to grasp the widest part of the gallbladder as steady traction on the organ is maintained. Once the gallbladder is caught by the blades of the speculum, traction on the speculum with to and fro rotation results in delivery of the bulky organ.

into contact with the rotating blades, resulting in their rapid fragmentation (Fig. 4.46). In one multicentre evaluation, successful lithotripsy with extraction of the gallbladder through the 1.0 cm incision was achieved in 85% of patients [12]. This technique of lithotripsy is ineffective in the presence of large calcified or impacted stones, and if the gallbladder is shrunken and

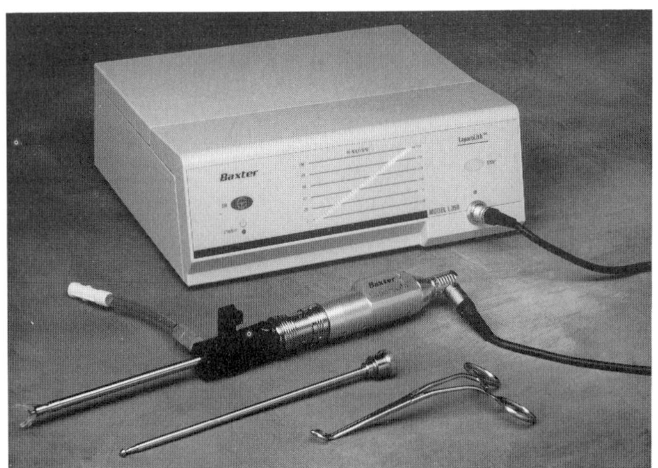

(a)

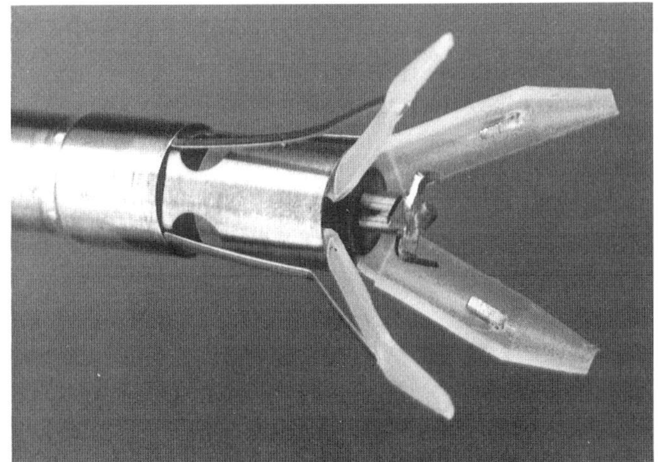

(b)

Fig. 4.45 (a) LaparoLith™ intraoperative lithotriptor (Baxter Health Care Corporation, California). This electromechanical device rotates a metal impeller inside a fixed protective cage. (b) Close-up view of the impeller.

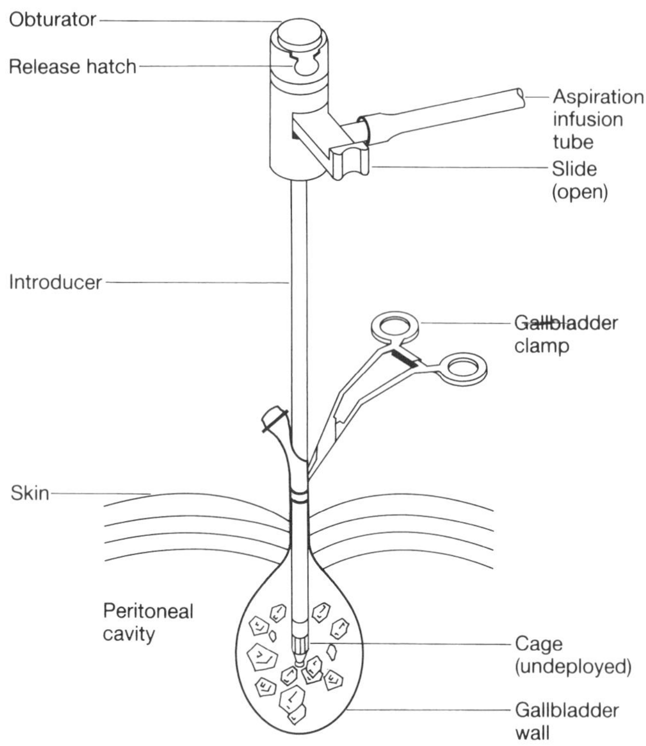

Fig. 4.46 When activated inside a dissected partially exteriorized gallbladder, the rotating impeller creates a fluid vortex which lifts the gallstones into contact with the rotating blades, resulting in their rapid fragmentation.

fibrotic such that it cannot be distended with saline to create a sufficient fluid vortex. If the gallbladder is perforated during dissection, it is placed within a plastic bag (Fig. 4.47) and the fundus opened once inside the bag. The neck of this is then exteriorized. As the opened gallbladder is extracted, the stones

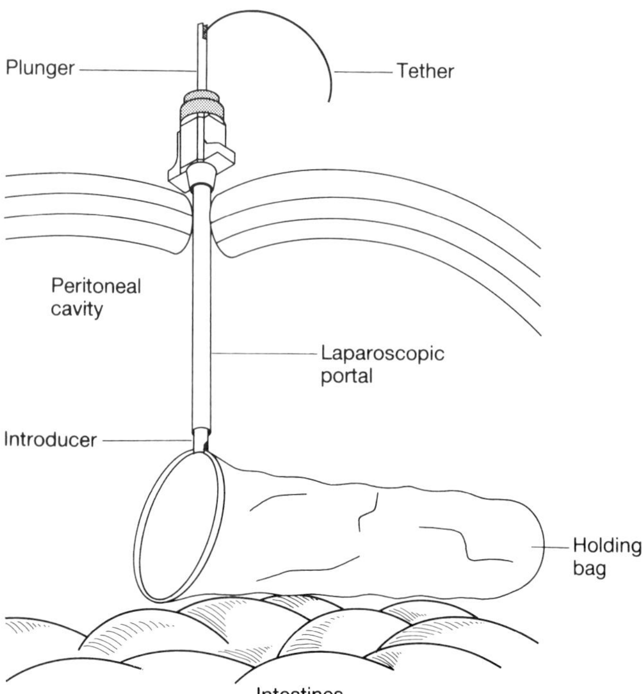

Fig. 4.47 Laparobag (Baxter Health Care Corporation, California).

fall into the bag which is then distended with saline prior to activation of the lithotriptor.

Cutdown. This is required for large (<3.0 cm), calcified or impacted stones. When a decision is made for this approach, the subumbilical route should be chosen. It is important that careful suture of the extended defect in the linea alba is performed after the gallbladder is extracted.

Final inspection, drainage, desufflation and suture of stab wounds

The pneumoperitoneum is restored and the telescope is reinserted. The suction/irrigation cannula is introduced through the upper left paramedian cannula.

Inspection, suction/irrigation and haemostasis

Any clots are evacuated. The subhepatic and the gallbladder bed are irrigated and suctioned dry. Any bleeding points in the gallbladder fossa are electrocoagulated to ensure a dry operative field. The liver surface is closely inspected for any accidental stab wounds or minor lacerations. Any hepatic bleeding is best controlled by argon beam spray coagulation, if available. The subphrenic space and the right paracolic gutter are next irrigated and suctioned until the fluid is clear and any debris has been evacuated. Finally the rest of the peritoneal cavity, including the pelvis is inspected.

Drainage

A subhepatic drain is not needed after routine laparoscopic cholecystectomy, unless the dissection has proved difficult, with oozing and some bile leakage, in which case a silicon subhepatic drain attached to a closed suction system is inserted.

Desufflation and removal of cannulae

It is important that the access cannulae are removed under vision to ensure that there is no abdominal wall bleeding from any of the wounds. Unless recognized and dealt with, this may result in significant postoperative blood loss. The technique for controlling abdominal wall bleeding is described earlier in this chapter. The desufflation of the pneumoperitoneum must be as complete as possible to reduce the amount of postoperative shoulder pain.

Suture of the stab wounds

The wounds are infiltrated with long-acting local anaesthetic (bupivacaine) before closure. Care is taken to suture the linea alba of the subumbilical wound to avoid subsequent hernia formation. The other small stab wounds require superficial approximation only (subcuticular absorbable sutures or skin tapes).

Immediate aftercare

Following the reversal of neuromuscular blockade and extubation, an oropharyngeal airway is inserted and oxygen is administered by mask for the first 3 hours. The patient is nursed on the side. Analgesia is administered as required. The majority of patients are ready for discharge the next day. Although day-case laparoscopic cholecystectomy is practised in some centres [13], this practice must be backed up with effective nursing care, otherwise it is unsafe.

References

1 Cuschieri A. Tissue approximation. In: Berci G (ed) *Problems in General Surgery (laparoscopic surgery)*. JB Lippincott, Philadelphia, 1991; pp. 366–377.

2 Dubois F, Berthelot G, Levard H. Cholecystectomy by coelioscopy. *Press Med* 1989; **18**: 980–982.

3 Dubois F, Icard P, Berthelot G, Levard H. Coelioscopic cholecystectomy. Preliminary report of 35 cases. *Ann Surg* 1990; **211**: 60–62.

4 Dubois F, Berthelot G, Levard H. Cholecystectomy with coelioscopy, 330 cases. *Chirurgie* 1990; **116**: 248–250.

5 Perissat J, Collet D, Belliard R. Gallstones: laparoscopic treatment, cholecystostomy, cholecystectomy, and lithotripsy. Our own technique. *Surg Endosc* 1990; **4**: 1–5.

6 Perissat J, Collet D, Vitale G, Belliard R, Sosso M. Laparoscopic cholecystectomy using intracorporeal lithotripsy. *Am J Surg* 1991; **161**: 371–376.

7 Reddick EJ, Olsen DO, Daniell JF, Saye WB, MacKernen B, Muller W, Hoback M. Laparoscopic laser cholecystectomy. *Laser Med Surg News* 1989; **7**: 38–40.

8 Reddick EJ, Olsen DO. Laparoscopic laser cholecystectomy. *Surg Endosc* 1989; **3**: 131–133.

9 Nathanson LK, Easter DW, Cuschieri A. Ligation of the structures of the cystic pedicle during laparoscopic cholecystectomy. *Am J Surg* 1991; **161**: 350–354.

10 Nathanson LK, Shimi S, Cuschieri A. Laparoscopic cholecystectomy: the Dundee technique. *Br J Surg* 1991; **78**: 155–159.

11 Cuschieri A. Variable-curvature shape-memory spatula for laparoscopic surgery. *Surg Endosc* 1991; **5**: 179–181.

12 Cuschieri A, Shimi S, Banting S, Nathanson LK, Garden OJ *et al.* Clinical evaluation of the LaparoLith intra-operative lithotriptor system. *Br J Surg* (in press).

13 Reddick EJ, Olsen DO. Outpatient laparoscopic laser cholecystectomy. *Am J Surg* 1990; **160**: 485–487.

5 : The difficult cholecystectomy

This chapter deals with the difficult laparoscopic cholecystectomy as well as the measures needed to overcome adverse situations encountered during the course of the operation. In some cases, the preoperative evaluation will indicate the possible difficulties and hence affect the decision on whether the operation should be performed laparoscopically or by the conventional open technique. To some extent, this elective decision is influenced by the experience of the surgeon in laparoscopic surgery, and the best advice that can be offered to surgeons taking up the laparoscopic approach is to gain the initial experience (the first 25 cases) on easy cases: thin patients with functioning gallbladders and normal liver function tests.

Other difficulties and problems, such as inadequate access, visceral injuries and bleeding, are encountered during the course of the operation. These may be coped with laparoscopically but in some cases enforced conversion to open surgery is necessary in the interests of patient safety.

Preoperative identification

There are both clinical and ultrasound/radiological criteria which suggest that the cholecystectomy is likely to be difficult or problematic in the individual patient. This evaluation is important for three reasons. Firstly, it indicates that the procedure should not be delegated to a trainee. Secondly, the patient is informed of the greater chance of conversion to open surgery, and thirdly it has a bearing on the scheduling of patients on a given operating list.

Clinical risk factors

These are shown in Table 5.1. Laparoscopic cholecystectomy is more difficult in stocky male patients (hypersthenic build). These individuals have a tightly packed internal anatomy which results in a reduced operating space, despite an adequate pneumoperitoneum.

The problems encountered in the morbidly obese vary considerably from patient to patient. Some indeed present fewer problems and better exposure of the cystic pedicle than in open surgery, as the thick abdominal wall is left behind by the optic. Others are less easy. In these patients the major problem relates to a fat-laden omentum, fatty deposition in the cystic pedicle which obscures the anatomy, and a heavy fatty liver which may be difficult to elevate and is easily lacerated. Special attention has to be paid to the siting of the access cannulae to ensure adequate reach to the operative region by the instruments, and to avoid impalement in the fat-laden falciform ligament. In these patients the laparoscopic telescope cannula should be sited above the umbilicus to the right of the midline.

The best evaluation of patients with previous abdominal surgery is obtained by the ultrasound visceral slide technique [1]. This technique has

Table 5.1 Clinical criteria indicative of a difficult laparoscopic cholecystectomy

Stocky male patients
Morbid obesity
Previous upper abdominal surgery
Cirrhosis and hepatomegaly
Inflammatory mass in the right hypochondrium (acute)
Previous severe acute cholecystitis
Previous percutaneous stone extraction/MTBE dissolution

been evaluated in a blind prospective fashion in the authors' institution and was found to be extremely reliable [2]. It can be performed in the radiological department during ultrasonography of the liver and gallbladder, or immediately preoperatively. In addition to precise localization of the adhesions to the anterior abdominal wall, this ultrasound assessment enables the identification of a safe window for the insertion of the Veress needle to create the initial pneumoperitoneum. In one centre, ultrasonic examination is performed after the creation of the pneumoperitoneum and prior to the insertion of the trocar cannula [3]. In the absence of adhesions, the CO_2 pneumoperitoneum produces a typical image consisting of a large conical shadow with dense hyperechogenic lines. Adhesions result in an amorphous picture with coarse echoes and loops of intestine, which are easily identified by their peristaltic movement. The major limitation of this technique is that it does not prevent injuries caused by the Veress needle.

Laparoscopic cholecystectomy is always difficult in patients with cirrhosis. In the first instance, the firm nodular enlarged liver lacks pliability and resists upward lift, resulting in limited exposure of the cystic pedicle and the triangle of Calot. This is especially difficult if the quadrate lobe is hypertrophied. In addition, the gallbladder is enlarged and is often surrounded by regenerative nodules, such that the fibrous plane of cleavage between the undersurface of this organ and the liver is difficult to find. Thus separation of the gallbladder from the hepatic parenchyma is difficult and bloody. The most adverse factor is the presence of portal hypertension. The risk of uncontrollable bleeding from the high-pressure variceal channels crossing the cystic pedicle renders laparoscopic cholecystectomy unsafe in these patients.

The clinical diagnosis of acute cholecystitis, based on physical findings, leucocytosis and ultrasonographic examination, covers a wide spectrum of disease severity. Table 5.2 outlines the findings of 60 consecutive patients with a diagnosis of acute obstructive cholecystitis subjected to laparoscopic inspection with a view to cholecystectomy by this route within 2 days of admission [4]. For the majority of these patients an early laparoscopic cholecystectomy (performed during the same hospital admission) is safe. Several previous randomized clinical trials on conventional open cholecystectomy had confirmed the undoubted benefits of early versus interval operation (delayed several weeks after resolution of the cholecystitis) [5–7]. However, in patients with established empyema and gangrenous cholecystitis, the risk of rupture of the gallbladder, with significant contamination of the peritoneal cavity, is significant and in the authors' opinion does not justify the use of the laparoscopic approach. Clinically this subgroup, which accounts for 15–20% of patients, is identified by an inflammatory mass in the right hypochondrium and overt signs of sepsis.

Patients who have undergone previous percutaneous treatment for gallstone disease, which involves cannulation of the gallbladder (percutaneous stone extraction or dissolution with MTBE), invariably have a gallbladder which is densely adherent to the hepatic flexure and anterior abdominal wall,

Table 5.2 Findings at laparoscopic inspection of patients with a diagnosis of acute obstructive cholecystitis ($n = 60$)

Finding	n
Tense obstructed gallbladder	15
Oedematous inflamed gallbladder	36
Severe disease: gangrenous patches, empyema, pericholecystic abscess	9

Table 5.3 Ultrasound/radiological criteria indicative of a difficult laparoscopic cholecystectomy

Gallbladder wall thickness >4.0 mm
Non-contracting gallbladder (ultrasound)
Stone load: packed gallbladder, large calcified stones (ultrasound)
Non-functioning gallbladder (oral cholecystogram/i.v. cholangiogram)

and is enwrapped by omental adhesions. However, with care and experience the majority of these cholecystectomies can be performed laparoscopically.

Ultrasound/radiological risk factors

The ultrasound/radiological findings which are suggestive of a technically difficult laparoscopic cholecystectomy are shown in Table 5.3.

Apart from its value in establishing the diagnosis, good and expert ultrasound examination of the gallbladder reliably predicts the degree of difficulty of the procedure. In this respect, the most important finding is a maximal gallbladder wall thickness >4.0 mm. This finding is indicative of a contracted fibrotic gallbladder which is difficult to grasp, and foreshortening of the cystic pedicle rendering dissection of the cystic duct and artery difficult. Other important findings are the absence of contraction after a fatty meal (or Mars Bar), a gallbladder which is packed full of stones, and large calcified stones (>2.5 cm). The main problem which is likely to be encountered in the presence of these ultrasound findings is difficulty in obtaining and maintaining a good hold on the gallbladder. Furthermore, a large stone impacted in Hartmann's pouch creates problems with dissection of the cystic artery and duct.

Non-function of the gallbladder on oral cholecystography is another reliable indicator of a shrunken fibrotic gallbladder, but this test is not performed routinely in X-ray departments nowadays and has been largely replaced by ultrasonography. Furthermore, non-opacification of the gallbladder requires confirmation with repeat testing, using a double dose of the oral contrast agent. In France, preoperative intravenous infusion tomographic cholangiography is performed. Non-visualization of the gallbladder by this test is indicative of either cystic duct obstruction or a fibrosed contracted gallbladder.

Difficult access due to adhesions

The measures needed to create a safe pneumoperitoneum in patients with previous abdominal surgery are outlined in Chapter 3. The purpose of the adhesiolysis is to expose the operative field and all regions within the subjacent areas of the access cannulae to enable unrestricted instrument manipulation.

The principles governing safe laparoscopic adhesiolysis are well established and generally follow those used in open surgery [8]. In the first instance, the exact anatomy of the adhesions in the individual case must be determined. This allows the formulation of an orderly plan of action necessary to achieve the objective of adequate exposure of the gallbladder and the cystic pedicle, and saves operating time. Adhesions to the anterior abdominal wall are divided first. Once the parietal peritoneum and the cannula access sites are freed, attention is directed to the adhesions within the operative area. These should be dealt with in the following order:

1 Adhesions between the superior surface of the right lobe of the liver and the diaphragm. These may be dense and multiple in patients with the Fitz-Hugh–Curtis syndrome.
2 Omental adhesions to the gallbladder and cystic pedicle.
3 Adhesions between the transverse colon/mesocolon and the gallbladder.
4 Adhesions between the duodenal bulb and the hepatoportal ligament and the cystic pedicle.

As adhesions are least vascular at their insertion this is the ideal plane for adhesiolysis. The insertion is outlined by grasping the adhesion and stretching it. Often, separation through this plane is best achieved by blunt teasing with the flat of the closed scissor blades. As fat-laden vascular adhesions may overlie intestinal loops, high-frequency electrocoagulation must be applied with great care, and only after the adhesion is tented well away from the bowel. Filmy avascular adhesions are best divided by sharp scissors, although they can be safely teased down with the atraumatic adhesion forceps (Fig. 5.1).

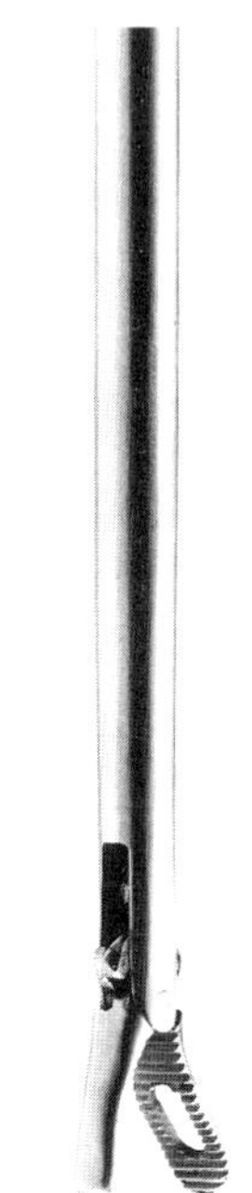

Fig. 5.1 Vancaillie adhesion forceps.

Exposure difficulties due to pathological anatomy of the liver and gallbladder

Abnormal liver

A problem is encountered if the liver is enlarged and diseased from fatty infiltration, cirrhosis or chronic hepatitis. The heavy pathological liver which is also firm is difficult to elevate and rotate. In these patients, the North American technique cannot be used to expose the cystic pedicle adequately. Another problem often encountered in the presence of a normal liver is a floppy left lobe or enlarged quadrate lobe. In all these instances adequate exposure requires an extra access cannula, which is inserted below and to the left of the xiphoid process (Fig. 5.2). Through this instrument is introduced a retractor (rod or expanding variety), which is passed underneath the round ligament and then used to elevate the quadrate lobe. As the retractor is beneath the round ligament, the entire central portion of the liver is elevated. A grasper is introduced through the right lower axillary cannula and is used to elevate the fundus of the gallbladder and lateral part of the right lobe of the liver.

An alternative technique to deal with the problem of a heavy liver or floppy quadrate lobe is the use of the dipping endoretractor. This lifts and pushes back the hepatic parenchyma ahead of the optic, providing excellent exposure (Fig. 5.3 a,b). It carries the added advantage of avoiding the need for the insertion of an extra cannula.

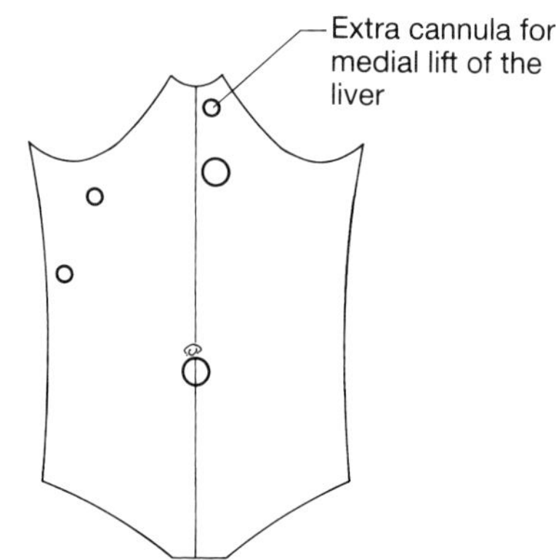

Fig. 5.2 Site of extra cannula for medial lift of the liver and round ligament.

Tense gallbladder

A gallbladder which is tense and distended due to the impaction of stones in the neck of the organ is difficult to grasp, and may be lacerated by the

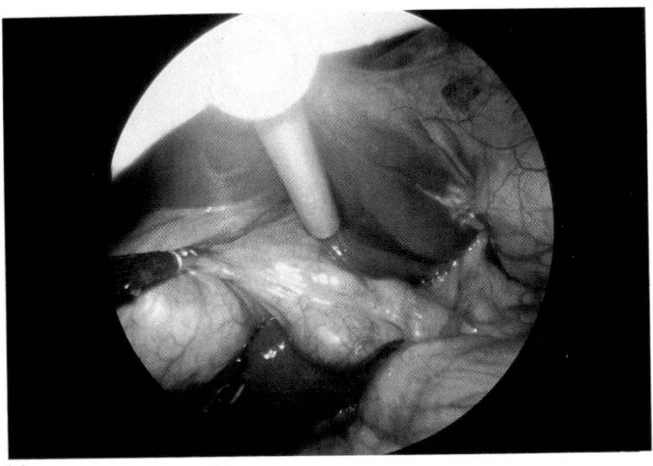
(a)

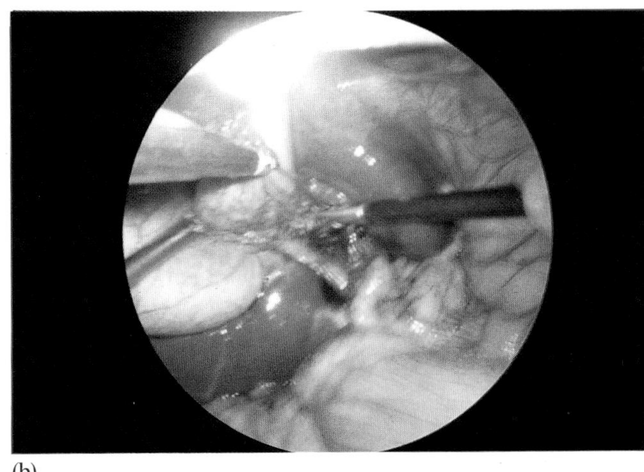
(b)

Fig. 5.3 (a) Dipping endoretractor in use to overcome exposure problems caused by a floppy quadrate lobe. (b) Dipping endoretractor used to overcome problems caused by a heavy fatty liver.

grasper jaws. This situation is often encountered in patients with mild acute cholecystitis, or after a recent attack of biliary colic. The correct step is aspiration of the gallbladder through the fundus. This may be performed using a specially designed cannula (Fig. 5.4) but the author now prefers to use a Veress needle attached to suction. The needle is inserted through the centre of the gallbladder fundus along the long axis of the organ using a stabbing movement (Fig. 5.5). The tap on the Veress needle is then opened and the bile aspirated. As the gallbladder is empty, the small perforation does not leak on withdrawal of the needle. As a precaution against leakage, the gallbladder fundus is grasped at the site of the perforation. Some surgeons secure the small perforation in the gallbladder with an endoloop at this stage, but this step is best delayed until just before extraction of the gallbladder through the parieties.

Packed gallbladder

A fibrotic leathery gallbladder packed full of stones poses a real problem. The situation may be approached by using an extra cannula to lift the medial aspect of the liver (see above). Alternatively, a small incision is made near the fundus and enough stones are removed using the spoon forceps to provide the necessary mural laxity. The incision is then closed by an endoloop and the grasper applied to the tissues distal to the ligature (Fig. 5.6).

Fig. 5.4 Gallbladder aspiration cannula.

Abnormal anatomy

Situs inversus

This should be discovered preoperatively, sometimes in association with Kartagener's syndrome [9]. The siting of the access cannula in the left upper quadrant reflects a mirror image of the usual positions (Fig. 5.7). In addition, the surgeon operates from the right side of the patient and the assistant stands on the left if the North American technique is used.

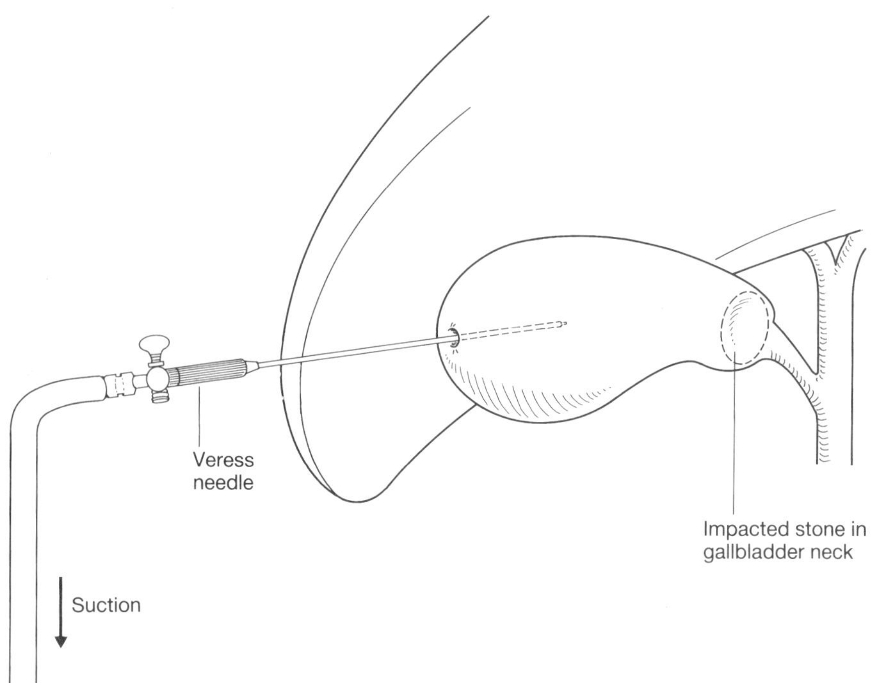

Fig. 5.5 Technique of aspiration of the distended gallbladder using Veress needle attached to suction. The fundus is impaled along the long axis of the organ.

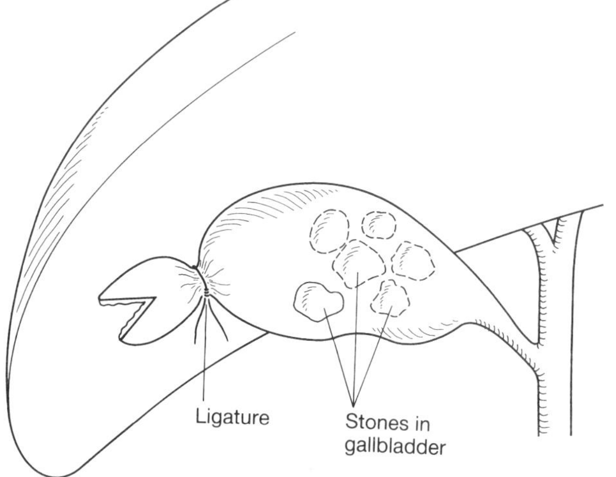

Fig. 5.6 A small incision is made near the fundus and enough stones are removed using the spoon forceps to provide the necessary mural laxity. The incision is then closed by an endoloop and the grasper applied to the tissues distal to the ligature.

Malposition of the gallbladder

There are two anomalies, both rare, which cause technical difficulties during the conduct of laparoscopic cholecystectomy. These are medioposition of the gallbladder, and the even rarer sinistroposition [10]. The author has encountered both anomalies and although the laparoscopic cholecystectomy was completed without complications in each case, both operations proved tedious.

In medioposition, the gallbladder is shifted medially towards the umbilical fissure and the ligamentum teres, the gallbladder fossa being situated on the anterior part of the quadrate lobe (segment iv) (Fig. 5.8). In sinistroposition

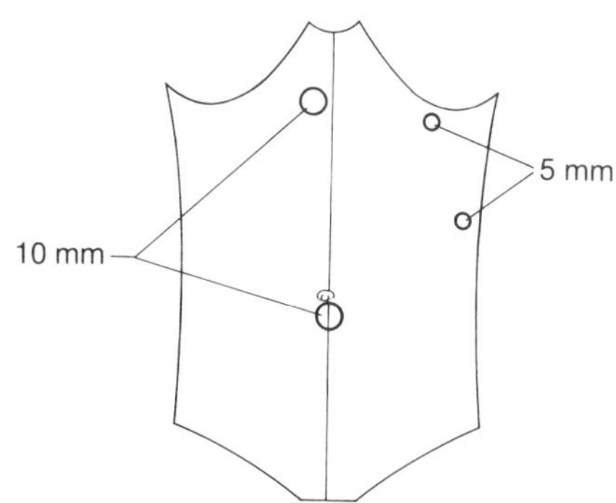

Fig. 5.7 Sites of trocars/cannulae in situs inversus.

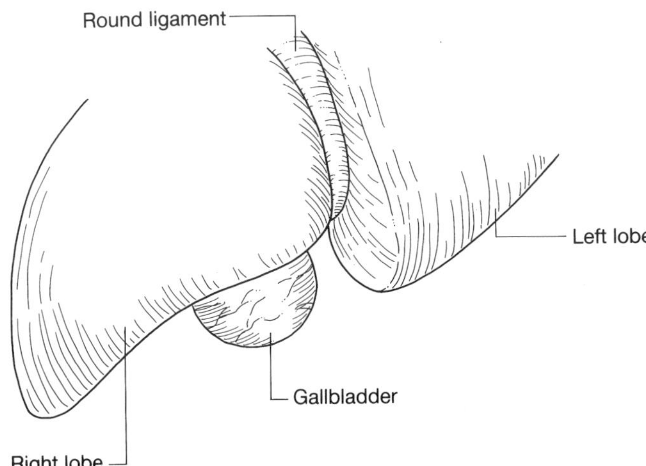

Fig. 5.8 In medioposition, the gallbladder is shifted medially towards the umbilical fissure and the ligamentum teres, the gallbladder fossa being situated on the anterior part of the quadrate lobe.

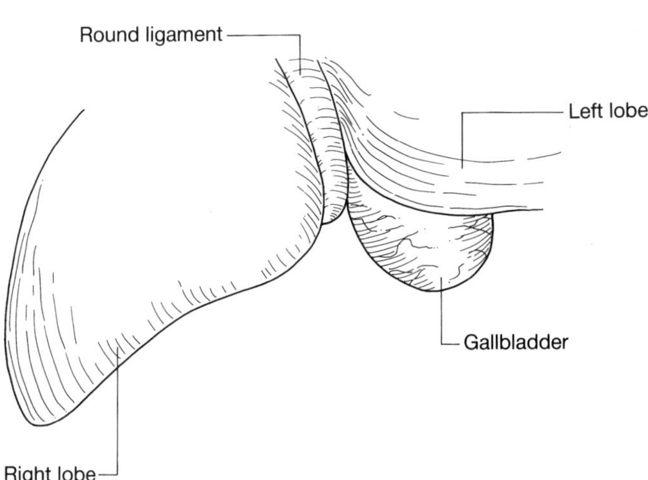

Fig. 5.9 In sinistroposition the gallbladder is situated to the left of the ligamentum teres underneath segment iii of the left lobe.

the gallbladder is situated to the left of the ligamentum teres underneath segment iii of the left lobe (Fig. 5.9). As the bile duct is in the normal position in both instances, the cystic duct and artery are long and have a tortuous course anterior to the structures of the porta hepatis. In both instances an extra cannula inserted near the xiphoid is required. An atraumatic forceps is introduced through this extra cannula and used to grasp the gallbladder, which is lifted upwards and slightly to the right. The dissection starts close to the neck of the gallbladder and both the cystic artery and duct are mobilized in a retrograde fashion (towards the bile duct). The main problem concerns the cystic artery, which closely simulates a looped right hepatic artery and has to be differentiated from this by adequate mobilization.

Parenchymatous, contracted and trabecular gallbladder

The problem relating to these abnormalities concerns the inability to grasp the gallbladder fundus. The parenchymatous organ is buried in the liver parenchyma to a variable extent. The shrunken contracted gallbladder results from recurrent episodes of inflammation, and is often accompanied

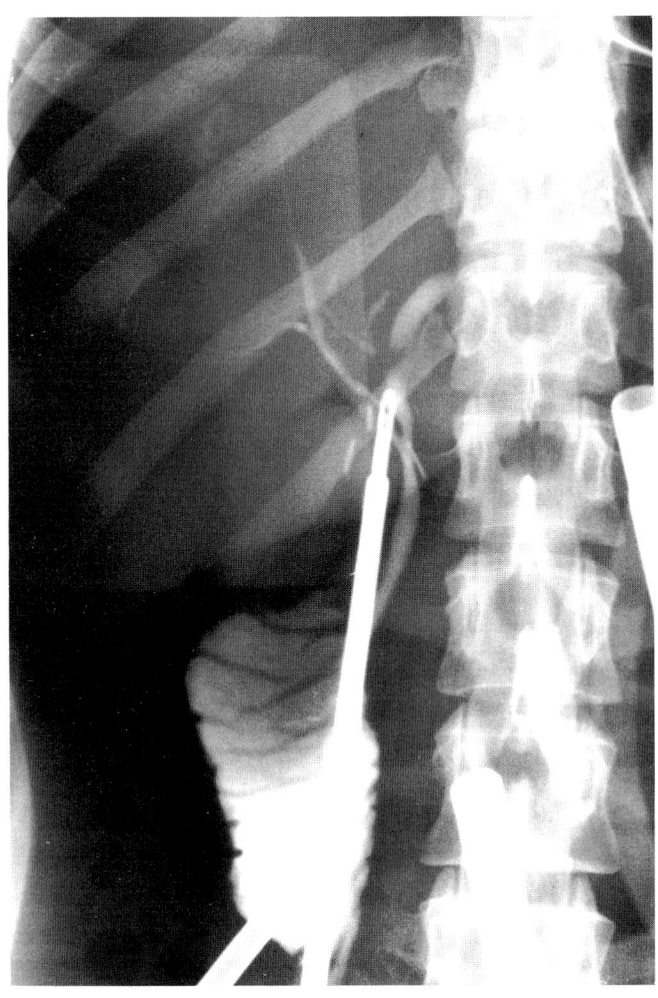

Fig. 5.10 Operative cholangiogram demonstrating short cystic duct entering the right hepatic duct.

by foreshortening of the cystic pedicle. The trabeculated gallbladder shows numerous criss-crossing strictures, which correspond to trabeculation in the gallbladder lumen. Often this type of gallbladder is associated with a significant gallstone load, which adds to the difficulties.

In all these situation, the French technique of medial liver lift (Chapter 4) provides better exposure of the cystic pedicle than the North American approach. Alternatively, the dipping endoretractor may be used.

Arterial abnormalities

Congenital anomalies are frequent and must be identified early on (Chapter 4). The most common variants are the anterior cystic artery, looped right hepatic artery and early division of the cystic artery. When suspected, the anterior cystic artery is confirmed by relaxing the traction on the gallbladder to restore pulsation. This artery is dissected, clipped and divided before mobilization of the cystic duct. The looped right hepatic artery is more problematic, as the cystic artery arises from the apex of the loop and is short. Again the cystic artery is secured first, with care to avoid inclusion of the right hepatic in the proximal clips. Once the cystic artery is divided, the looped right hepatic is teased medially and above the cystic duct.

If the cystic artery appears small, this may indicate early division in which case the posterior branch is usually located near the hepatic substance behind the cystic duct and the neck of the gallbladder. This branch must be sought for before the detachment of the gallbladder from the liver is commenced.

Another important acquired abnormality is a cystic artery which is densely adherent to the cystic duct as a result of chronic inflammation. The separation of the two structures may be very difficult. This is one of the common causes of bleeding during dissection of the cystic pedicle. The separation of the artery from the duct has to be undertaken slowly and with great gentleness. The creation of the window between the two structures is considerably helped in this situation by the use of curved dissecting graspers or the variable-curvature shape-memory dissecting spatula.

Biliary tract abnormalities

These are either congenital anomalies or acquired abnormalities secondary to chronic calculous disease. The various anomalies of the extrahepatic biliary tract are dealt with in Chapter 6.

Short cystic duct entering common hepatic duct

From a practical standpoint, the most important anomaly is a short cystic duct which joins the right hepatic duct, since this is the anomaly that is most often missed and the right hepatic duct is mistaken for the continuation of the cystic duct, with disastrous consequences. The only way in which this condition can be identified is by operative cholangiography (Fig. 5.10). The medial end of such a duct must be secured by ligature in continuity using the Roeder slip knot. The application of clips is extremely hazardous in this situation, as the risk of total or partial occulsion of the right hepatic duct is substantial.

Large stone impacted in Hartmann's pouch

A large stone impacted in Hartmann's pouch causes difficulties because the gallbladder neck cannot be grasped. Sometimes it is possible to dislodge the stone into the body of the gallbladder. When this proves impossible, the grasper is used as a probe to depress and lift Hartmann's pouch as the dissection alternates from above and below the cystic pedicle (Fig. 5.11).

Hartmann's pouch adherent to common duct

This operative finding always causes concern as the cystic pedicle is completely obscured. If the operator is experienced, a trial dissection is

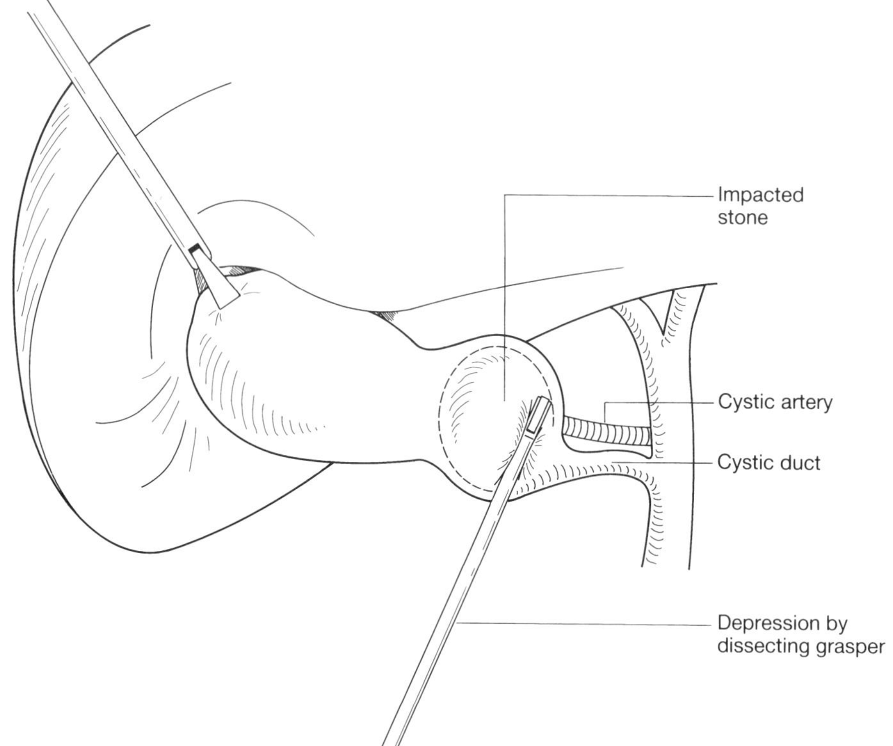

Fig. 5.11 The dissecting grasper is used as a probe to depress and lift Hartmann's pouch as the dissection alternates from above and below the cystic pedicle.

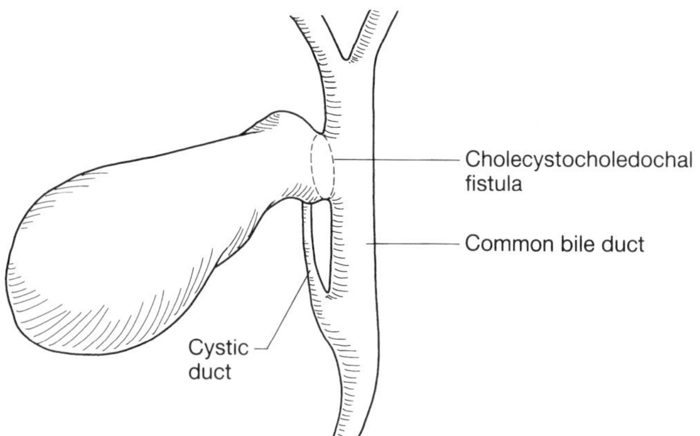

Fig. 5.12 Mirizzi syndrome. There is a fistula between the gallbladder neck and the common hepatic duct, overlying the cystic duct.

indicated to determine whether the gallbladder is simply loosely adherent to the bile duct and can thus be separated from it, or is connected to it by the establishment of a cholecystocholedochal fistula (Mirizzi syndrome) (Fig. 5.12). If the latter is confirmed, the case should be converted to open surgery irrespective of the experience of the operator, as the dissection is hazardous and the risk of bile duct and hepatic arterial damage is high.

During the trial dissection, the neck of the gallbladder is grasped anteriorly and held on traction in a lateral and downward direction to display the adhesion plane with the common duct. This is gently separated

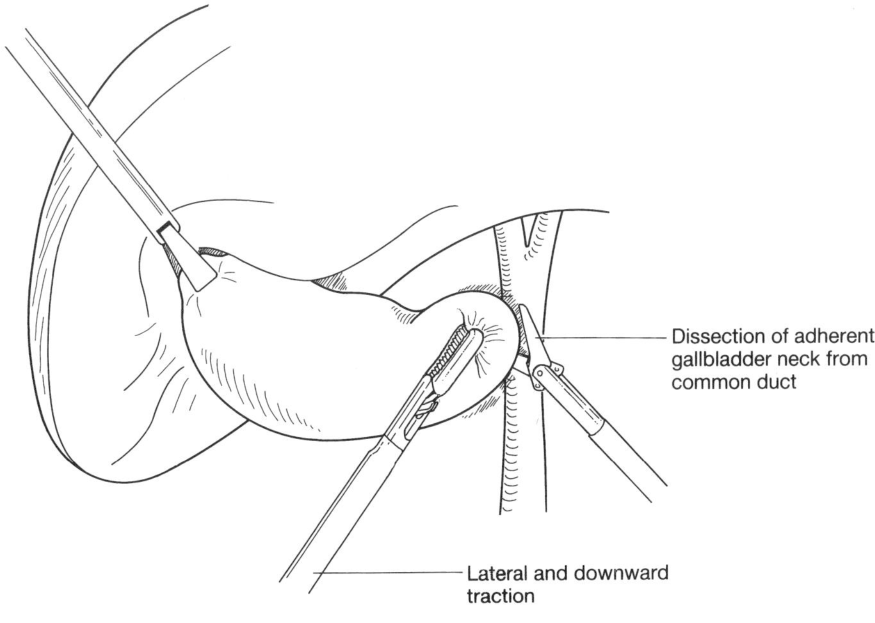

Fig. 5.13 During the trial dissection, the neck of the gallbladder is grasped anteriorly and held on traction in a lateral and downward direction to display the adhesion plane with the common duct. This is gently separated with scissors and blunt dissection.

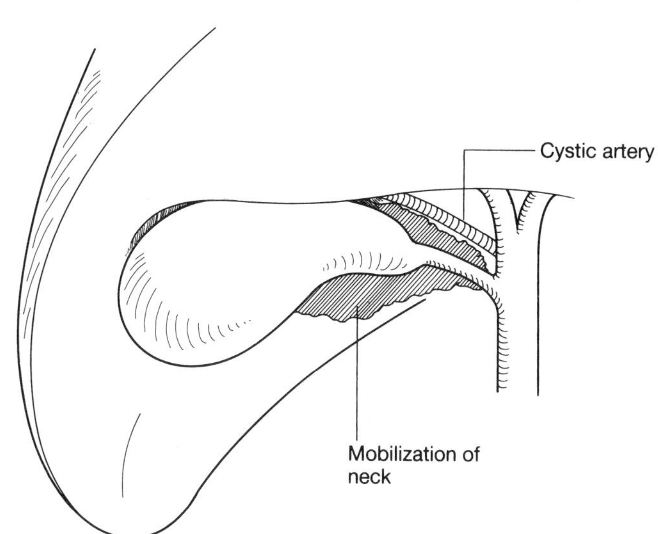

Fig. 5.14 Foreshortening of the cystic pedicle is remedied by lateral mobilization of the neck of the gallbladder. This creates the space required for the dissection of the cystic duct to proceed, and enough length of cystic duct can be mobilized for safe ligature or clipping, especially if the lateral end is secured across the neck of the gallbladder, preferably by a ligature.

with scissors and blunt dissection (Fig. 5.13). On no account must high-frequency electrosurgery be used during this trial separation of the neck of the gallbladder from the common duct.

Foreshortened cystic pedicle

This is a frequent finding in patients with chronic cholecystitis and a contracted or trabecular gallbladder. The space between the gallbladder neck and the common duct is reduced due to shortening and thickening of the cystic pedicle. Although the anatomy is not grossly disturbed, the operating space is limited and there is insufficient length of the cystic duct at the start

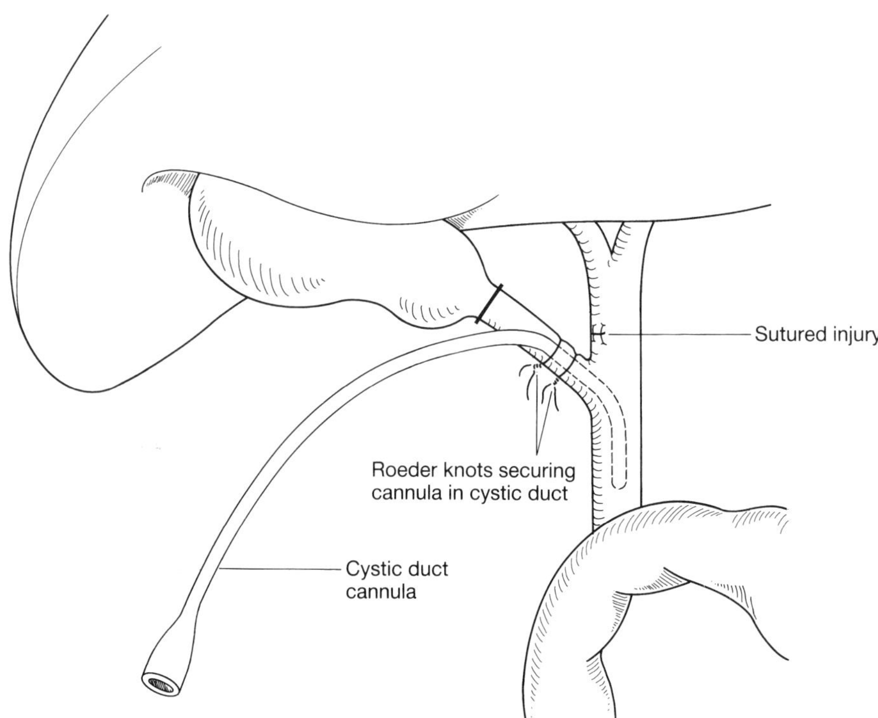

Fig. 5.15 If the injury is minor and lateral, it is sutured with one 5/0 atraumatic interrupted suture. The laparoscopic operation is continued but a cannula (infant feeding tube) is inserted through the cystic duct, to which it is secured by two Roeder catgut slip knots.

of the dissection. This problem is remedied by lateral mobilization of the neck of the gallbladder (Fig. 5.14). This creates the required space for the dissection of the cystic duct to proceed and enough length of cystic duct can be mobilized for safe ligature or clipping, especially if the lateral end is secured across the neck of the gallbladder, preferably by a ligature.

Complications during dissection

The complications which may be encountered during the course of the dissection are hepatic injuries, bleeding, bile duct damage, visceral damage, perforation of the gallbladder and stone loss. It is important to stress that with care and the right technique the vast majority of these complications can be avoided, but mishaps do happen.

Bleeding

Bleeding is undoubtedly a problem during laparoscopic surgery: it used to be the commonest cause for enforced conversion [11]. It is important to realize that the extent of haemorrhage is substantially magnified by the optic and a small arterial spurter may appear to the inexperienced as a torrential haemorrhage. Bleeding during laparoscopic cholecystectomy may consist of oozing, minor arterial bleeding, major arterial haemorrhage and venous welling. There are certain risk factors which predispose to a slow oozy procedure; the most important are difficult dissection, cirrhosis, coagulation defects, acute cholecystitis and gross obesity.

The main problem with oozing is light absorption and loss of detail of the visual field. The most effective practical adjunct is peanut (pledget) swab compression for a few seconds. Irrigation followed by aspiration is often necessary to clear the field.

Minor arterial bleeding requires the insertion of a sucker close to the bleeding site, with active aspiration to visualize the bleeding vessel. This is then grasped by an insulated grasper and either coagulated (through the grasper) or clipped. More serious arterial bleeding is approached in the same way. Often it is possible to grasp an adjacent organ (gallbladder or duodenum) and use overlay compression to achieve control until an extra cannula is inserted to enable the simultaneous use of sucker and insulated grasper. If control is not achieved within 1–2 minutes, or there is a persistent 'red out', then conversion to open surgery is necessary and should not be delayed.

Venous welling encountered during dissection of the cystic pedicle is due to cut venules in the cystic pedicle fat. It requires compression by adjacent tissues or pledget swab for a few minutes, followed by irrigation and suction. If the vessels can be identified, which is difficult because they retract within the surrounding fat, they are secured by electrocoagulation. More serious or persistent venous bleeding from the cystic pedicle requires conversion to open surgery.

Bleeding during detachment of the gallbladder from the liver is largely preventable by keeping the plane of separation above the fascial layer which separates the hepatic parenchyma from the undersurface of the gallbladder. If this is breached the hepatic parenchyma is torn, with bleeding and the added risk of postoperative bile leakage. Bleeding from the hepatic parenchyma is controlled by either electrocoagulation using the Berci spatula, or by use of the argon beam spray. In the author's experience the argon spray coagulation is the most effective and safest technique for control of bleeding from the liver parenchyma, whether this results from separation of the gallbladder from the liver parenchyma or is due to accidental instrumental lacerations of the liver substance.

A subhepatic drain should be inserted at the end of an oozy dissection.

Bile duct injury

The prophylactic measures are careful dissection and display of the anatomy and the use of operative cholangiography. The lesion is first identified by the escape of bile during the dissection of the cystic pedicle. When this is encountered, the following steps are essential:

1 Adequate laparoscopic exposure with constant suction of the area. This may necessitate the insertion of an extra trocar cannula just below the xiphoid to achieve medial lift of the liver over the porta hepatis. If the hole is identified, a soft catheter (infant enteral feeding tube Fr 5–8) is inserted in a proximal position as far as it can go, and is held in place by an atraumatic grasper until a cholangiogram is performed. This will outline the pathological

anatomy: minor lateral breach in the common hepatic or common bile duct or more serious injuries (loss of continuity, near complete transection, etc.).

2 If the injury is minor and lateral, it is sutured with one 5/0 atraumatic interrupted suture. The laparoscopic operation is continued but a cannula (infant feeding tube) is inserted through the cystic duct, to which it is secured by two Roeder catgut slip knots (Fig. 5.15). The cholangiogram is then repeated and if satisfactory ductal integrity is confirmed, the gallbladder is detached from the liver and a subhepatic drain is inserted. The cystic duct drainage cannula is used to decompress the biliary tract for 7–10 days, and is then removed if the postoperative cholangiogram is satisfactory. In the absence of complications or abnormal liver function tests, no further measures are required but an ERCP may be considered 6 months later.

3 If the injury is major, conversion to open surgery is essential.

Gallbladder perforation and stone loss

Perforation of the gallbladder is common and occurs in 15–20% of cases [11]. It is of little consequence and does not increase the morbidity, provided the extravasated bile is aspirated and the gutters are irrigated and sucked dry at the end of the procedure. When encountered, a small perforation is best secured by an endoloop.

The escape of stones is a problem, especially when multiple, as these are easily lost amongst the loops of the small intestine. The best instrument for picking up loose stones is the Semm spoon forceps. When several stones have escaped, a plastic bag may be inserted and all the stones (both extravasated and those still inside the gallbladder) transferred to the bag, which is then closed and removed.

There is insufficient information on the morbidity following lost intraperitoneal gallstones. It is often stated that the majority of these patients come to no harm, but it is known that some of these calculi harbour bacteria and the author has been involved as an expert witness in one court case involving a patient who developed a major intraperitoneal abscess around a 1.5 cm cholesterol stone several weeks after a laparoscopic cholecystectomy. Another patient developed an abscess and a CT scan confirmed the collection to be around a calcified stone (Scott-Conner, personal communication). In practice, every effort should be made to find and retrieve escaped stones, and those patients in whom stones have been lost should be put on a 5-day course of antibiotics and informed of the situation.

Visceral injuries

All hollow visceral injuries during dissection are preventable by careful dissection and avoidance of unnecessary electrocautery. When they occur, they usually involve the transverse colon, duodenum or upper small bowel. All can be sutured laparoscopically if the surgeon has acquired this basic skill. Thorough lavage with irrigation and aspiration is necessary after the injury is closed, and these patients should be put on a 5-day course of antibiotics.

Stab injuries to the liver may result from the sudden give of an instrument as increased force is applied to overcome resistance to slide caused by a trumpet valve. It is for this reason that cannulae with flap valves are preferred by the authors. Stab injuries should be carefully inspected and, if deep, are best packed with absorbable cellulose or microfibrillar collagen. These cases should be drained and watched carefully for the development of a subcapsular haematoma in the postoperative period. More superficial injuries are simply electrocoagulated, preferably by argon spray coagulation.

References

1 Sigel B, Golub RM, Laurie A *et al.* Technique of ultrasonic detection and mapping of abdominal wall adhesions. *Surg Endosc* 1991; **5**: 161–165.

2 Ravintharan T, Shimi S, Banting S, Hassan AK, Sinclair DJ, McCullough AS, Cuschieri A. Prospective blind evaluation of the ultrasound visceral slide technique in the location of adhesions in patients undergoing laparoscopic cholecystectomy. *Surg Endosc* (in press).

3 Marin G, Bergamo S, Miola E, Caldorini MW, Dagnini G. Prelaparoscopic echography used to detect abdominal adhesions. *Endoscopy* 1987; **19**: 147–149.

4 Cuschieri A. Approach to the treatment of acute cholecystitis: open surgical, laparoscopic or endoscopic. *Endoscopy* (in press).

5 McArthur P, Cuschieri A, Sells RA, Shields R. Controlled clinical trial comparing early with interval cholecystectomy for acute cholecystitis. *Br J Surg* 1975; **62**: 850–852.

6 Jarvinen JH, Hastbacka J. Early cholecystectomy for acute cholecystitis. A prospective randomized study. *Ann Surg* 1980; **191**: 502–505.

7 Norrby S, Herlin P, Holmin T, Sjodhal R, Tagesson C. Early or delayed cholecystectomy for acute cholecystitis? A clinical trial. *Br J Surg* 1983; **70**: 163–165.

8 Weibel MA, Majno G. Peritoneal adhesions and their relation to abdominal surgery. *Am J Surg* 1973; **126**: 345–353.

9 Campos L, Sipes E. Laparoscopic cholecystectomy in a 39-year-old female with situs inversus. *J Laparoendosc Surg* 1991, **1**: 123–125.

10 Beck K. *Colour Atlas of Laparoscopy.* W B Saunders, Philadelphia 1984; pp. 50–51.

11 Cuschieri A, Dubois F, Mouiel J, Mouret P *et al.* The European experience with laparoscopic cholecystectomy. *Am J Surg* 1991; **161**: 385–387.

6 : Laparoscopic cholangiography

Since the introduction of intraoperative cholangiography (IOC) by Mirizzi and the advocation of its use in the USA by Hickens in 1936, a debate began which has since continued on whether this intraoperative diagnostic modality should be used during cholecystectomy routinely, selectively or not at all. The controversy has, if anything, increased with the advent of laparoscopic cholecystectomy. At present, opinion remains sharply divided and practice concerning the use of IOC during laparoscopic cholecystectomy differs as follows:

1 Preoperative infusion tomographic cholangiography with selective IOC.

2 No IOC unless dictated by operative findings.

3 Routine IOC even in the presence of normal liver function tests and apparently normal intraoperative anatomy.

Case for routine intraoperative cholangiography during laparoscopic biliary surgery

Cholecystectomy

The arguments for routine IOC during conventional open cholecystectomy are that it provides an accurate anatomical 'map' of the biliary tract, which

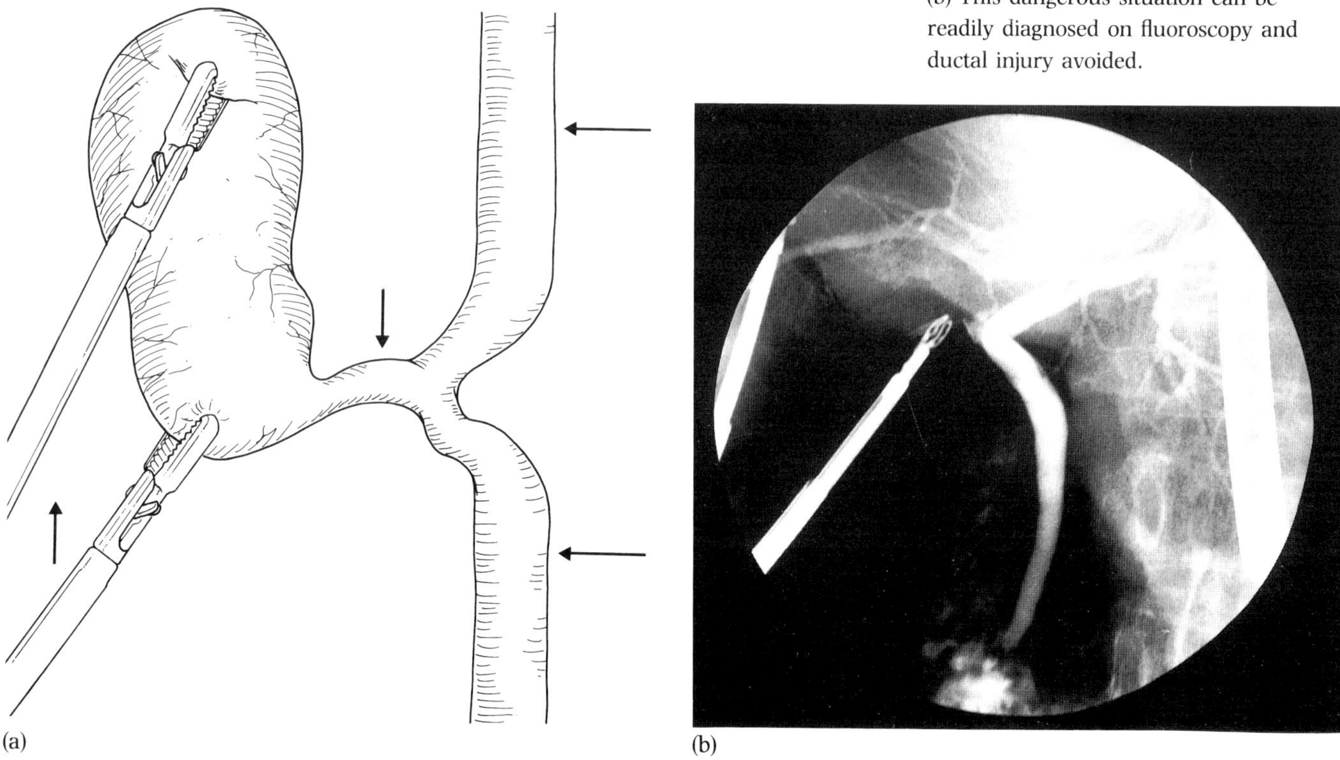

Fig. 6.1 (a) Diagrammatic representation of the stretched cystic–common duct junction as a result of the traction applied on the gallbladder fundus during laparoscopic cholecystectomy. The tented common hepatic or common bile duct may be mistaken for the continuation of the cystic duct and mistakenly clipped. (b) This dangerous situation can be readily diagnosed on fluoroscopy and ductal injury avoided.

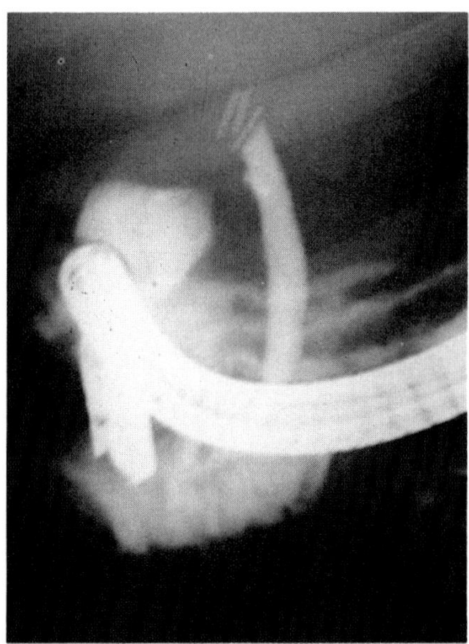

Fig. 6.2 Occlusion of the common hepatic duct by clips. (Kind permission of Prof. P. Bormann, Groote Schurr Hospital, Cape Town.) This patient was referred to Prof. Bormann with jaundice and cholangitis after laparoscopic cholecystectomy.

is essential in the prevention of iatrogenic bile-duct injuries; it detects unsuspected stones and can identify and characterize injuries during surgery when primary repair can be undertaken [1,2]. The routine use of IOC ensures experience with the technique, optimizing results and interpretation to a much greater extent than when IOC is employed occasionally as dictated by the selective policy.

The case for routine IOC during laparoscopic cholecystectomy is even stronger, since the termination of the cystic duct and indeed the common hepatic and common bile ducts are not well displayed [3–5]. It is true that the identity of the cystic duct can be established during laparoscopic cholecystectomy by tracing it back during the dissection to the gallbladder, but what is important is the drainage configuration of the cystic duct, to enable the selection of the safe site for medial clipping or ligature without compromise of the integrity of the extrahepatic ductal system. This is especially important as the traction on the gallbladder (necessary for exposure of the triangle of Calot) may result in tenting of the cystic–common duct junction (Fig. 6.1), which if ignored can lead to partial or total occlusion by the medial clips (Fig. 6.2). *There is no substitute diagnostic modality, including infusion tomographic cholangiography and ERCP performed preoperatively, which provides this essential information.*

Ductal calculi and bilioenteric bypass

There is no argument concerning the absolute necessity of IOC during these laparoscopic interventions (Chapters 9 and 10). The extraction of ductal calculi via the cystic duct or by means of supraduodenal exploration of the common bile duct requires the performance of fluoroscopic imaging, both during the execution of these procedures and as a completion check to ensure that complete ductal clearance has been achieved.

In patients with inoperable cancer of the head of the pancreas, a cholecystocholangiogram to determine safe clearance between the entry of the cystic duct and the upper limit of the tumour is essential for the appropriate decision as to the correct bilioenteric bypass in the individual patient. In the presence of a safe distance (1.0 cm or more), a laparoscopic cholecystojejunal anastomosis will provide excellent palliation, but if the tumour encroaches on the termination of the cystic duct, a choledochojejunostomy is required.

Radiological equipment

Mobile X-ray machines

The arguments which have been put forward against the routine use of IOC have been several: it is unnecessary in the majority, time-consuming, blind exposures and poor-quality/misleading films [6, 7]. These objections are valid when cholangiography is performed using mobile X-ray equipment with three blind exposures after the injection of varying amounts of contrast material. Indeed, the resolution of these films is often poor, especially in the obese patient. The blind exposure has three significant drawbacks: sections of the relevant biliary tract anatomy are at times inadvertently left out of the picture, the important early filling phase of the common duct is missed and the exact anatomy of the cystic duct and its distal drainage is not outlined adequately. These mishaps contribute to significant irritation and frequent delays as the surgeon often has to repeat the entire process after 20–30 minutes, because of unsatisfactory exposures.

Modern C-arm imaging

All these disadvantages have been overcome with the advent of the mobile C-arm with digital facilities and an expanded surgical software package (Fig. 6.3a,b), which enables image storage and advanced image processing through the use of sophisticated digital processing algorithms. Of particular benefit to operative cholangiography are the real-time subtraction and roadmapping modes. The former allows a dynamically subtracted view during contrast studies. Roadmapping is especially useful during interventional operative cholangiography, since live images are subtracted from an opacified contrast image, such as the contrast-filled common bile duct, thereby providing a precise map for the manipulation of balloon catheters or Dormia baskets during stone extraction. When needed for defining details of minor abnormalities, boosted fluoro- and peak opacification are employed to provide superb image quality with high-grade resolution. Apart from control of the image processing, the keyboard allows patient information to be inserted on the fluoroscopic image and any hard copies produced.

With this system screening is commenced just before the injection of contrast and the entire process lasts 2–3 minutes. By means of a foot-operated switch, the desired images are selected as they appear on the screen and stored on the hard disk. On completion of the screening (fluoro, subtraction, roadmapping), the images stored on disk can be recalled to the screen for review, and when desired, subjected to postprocessing. Hard copies are obtained on X-ray film cassettes within minutes by exposure of the image to the multiformat camera. Alternatively, the entire screening process can be stored in video format on a video cassette recorder.

The case for IOC during open and laparoscopic biliary surgery assumes the availability of this modern C-arm image intensifier. In particular, laparoscopic IOC cannot be performed expeditiously and with reliability with outdated mobile X-ray equipment.

Technique of laparoscopic cholangiography

There are two techniques of laparoscopic cholangiography: cystic duct cannulation and cholecystocholangiography. In both instances Hypaque (sodium diatrizoate) diluted to a concentration of 30% is the contrast agent

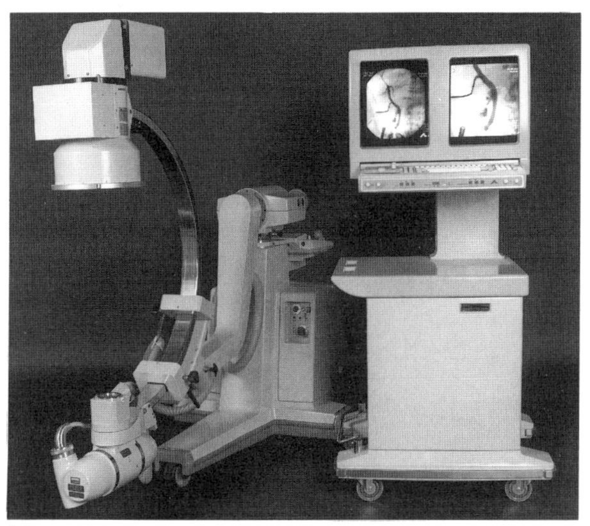

(a)

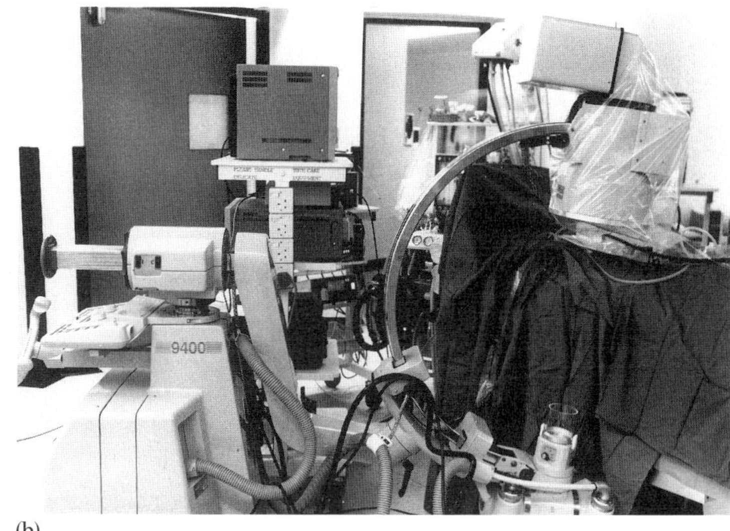

(b)

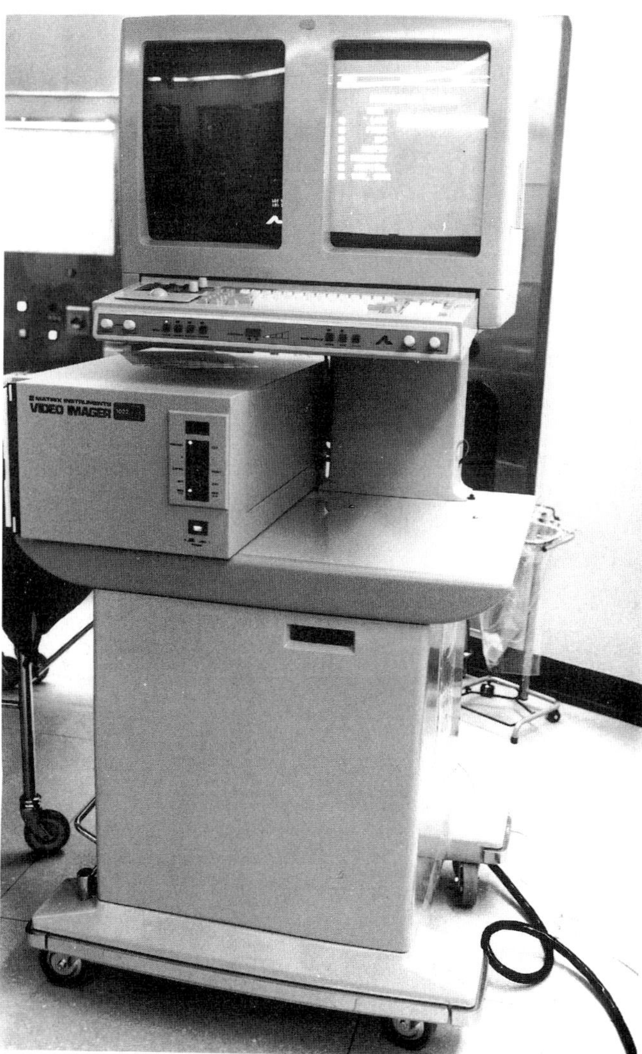

(c)

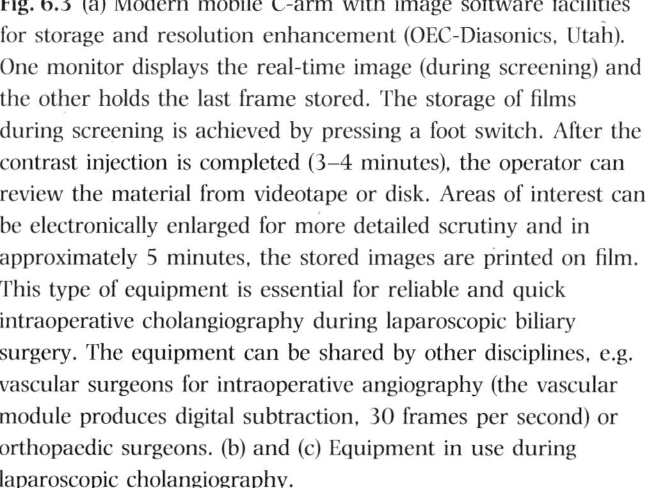

Fig. 6.3 (a) Modern mobile C-arm with image software facilities for storage and resolution enhancement (OEC-Diasonics, Utah). One monitor displays the real-time image (during screening) and the other holds the last frame stored. The storage of films during screening is achieved by pressing a foot switch. After the contrast injection is completed (3–4 minutes), the operator can review the material from videotape or disk. Areas of interest can be electronically enlarged for more detailed scrutiny and in approximately 5 minutes, the stored images are printed on film. This type of equipment is essential for reliable and quick intraoperative cholangiography during laparoscopic biliary surgery. The equipment can be shared by other disciplines, e.g. vascular surgeons for intraoperative angiography (the vascular module produces digital subtraction, 30 frames per second) or orthopaedic surgeons. (b) and (c) Equipment in use during laparoscopic cholangiography.

most commonly used. There are basic principles which are common to both techniques and these are:

1 The adequate protection of staff against radiation exposure. This is best achieved by a portable lead screen. If this is not available, the surgeon and his assistant should wear lead aprons and use double gloves during injection and fluoroscopy.

2 The screened area must not be overlaid with radio-opaque instrumentation: metal cannulae, electrosurgical cables, metal ends of nasogastric tubes etc.

3 The operating table should be tilted slightly head down and 20° to the right. This position encourages proximal filling of the biliary tract and overcomes the problem of superimposed shadows caused by the spinal column and the transverse processes.

4 The delivery system used (see below) should be connected via a three-way tap to two 30 ml syringes, one containing isotonic saline and the other the contrast material.

5 The delivery system must be completely primed with isotonic saline, ensuring that there are no air bubbles in the system.

6 Injection of the contrast should be slow and screening commence with the start of the injection, so that the important early phase of ductal filling is observed.

7 No cholangiogram should be considered satisfactory unless the intrahepatic as well as the extrahepatic system has been outlined.

Cystic duct cholangiography

This is the method of choice for routine IOC during laparoscopic cholecystectomy. The authors use a Fr 4–5 Cook ureteric catheter with a terminal hole inside the Storz cholangiograsper (Fig. 6.4) introduced through the midclavicular right subcostal cannula. Our technique, which achieves successful cannulation in 95% of cases, is as follows: once the cystic duct has been dissected, a clip is applied at the lateral end close to the infundibulum. The optic is advanced close to the cystic duct to achieve the desired magnification and the duct is opened anterosuperiorly by the curved microscissors (Fig. 6.5). In some instances, bleeding from the cut cystic duct wall may be encountered. This usually stops rapidly if compression is applied by the flat of the scissor blades for a few seconds, but it often requires saline injection through the cholangiography catheter to clear the field. Entry of the cystic duct lumen is detected by the escape of bile only if the traction on the gallbladder is momentarily released. The curved microscissors are then introduced closed inside the lumen and the blades are gently opened to dilate the orifice. The catheter is then introduced into the cystic duct over a distance of 1.0 cm and the jaws of the cholangiograsper are then advanced and closed, holding the catheter in a watertight grip (Fig. 6.6). Sometimes catheter insertion is hindered by prominent folds of the Heister valve. This can often be overcome by saline injection as the catheter tip is advanced

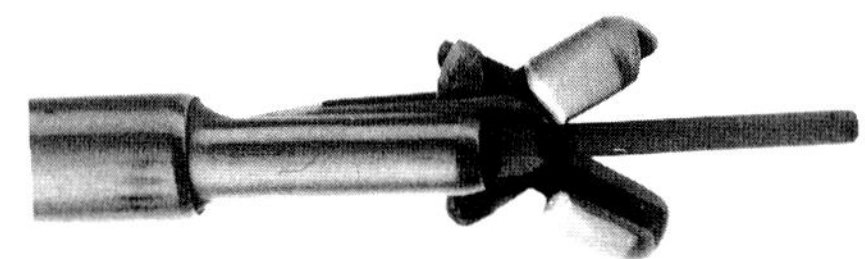

Fig. 6.4 Ureteric catheter inside Storz cholangiograsper.

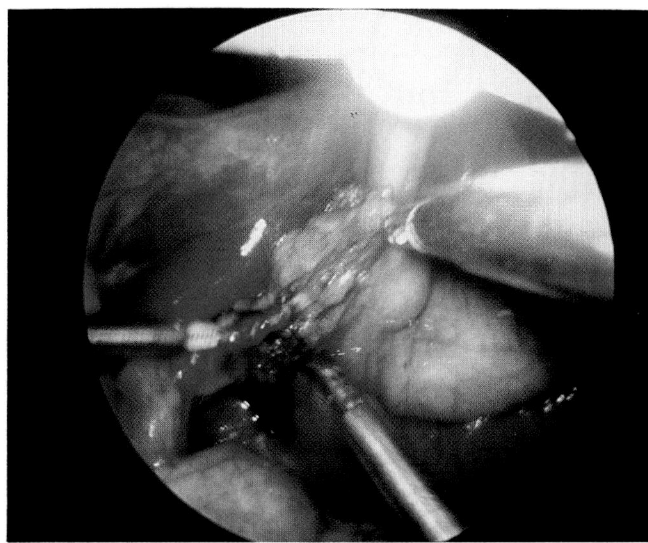

Fig. 6.5 After ligature or clipping of the lateral end, the cystic duct is opened anterosuperiorly with curved microdissecting scissors.

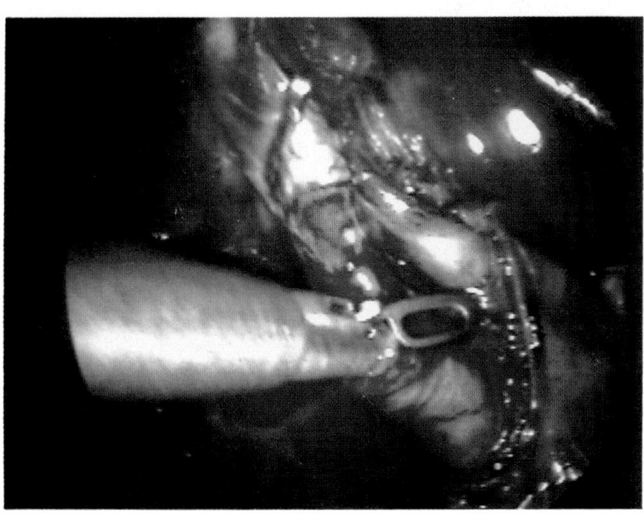

Fig. 6.6 Cholangiography catheter inside the cystic duct held a watertight grip by the closed jaws of the cholangiograsper.

inside the lumen. If this measure fails, a guidewire is first introduced into the cystic duct lumen and the catheter is railroaded over it. The guidewire is then removed and the catheter affixed by closing the jaws of the cholangiograsper.

Other techniques and catheters are available for cystic duct cholangiography. One popular alternative technique is the use of an Intracath type of guidewire sheathed cannula, which is introduced percutaneously under the right costal margin above and in line with the cystic duct. In practice, familiarization with one technique is important to ensure quick and successful cannulation in the majority of patients.

Once the duct is cannulated, the large metal trocar/cannula is removed over a radiolucent plastic rod, which is two and a half times the length of the cannula (Fig. 6.7). This rod is left in place until the IOC is completed, when the cannula is reinserted over it. If disposable radiolucent cannulae are used, this step is of course unnecessary. On completion of the IOC, the

(a)

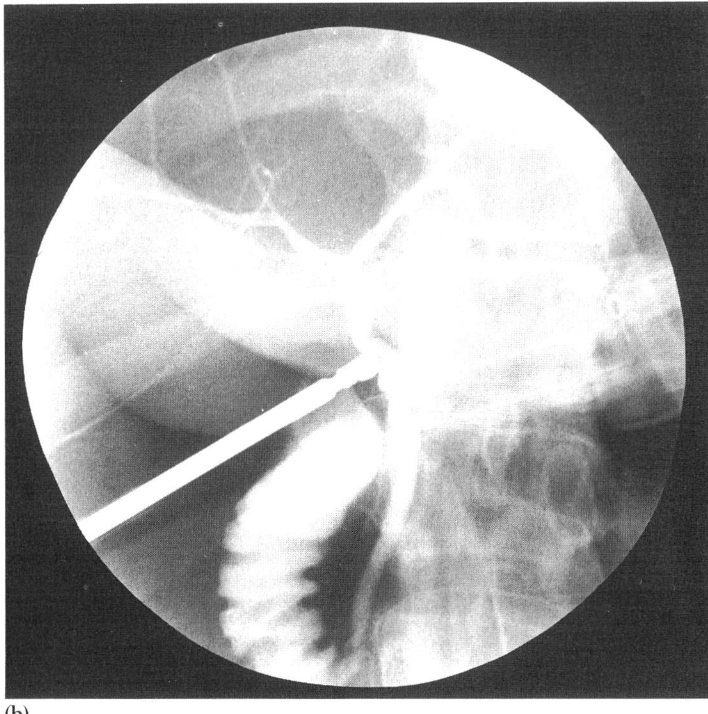

(b)

Fig. 6.7 (a) Transparent plastic rod inside 11.0 mm cannula. (b) Superimposed over the common bile duct during cholangiography.

cholangiograsper is opened and withdrawn, together with the ureteric catheter. Although most surgeons use metal clips to close the medial end of the cystic duct, this practice is unwise, as there have been sporadic reports of internalization of these clips leading to the formation of ductal calculi. In the authors' view, the best technique for securing the medial end of the cystic duct is by ligature using the external Roeder knot with dry catgut (Chapter 4). A

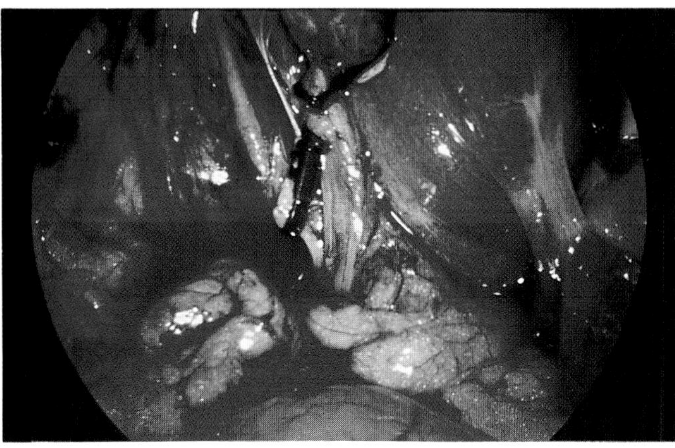

Fig. 6.8 Polydioxanone absorbable clip (Absolok, Ethicon) applied to the medial end of the cystic duct.

good alternative is clipping with absorbable polydioxanone clips (Absolok, Ethicon) (Fig. 6.8).

Cholecystocholangiography

Laparoscopic cholecystocholangiography has been established for several years [8–11] and is a well-validated technique. Apart from being easy to perform, laparoscopic cholecystocholangiography provides an entire picture of the biliary tract and does not commit the surgeon to any particular procedure. In this respect it carries an undoubted advantage over cystic duct cholangiography, which has to be followed by cholecystectomy. However, it has certain intrinsic disadvantages in relation to laparoscopic cholecystectomy, and for this reason it is not the method of choice for IOC during this procedure. The important limitations of cholecystocholangiography during laparoscopic cholecystectomy are:

1 The technique is not feasible in contracted fibrotic gallbladders.

2 It carries the risk of flushing small calculi into the common bile duct. As the amount of contrast which has to be injected is substantial, this is a real risk in patients with multiple small gallstones.

Within the context of laparoscopic biliary surgery, the indications for cholecystocholangiography are:

1 Selective use in patients undergoing laparoscopic cholecystectomy. There are three situations which may be encountered. The first concerns patients with biliary symptoms and equivocal findings on the routine work-up. The laparoscopic cholecystocholangiogram may detect small calculi/debris which would dictate the need for laparoscopic cholecystectomy. The second concerns the detection of intrinsic gallbladder disease, especially neoplasia, which would alter the surgical management and approach. The third is adherence of the gallbladder neck to the common duct, observed during the initial laparoscopic inspection. The cholecystocholangiogram is the best method available for excluding a fistulous communication between the gallbladder and the common hepatic duct (Mirizzi syndrome), the documentation of which necessitates conversion to open cholecystectomy.

2 As an alternative to percutaneous transhepatic cholangiography in the investigation of patients with large bile duct obstruction when the ERCP demonstrates complete occlusion of the common duct with no proximal filling.

3 In patients undergoing laparoscopic bilioenteric bypass for advanced inoperable cancer of the pancreas.

Although several disposable and non-disposable cannulae can be used, the best and safest technique is the use of a Veress needle connected by a three-way tap to the contrast and saline syringes. The main advantage of the Veress needle is the prevention of through-and-through perforation of the gallbladder as the needle is advanced through the lumen of the organ, because of the spring-loaded protective mechanism. Furthermore, the position of the needle can be ascertained readily by tenting the gallbladder wall with the round end of the needle without risk of damage (Fig. 6.9).

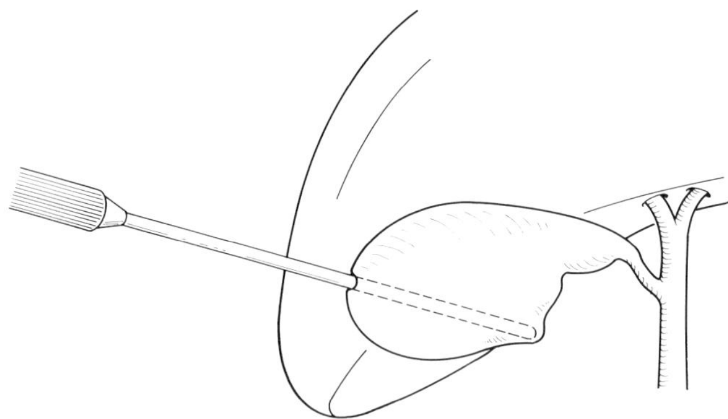

Fig. 6.9 The exact position of the Veress needle inside the gallbladder can be ascertained readily by tenting the gallbladder wall with the round end of the needle without risk of damage.

The gallbladder can be entered through the edge of the right lobe of the liver or directly by fundal puncture (Fig. 6.10). In the presence of an extrahepatic bile duct obstruction (jaundice), the former technique prevents bile leakage by tamponade of the liver substance on withdrawal of the needle. The direct puncture is, however, easier to perform and does not leak in the absence of ductal obstruction, provided the gallbladder is aspirated prior to withdrawal of the needle. The technique requires prior grasping of the fundus by a self-holding forceps. The Veress needle is inserted through the abdominal wall at a point in line with the long axis of the gallbladder. Under visual guidance, the fundus is pierced as counter-traction is maintained with the gallbladder-holding forceps. The luminal location of the needle is checked by aspiration, and if bile is obtained the needle is advanced further and tilted momentarily to check its final position within the gallbladder lumen. Ideally, the tip of the needle should be placed near the neck of the gallbladder. On average, some 40 ml of contrast medium are needed to fill the gallbladder before opacification of the cystic duct and the biliary tract is achieved (Fig. 6.11). Fluoroscopy is commenced at the start of

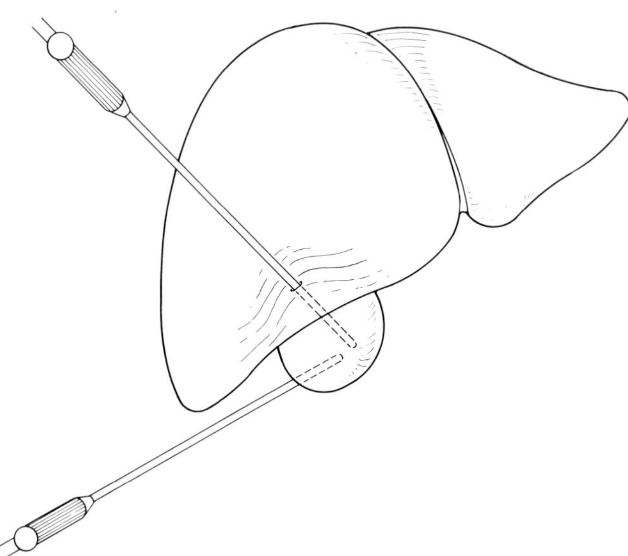

Fig. 6.10 Cholecystocholangiography—the gallbladder can be entered through the edge of the right lobe of the liver, or directly by fundal puncture.

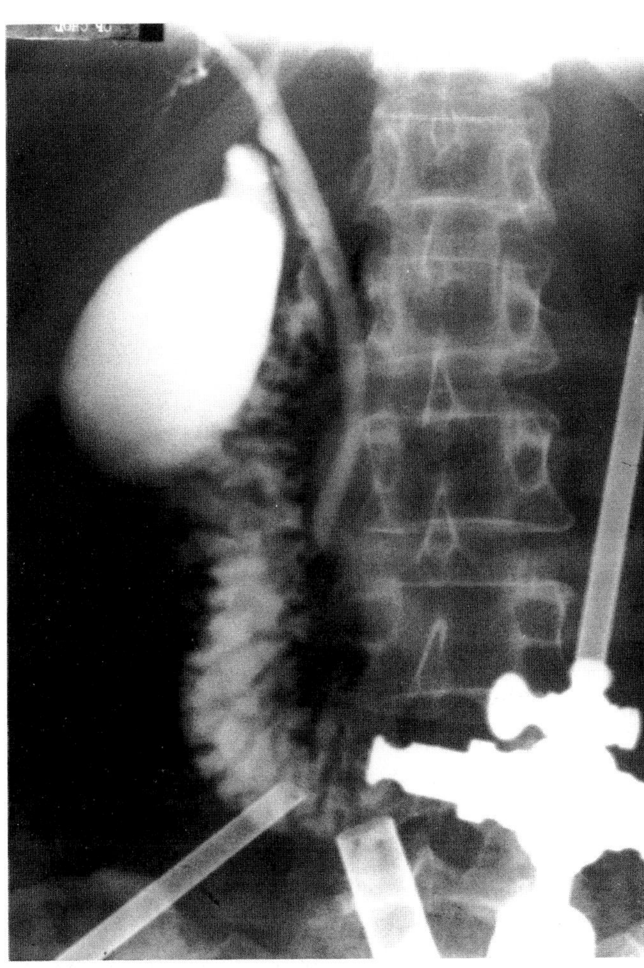

Fig. 6.11 Laparoscopic cholecystocholangiogram obtained by direct puncture of the gallbladder.

the injection. On completion, the gallbladder is aspirated and the needle is withdrawn. The elasticity of the gallbladder wall seals the hole so that leakage is not a problem. However, ligature of the site by an endoloop is required at some stage before the gallbladder is exteriorized through the parieties, as the pressure exerted by compression against the abdominal wall will result in bile leakage from the fundal perforation. *If the gallbladder is not removed after a direct-puncture cholecystocholangiogram, on no account must an endoloop be applied to the puncture site, as the author has encountered biliary peritonitis due to necrosis of the ligatured area.* If there is no obstruction and the site is dry, no further measures are required; otherwise the site of puncture is closed by a single interrupted suture.

Ductal anatomy

The cystic duct anatomy, particularly its drainage into the main ductal system, is best outlined during the early (injection) phase. Although many standard surgical textbooks describe an angled lateral entry of the cystic duct into the common duct, this configuration is only found in 17% of patients [1]. The various configurations of this part of the biliary tract anatomy are shown

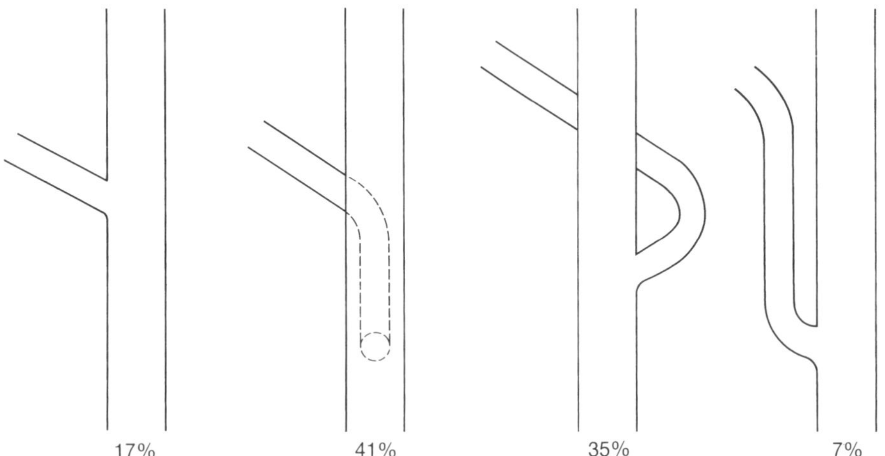

Fig. 6.12 Schematic representation of cystic duct drainage in the human. Lateral drainage occurs in only 17%. The most common configuration is posterior entry (41%).

schematically in Fig. 6.12. The commonest termination of the cystic duct (41%) is on the posterior wall of the common duct. A spiral course with entry of the cystic duct into the medial aspect of the common duct is found in 35% of cases (Fig. 6.13), and in 7% the cystic duct runs parallel to the common duct before joining it lower down (Fig. 6.14). An important anomaly— the short cystic duct—is encountered in 5–10% of patients. This may enter the common hepatic (Fig. 6.15) or the right hepatic duct (Fig. 6.16). It is vitally important that this abnormality be detected early, and certainly before the duct is clipped or ligatured medially. When the distance between the opening in the cystic duct and the common duct is very short (<2 mm), the safest technique is to divide the duct across the cystic duct hole and suture the medial end (Fig. 6.17). This is especially indicated when the short cystic duct enters the right hepatic duct. An alternative technique consists of double-

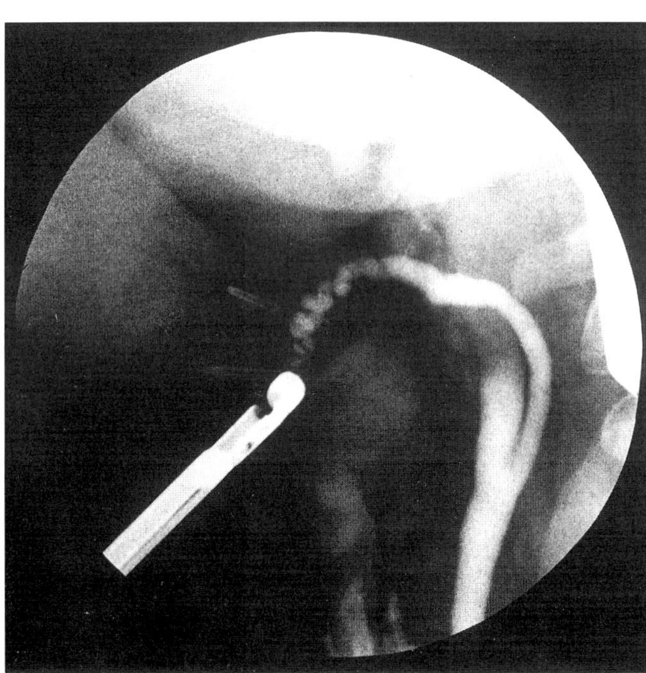

Fig. 6.13 Cystic duct with pronounced Heister valve and spiral drainage into the left side of the common bile duct.

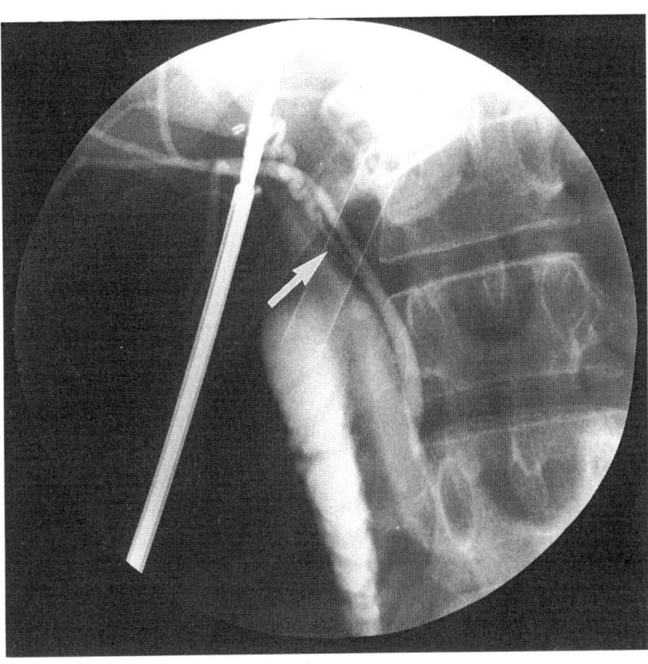

Fig. 6.14 Extreme close parallel run of the cystic duct to the common bile duct (arrow).

clipping the cystic duct at the incision site. Though less satisfactory, this method is used by some surgeons with apparent safety.

If the short cystic duct is overlooked—usually because a cholangiogram is not performed—the tented common hepatic duct may be misinterpreted as the medial continuation of the cystic duct, and thus clipped, transected and in some cases excised, with disastrous consequences. Another complication which may arise in this situation is the inclusion of a segment of the wall of the common hepatic or common bile duct in the clip. This will lead to a

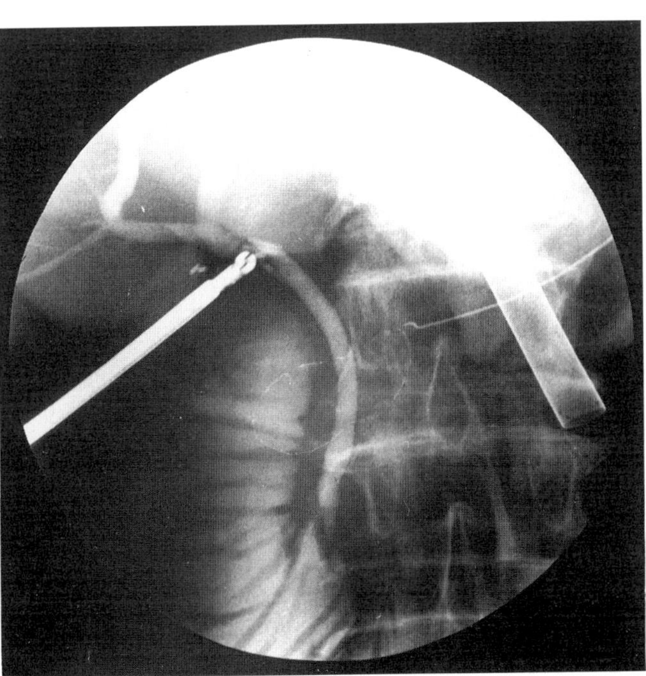

Fig. 6.15 Short cystic duct draining into the common hepatic duct.

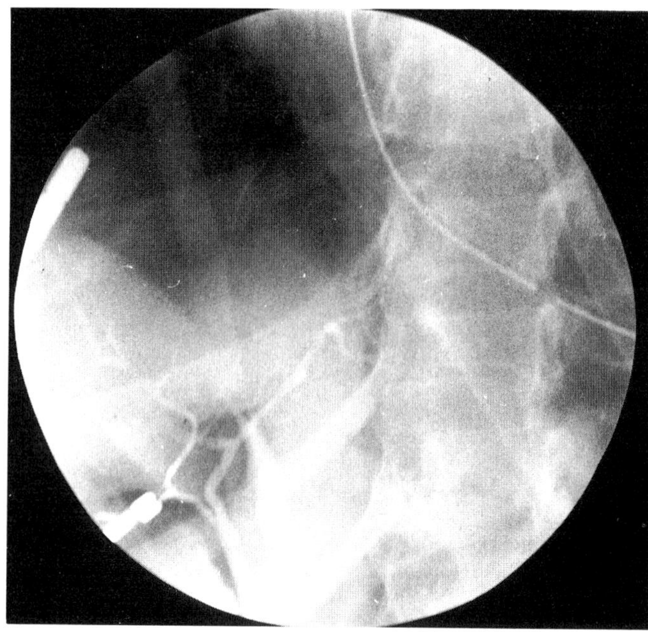

Fig. 6.16 Short cystic duct entering the right hepatic duct.

localized area of pressure necrosis over a few days, with the development of a postoperative biliary fistula and subsequent stricture formation.

Another problem may be encountered with cystic ducts which run parallel to the common duct and are so closely applied to this structure that they appear to share a common wall with it. Unless recognized, this abnormality can lead to ductal injury (see Fig. 6.14). Often the duct can be teased off the common bile duct for an adequate distance (5 mm) to enable safe ligature or clipping without lateral encroachment of the bile duct. Otherwise the cystic duct is either sutured, ligated or double-clipped at the incision site.

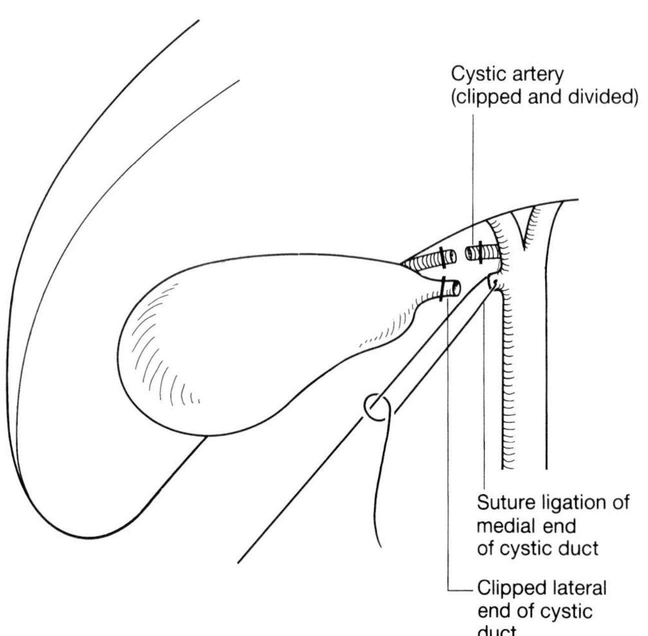

Fig. 6.17 When the distance between the opening in the cystic duct and the common duct is very short (<2 mm), the safest technique is to divide the duct across the cystic duct hole and suture the medial end. This is especially indicated when the short cystic duct enters the right hepatic duct.

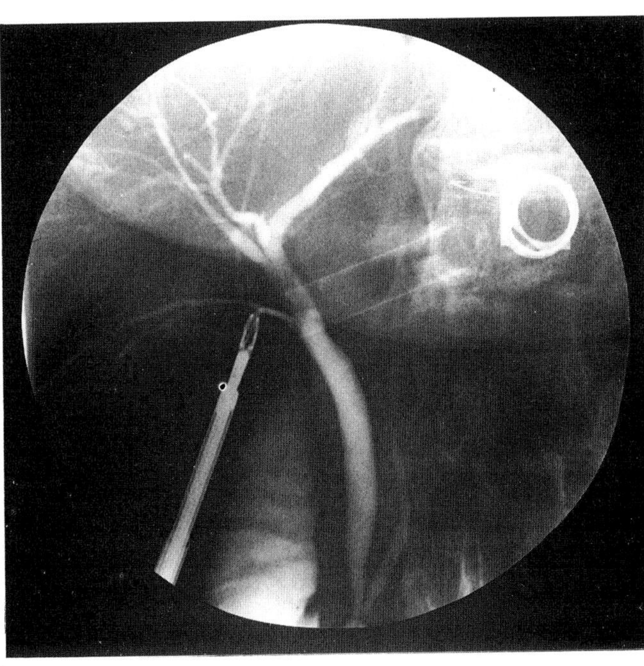

Fig. 6.18 Accessory duct draining into the cystic duct.

An infrequent anomaly consists of the presence of accessory ducts (Fig. 6.18); these occur in 2% of patients and unless recognized they will lead to postoperative bile leakage. Other problems may arise from the placement of clips on the cystic artery. The most common variation is a cystic artery which runs very close to the right hepatic duct (Fig. 6.19), when there is a risk of partial or total occlusion of the right hepatic duct. This eventuality can only be detected if the cholangiogram is performed after the cystic artery has

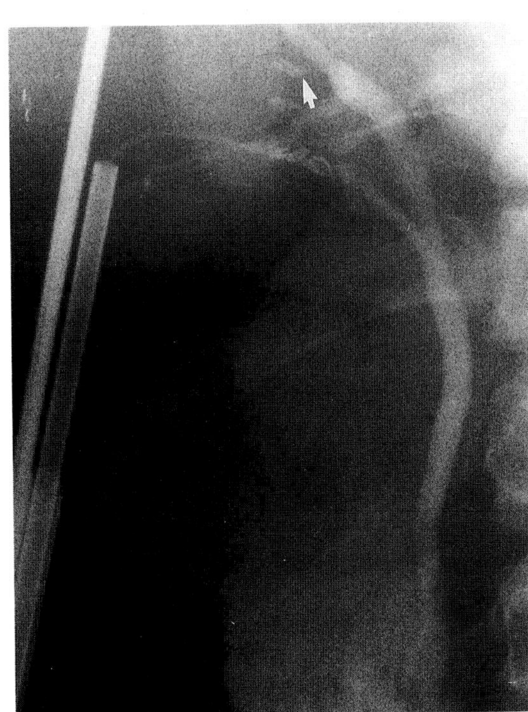

Fig. 6.19 Other problems may arise from the placement of clips on the cystic artery. The most common variation is a cystic artery which runs very close to the right hepatic duct, when there is a risk of partial or total occlusion of the right hepatic duct. This eventuality can only be detected if the cholangiogram is performed after the cystic artery has been secured. It is prevented by ensuring that the cystic artery is dissected well clear of any ductal elements before it is clipped and divided.

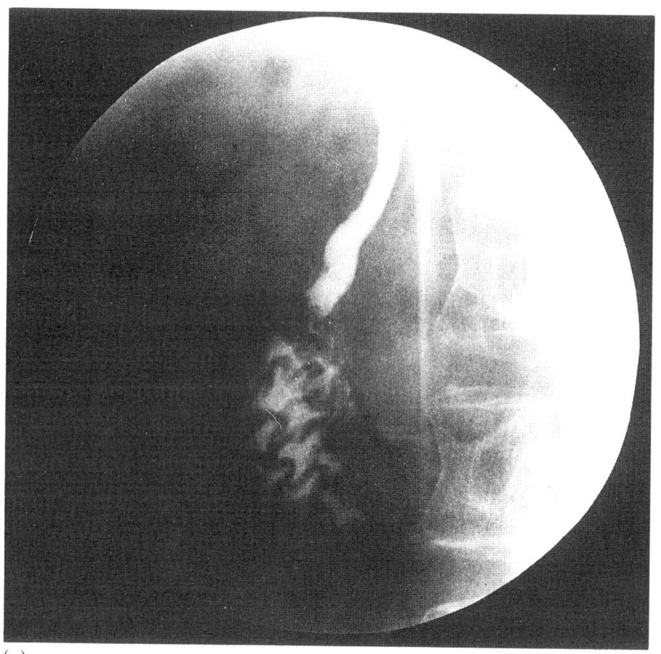
(a)

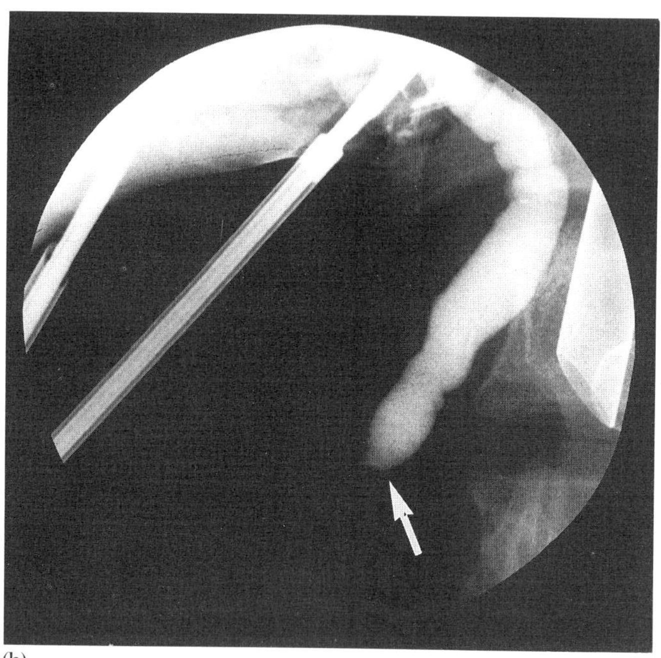
(b)

Fig. 6.20 (a & b) Unsuspected stone in the distal common bile duct. Both patients had normal liver function tests and normal common bile duct appearance on ultrasound.

been secured. It is prevented by ensuring that the cystic artery is dissected well clear of any ductal elements before it is clipped and divided.

Unsuspected stones

These are encountered in 5–7% of patients [12] in whom the preoperative work-up is normal (Fig. 6.20). IOC is the most accurate technique for detecting these unsuspected stones, although early results with laparoscopic biliary ultrasonography are promising though not conclusive as yet. If stones are discovered during laparoscopic cholecystectomy, ductal clearance should be performed either through the cystic duct or by supraduodenal bile duct exploration (Chapter 9). This surgical treatment strategy avoids the uncertainties and disadvantages of postoperative ERCP and endoscopic sphincterotomy. The suggestion made recently that these calculi can be left [13] is unacceptable because of the known pathological potential of ductal calculi in terms of jaundice and cholangitis. Indeed, over 90% of patients requiring endoscopic sphincterotomy and stone extraction have had previous cholecystectomy.

Ductal injuries

In a seminal report by Moossa *et al.* [14] of 81 patients undergoing remedial surgery for iatrogenic bile duct injuries, only four cases were discovered at the time of the cholecystectomy, and all four had had an intraoperative cholangiogram. This is another reason for IOC during cholecystectomy, as it identifies ductal injuries and therefore enables primary correction or repair.

At Ninewells, 520 consecutive laparoscopic cholecystectomies have now been performed without ductal injuries. In this series the following were identified by IOC and appropriate action taken to avoid ductal injury: 11 patients with short cystic duct entering the right hepatic duct; 29 with short cystic duct entering the common hepatic duct; and 15 common bile ducts juxtaposed to a parallel-running cystic duct. At the Cedars–Sinai Medical Center, over 1400 laparoscopic cholecystectomies have been performed by 11 surgeons. One duct was transected, but this injury was discovered by IOC and the duct repaired after conversion to open surgery. Two cystic ducts were torn due to excessive traction. In both instances the cystic duct stump was repaired. In three additional cases the common bile duct was cannulated. Again this was discovered by IOC and the small lateral hole sutured.

There is one important rule which must not be forgotten. This concerns the importance of opacification of the entire biliary tract during IOC. If during laparoscopic cholecystectomy proximal filling is not achieved in a non-jaundiced patient, the cholangiogram should be repeated with a steeper Trendelenburg tilt. *Should the repeat cholangiogram after this measure fail to outline the proximal biliary tract, the case should be converted to open surgery, since the risk of duct transection or obstruction by a misplaced clip having been inadvertently enacted is unacceptably high.*

References

1 Berci G, Hamlin JA. *Operative Biliary Radiology.* Williams and Wilkins, Baltimore 1981.
2 Cuschieri A, Berci G. *Common Bile Duct Exploration.* Martinus Nijhoff, Boston 1984.
3 Hunter J. Avoidance of bile duct injury during laparoscopic cholecystectomy. *Am J Surg* 1991; **162**: 71–76.
4 Berci G, Sackier JM, Paz-Partlow M. Routine or selected intraoperative cholangiography during laparoscopic cholecystectomy? *Am J Surg* 1991; **161**: 355–360.
5 Phillips EH, Berci G, Carroll B *et al.* The importance of intraoperative cholangiography during laparoscopic cholecystectomy. *Am Surg* 1990; **56**: 792–795.
6 Greeg RD. The case for selective cholangiography. *Am J Surg* 1988; **155**: 540–544.
7 Pasquale MD, Nauta RJ. Selective versus routine use of intraoperative cholangiography. *Arch Surg* 1989; **124**: 1041–1042.
8 Berci G, Morgenstern L, Shore JM, Shapiro S. A direct approach to the differential diagnosis of jaundice. Laparoscopy with transhepatic cholecystocholangiography. *Am J Surg* 1973; **126**: 372–378.
9 Cuschieri A. Value of laparoscopy in hepatobiliary disease. *Ann Roy Coll Surg Engl* 1975; **57**: 33–38.
10 Irving AD, Cuschieri A. Laparoscopic assessment of the jaundiced patient. *Br J Surg* 1978; **65**: 678–680.
11 Berci G, Cuschieri A. *Practical Laparoscopy.* Baillière Tindall, London 1986.
12 DenBesten L, Berci G. The current status of biliary tract surgery: an international study of 1072 consecutive patients. *World J Surg* 1986; **10**: 116–122. IBA study.
13 McEntee G, Grace PA, Bouchier-Hays D. Laparoscopic cholecystectomy and the common bile duct. *Br J Surg* 1991; **78**: 385–386.
14 Moossa AR, Mayer AD, Stabile B. Iatrogenic injury to the bile duct. *Arch Surg* 1990; **125**: 1028–1030.

7 : Clinical aspects of laparoscopic cholecystectomy

Overall results

There are now several large reported series of laparoscopic cholecystectomy for symptomatic gallstone disease [1–6] and recently the Society of American Gastrointestinal Endoscopic Surgeons (SAGES) has completed its prospective survey on 1771 cases [7]. The message from all these reports has been consistent: when performed by the fully trained, laparoscopic cholecystectomy is a safe procedure with low morbidity and negligible mortality. It has unequivocal benefits over conventional open cholecystectomy: diminished postoperative pain, discomfort and ileus; significant reduction in the postoperative hospital stay; accelerated recovery with return to full activity or work within 7–10 days of discharge; and virtual absence of wound-related complications, early or late. Within the remarkably short period of 3 years, laparoscopic cholecystectomy has become the 'gold standard' in the treatment of symptomatic gallstone disease. No other surgical advance in the history of the profession has ever achieved this stage of universal acceptance and usage within such a short interval from its introduction into surgical practice.

There are other perceived, though yet unproven, advantages following the use of laparoscopic rather than open cholecystectomy. Some of these merit close attention. The early ambulation is likely to be accompanied by a lowered incidence of complications related to recumbency and diminished physical activity, such as deep vein thrombosis, pulmonary embolism, postoperative pulmonary collapse and chest infections. The markedly diminished contact of blood between patient and operating staff is likely to diminish the risk of transmission of viral disease such as hepatitis B and HIV. Finally, those who have practised laparoscopic surgery for several years and have had a number of patients who needed subsequent surgical interventions have been impressed by the virtual absence of intraperitoneal adhesions following laparoscopic surgery. Though likely on the basis of the clinical observations to date, all these perceived benefits require confirmation by prospective studies.

Applicability of laparoscopic cholecystectomy

All the large reported series have outlined a similar applicability rate, which averages 95% in experienced hands. This oft-quoted figure must be interpreted carefully, and refers to the group of patients who have been assigned preoperatively to laparoscopic cholecystectomy. Although there are no exact figures it is likely that this group represents some 80% of the total population of patients with symptomatic gallstone disease.

Preoperative work-up and patient management

In both the European and SAGES studies [1,7] differences were observed.

Table 7.1 Preoperative work-up and management

Liver function tests
Gallbladder/liver/bile duct ultrasound examination
Group and save
Single-shot antibiotic prophylaxis (with induction)
Heparin prophylaxis against DVT in the high-risk groups

The generally adopted preoperative schedule is outlined in Table 7.1. Some surgeons, predominantly the French, use preoperative intravenous tomographic cholangiography routinely, and on the basis of their experience, maintain that this radiological investigation provides sufficient anatomical information on the extrahepatic biliary tract as to dispense with the need for the routine use of intraoperative cholangiography. However, a recent report from France [8] expressed considerable doubt on the value of preoperative intravenous cholangiography and, in particular, demonstrated its unreliability in the detection of ductal calculi. The contrast agent used was iotroxate megulamine and this caused a serious hypersensitivity reaction. Preoperative ERCP is only indicated in those patients (3–5%) who exhibit abnormal liver function tests or demonstrate suspicious ductal features on the ultrasound examination.

In patients with previous surgery, ultrasound scanning of the abdomen using the technique of visceral slide accurately localizes the site of the adhesions, and more importantly, indicates a safe site for the insertion of the Veress needle. This examination can be carried out by the radiologist at the same time as the gallbladder/ductal ultrasound scanning.

Nearly all surgeons use single-dose antibiotic prophylaxis at the time of induction of anaesthesia. There has been no survey on the practice regarding chemical prophylaxis against deep vein thrombosis. The authors use subcutaneous heparin in patients at risk of this complication. Cross-matching of blood is unnecessary as the need for perioperative transfusion is rare—blood-grouping with specimen saving is sufficient.

Operative practice

Apart from the positioning of the patient, there are differences in operative management and practice. Nasogastric intubation is used routinely by some and selectively by others. Those, like the authors, who advocate nasogastric suction consider it a useful adjunct to enhance the exposure of the operative field, and remove it after recovery from anaesthesia. Not all catheterize the urinary bladder before creating the pneumoperitoneum. If this step is omitted, it is essential for the surgeon to percuss the suprapubic region for dullness before inserting the Veress needle, as when the bladder is full, injuries are a well-known complication [9].

Only a small percentage use an adjustable camera-holder, the majority relying on the service of a surgeon assistant or scrub nurse for this purpose. It is true that a trained camera operator is invaluable, particularly in difficult cases, but for the average situation a good camera-holder which the surgeon can adjust quickly offers advantages in terms of increased elbow room around the immediate vicinity of the operating table. The main benefit of the routine use of a camera operator relates to training in laparoscopic surgery. High-frequency electrosurgery is used by the majority of American and European surgeons (80–90%) in preference to laser [1,7,10,11]. The reasons are several: familiarity with this equipment, less crowding of the operating theatre and substantially lower costs. The original laser hype for laparoscopic cholecystectomy, with good reason, has not been vindicated by subsequent well-audited experience. There is a danger that the outcome of this controversy will be misinterpreted as indicating that there is no place for lasers in laparoscopic surgery; this would be unfortunate, as certain laparoscopic procedures are considerably facilitated by the use of laser light energy, but these do not include cholecystectomy. The current intensive research on the production of the next generation of laser devices—hand-held tuneable lasers based on diode arrays and non-linear crystals—will solve all the existing problems and lead to their useful application in various laparoscopic operations.

Contraindications

Initially several contraindications to laparoscopic cholecystectomy were listed, but as experience has increased many of these have been dropped. There are, however, considerable reported differences in the criteria for eligibility between the various centres. To some extent these reflect different interpretations of pathological nomenclature. On a more practical level, contraindications are relative to the experience of the surgeon. The beginner would do well to heed the advice that he should gain initial experience with 20–30 easy cases with functioning gallbladders, before tackling more demanding pathology. Because of the apparent controversy, it is best to consider each situation separately in an attempt to establish the prevalent view based on the surgical literature.

Acute cholecystitis

As outlined in Chapter 5, acute cholecystitis is a clinical diagnosis which covers a spectrum of pathology when the area is inspected laparoscopically. In the majority, some 70% of patients with this diagnosis, laparoscopic cholecystectomy can be performed with safety. Severe disease characterized by gangrenous patches or established empyema carries a significant risk of rupture, with peritoneal contamination, and for this reason must still be regarded as a contraindication. In the author's view, acute cholecystitis in the elderly, the immunocompromised and in patients with significant cardiorespiratory disease, is best managed in the first instance by percutaneous or laparoscopic drainage (Chapter 8).

Acute gallstone-associated pancreatitis

Several clinical studies have shown that early cholecystectomy (performed during the same hospital admission) carries no added risk in patients with mild to moderate acute pancreatitis [12], and this policy applies equally to laparoscopic cholecystectomy. However, patients with severe acute necrotizing disease should not be treated by early cholecystectomy, as this management policy is accompanied by an increased mortality; these patients are best managed with delayed-interval cholecystectomy. The feasibility of laparoscopic cholecystectomy at this stage depends on the state of the supracolic compartment following resolution of the pancreatic disease. In those patients who survive after a prolonged period of recurrent intra-abdominal sepsis requiring repeated open drainage, attempts at laparoscopic cholecystectomy are ill-advised.

Obstructive jaundice

There are well-established ground rules concerning the management of jaundiced patients and these have not changed with the advent of laparoscopic cholecystectomy. In the first instance, the exact cause must be established and this usually entails an ERCP. If ductal calculi are found to be the cause of the jaundice, then the management depends on the condition of the patient. There is no doubt that in the poor-risk patient and those with overt cholangitis, the appropriate treatment is endoscopic sphincterotomy and stone extraction. Laparoscopic cholecystectomy is performed after resolution of the acute episode. The authors and others have observed that, following endoscopic sphincterotomy, gross oedema of the hepatoportal ligament develops after 24 hours, and may last several days. It is therefore wise either to perform the operation next day or delay it for 2 weeks after the endoscopic sphincterotomy and ductal clearance.

In patients who are fit and show no evidence of cholangitis, there are two options: preoperative endoscopic sphincterotomy and stone extraction followed by laparoscopic cholecystectomy, or laparoscopic cholecystectomy with laparoscopic stone extraction. To a large extent, the treatment adopted depends on local expertise and experience at laparoscopic stone extraction. These two options are covered in Chapter 9.

Cirrhosis

Cholecystectomy can be a formidable operation in the presence of cirrhosis and is accompanied by an increased mortality [13]. Although some of the large reported series have contained a few patients with cirrhosis (1–2%), this condition, if accompanied by portal hypertension and advanced disease (Child's B or C) must be regarded as a contraindication to laparoscopic cholecystectomy. The risk of uncontrollable haemorrhage in the presence of varices is substantial, and there has been one reported death consequent on this eventuality from one German centre [14].

Biliary fistulae

Provided the surgeon is experienced and familiar with laparoscopic suturing technique, a cholecystoduodenal fistula is not a contraindication to laparoscopic cholecystectomy. Although difficult and requiring careful dissection, these cases can be undertaken with safety. At operation, the disconnection of the fistula and closure of the duodenal perforation is performed before the cholecystectomy (Chapter 11). By contrast, the presence of a fistulous communication between the neck of the gallbladder and the common hepatic duct (Mirizzi's syndrome) is an absolute contraindication to laparoscopic cholecystectomy, as is a gallbladder which is densely adherent to the common duct. The guiding common-sense principle underlying safe laparoscopic cholecystectomy is that the structures in the triangle of Calot must be capable of being displayed and dissected with safety from the common duct and the hepatic artery. If not, the best interest of both the patient and the surgeon is met by elective conversion to open surgery.

Pregnancy

Laparoscopic cholecystectomy has been performed in pregnant females without any apparent problems to the mother and child. In the SAGES survey [7], it accounted for 0.2% of the total cohort. There is no information available on the effect of a sustained high-pressure CO_2 pneumoperitoneum on the developing fetus. The mental ability and IQ of children born of mothers who have undergone laparoscopic cholecystectomy during pregnancy will have to be appraised before any definite conclusion as to the safety of the procedure in pregnancy can be reached. Until then, it would seem prudent to delay the operation until after delivery whenever possible. In those patients who require intervention because of severe disease or acute complications, consideration should be given using a low-pressure pneumoperitoneum and the abdominal wall lift (Chapter 3).

Obesity

This is no longer regarded as a contraindication to laparoscopic cholecystectomy, even when extreme. Extra-long instruments may be needed in the morbidly obese. Many of these patients turn out to be surprisingly easy compared to the open operation, as the deep parieties are 'left behind' by the optic.

Complications

The overall results in terms of mortality and morbidity have compared very favourably with those following open cholecystectomy [1,5,7,15]. Significant reduction of postoperative ailments and discomfort has been observed. Postoperative ileus has been encountered in about 1–10% of patients. Undoubtedly the postoperative disturbance of pulmonary function is less when compared to open surgery [16]. None the less, complications have occurred and many tragedies, including preventable ones, have undoubtedly not been reported. The fact remains, however, that in experienced hands the laparoscopic procedure is as safe if not safer than open cholecystectomy.

Bleeding

Intraoperative haemorrhage occurs either during the dissection of the cystic pedicle or when the gallbladder is detached from the liver. The risk factors include difficult dissections, acute cholecystitis and parenchymatous gallbladder. Bleeding used to be the commonest cause for enforced conversion to open surgery [1]. There is no doubt that haemorrhage is grossly magnified by the optic, and what appears as a torrential gush may turn out to be a minor spurting arteriole when the case is explored. None the less, if control is not achieved rapidly with the measures described in Chapter 4, conversion is sensible and prudent.

The biggest problem is a cut cystc artery which retracts inside the tissue of the cystic pedicle and porta hepatis. Although compression is safe in this situation, blind clamping must be avoided at all costs. Bleeding from the hepatic parenchyma is largely avoidable by keeping the plane of dissection of the gallbladder above the fascial plate covering the hepatic parenchyma. When encountered, the most efficient control is achieved by argon spray coagulation. Otherwise, standard high-frequency electrocoagulation with the Berci spatula is used.

Bleeding may occur postoperatively, when it is most commonly due to liver lacerations or instrumental stab injuries to the hepatic parenchyma. Less frequently, slippage of the cystic artery clip is the cause. Haemorrhage is one of the reported complications necessitating laparotomy in the postoperative period.

To date, major arterial trocar or Veress needle injuries (aortoiliac), which are well-documented albeit rare complications of laparoscopy [17], have been rare during laparoscopic cholecystectomy. The probable reason for this is the increased awareness of this lethal complication, which has resulted in extreme care with the creation of the pneumoperitoneum and ready recourse to open laparoscopy in the event of difficulties [18].

Bile leakage

Postoperative bile leakage is reported in 1–2% [1–7]. In the prospective SAGES study, it occurred in 14/1771 patients (0.8%). This is contrary to the author's experience at Ninewells, where this complication was encountered only once in 500 consecutive patients. The main difference between the Ninewells technique and other centres is that here the medial end of the cystic duct is routinely ligated in continuity, with dry chromic catgut using the Roeder slip knot [19,20], whereas most centres clip the duct. The most common cause of postoperative bile leakage has been slippage of the cystic duct clips. It is the authors' view that this complication can be largely avoided by ligation of the medial end of the cystic duct. If the surgeon is not familiar with tying the cystic duct in continuity, the application of the preformed endoloop after the cystic duct has been divided is recommended. If a clip has been applied, the endoloop must be placed medial to it, provided this does not encroach on the common duct. There is another potential danger to the application of clips on the medial end of the cystic duct. This relates to evidence in the literature that clips may in time become internalized and then act as a nidus for stone formation [21,22].

A less frequent cause of postoperative bile leakage is damage to the hepatic parenchyma during separation of the gallbladder from the liver bed. This can be prevented by keeping the dissection above the fascial layer between the hepatic parenchyma and the gallbladder (Chapter 4).

Bile leakage after laparoscopic cholecystectomy requires investigation in all patients. Although some information regarding the site of extravasation can be obtained by biliary scintiscanning, more precise definition is required and this can only be achieved by ERCP. This will establish ductal integrity and outline the extravasation site, which is usually the cystic duct and less commonly the gallbladder bed. In the absence of bile duct injury, several options are available: endoscopic insertion of a stent, laparoscopic suture ligation of the cystic duct, or simple insertion of a drain if the leakage is from the liver bed.

Bile duct injury

It is not possible to arrive at a reliable figure for this iatrogenic complication: the reported incidence varies from 0.2 to 1.0%. In the European survey of seven centres there were four ductal injuries out of 1236 operations (0.3%). Two of these were discovered at operation and the other two postoperatively. In the prospective SAGES study, four ductal injuries were encountered in 1771 cases (0.2%). Only one patient in this study was discovered during the operation. Intraoperative cholangiography (IOC) was not performed in any of these eight instances of iatrogenic ductal damage, according to these two reports. Apart from their possible prevention, the five patients who were missed would certainly have been identified by IOC during the laparoscopic procedure if this intraoperative investigation had been performed. There is little doubt that good IOC is an important factor in the prevention of bile duct damage during laparoscopic cholecystectomy (Chapter 6). Laser dissection of the cystic pedicle and gallbladder, because of the past-pointing phenomenon and deflections of the laser beam, may be a particularly conducive to bile duct damage as is excessive use of electrosurgery in this region [23,24].

The above incidence of bile duct damage during laparoscopic cholecystectomy is likely to be an underestimate, as only 70% of ductal injuries are diagnosed within the first 6 months and some may not manifest until several years after the operation [25]. The follow-up to date does not allow a firm estimate of the incidence of bile duct strictures after this surgical intervention. The risk appears highest during the first 12 cases [5]. A recent report suggested that the risk factors for bile duct damage are: inexperience, bleeding, failure to expose the anatomy or to perform operative cholangiography and excessive use of thermal energy (laser or electrosurgery) in the region of the porta hepatis [26].

Bile duct injuries discovered during laparoscopic cholecystectomy must be repaired immediately. The exact procedure depends on the nature and severity of the injury: major lesions require conversion and expert biliary reconstruction, injuries discovered postoperatively require urgent investigation with ERCP and referral to a specialist centre.

Gallbladder perforation and stone loss

Perforation of the gallbladder during laparoscopic cholecystectomy is common, and in the reported literature varies from 9 to 20%. It usually occurs during separation of the gallbladder from the liver. Provided the escaping bile has been aspirated and adequate lavage of the peritoneal gutters performed at the end of the operation, perforation of the non-inflamed gallbladder has not resulted in any adverse consequences in the immediate outcome in any of the large reported series. Rupture of the gallbladder in patients with severe acute cholecystitis is a separate issue. In the first instance it is caused by the forceps used to hold and lift the fundus of the gallbladder, and therefore occurs early during the operation. If contamination of the peritoneal cavity and contents is substantial, the risk of both early and delayed intraperitoneal sepsis cannot be ignored.

Another consequence of gallbladder perforation is the escape of gallstones, which can easily be lost amongst the loops of the small intestine. There are no published figures to document the incidence of this eventuality. Its exact pathogenic potential is unknown but studies have confirmed that some at least of these stones harbour bacteria [27], and abscesses may form around residual intraperitoneal stones. The author has been involved as an expert witness in one such instance, which led to medicolegal litigation. In practice, all extravasated calculi should be retrieved whenever possible. When this is unsuccessful, the patient should be put on a full course of antibiotics and informed of the situation. Currently, the view generally held is that stone loss is not a reason for conversion to open surgery.

Perforation of the gallbladder should be dealt with immediately it is identified, as in addition to the risk of stone escape, delay in closure is likely to result in extension of the tear because of the constant traction on the gallbladder. The best and quickest way to deal with a small perforation is ligation with a preformed endoloop. However, a large rent is difficult to close without suturing. Thus in this eventuality, the best approach is to introduce a laprobag and transfer all the gallstones into it; the bag is then closed and retrieved. Although the dissection of the collapsed gallbladder from the liver bed is more difficult, it should not pose any major problems.

Intestinal trauma

Intestinal injury (duodenum, colon and small bowel) has been reported in 0.2–0.3% of cases. The majority have been caused by trocar injuries but others have been due to electrosurgery and direct mechanical damage by instruments. The majority (70–75%) have been recognized at operation, but the rest have been missed, with the development of peritonitis within days of the procedure. All the reported deaths from this cause (including two out of the three deaths in the prospective SAGES study) have occurred in this subgroup. This information stresses the importance of the final inspection of the entire peritoneal cavity after completion of the cholecystectomy, and before desufflation of the pneumoperitoneum.

If the injury is recognized at operation, laparoscopic suturing of the tear is safe but should only be attempted by those who are experienced at endoscopic suturing. Otherwise the safest course is conversion to open surgery. All these patients must be put on a full course of antibiotics and should be kept in hospital for at least 5 days after the operation.

Minor infections

Common postoperative infections, such as chest infections, including pneumonia, and urinary tract infections are rare (below 1.0%) although short-lived postoperative pyrexia is not infrequent (2–3%). Wound infection has been reported in 0.5–1.0%, usually at the site of extraction of the gallbladder. The majority of these have become clinically apparent after discharge from hospital. It thus seems likely that many are missed and the published figures probably underestimate the true incidence of this complication. Data are not available for the incidence of late hernia formation following laparoscopic cholecystectomy, largely because the follow-up to date has not been long enough.

Late intra-abdominal abscess formation has been reported occasionally from a number of centres. Most have been instances of subhepatic abscess formation. The aetiology of this rare complication is likely to be multifactorial.

Cardiovascular

The majority of deaths following laparoscopic cholecystectomy (0.1%) have been caused by myocardial infarctions, or cerebrovascular accidents in patients above the age of 65 years. There have been very few reports of deaths from pulmonary embolism, and the incidence of deep vein thrombosis has not been evaluated by objective testing. This is important, as the majority of calf vein thromboses are silent, and because these patients are discharged home early, it is extremely likely that this complication still occurs but is being missed. Although the early ambulation and accelerated recovery to full activity may be a factor in the reduction of deep venous thrombosis after laparoscopic cholecystectomy, the longer operating time may be resulting in enhanced compression trauma to the vascular endothelium. This is especially likely when the lithotomy position is used.

Unresolved problems

There are a number of unresolved problems. The two that are generally recognized are the need or otherwise for routine intraoperative cholangiography (Chapter 6) and the management of ductal calculi (Chapter 9). Others, such as gallbladder extraction, still require further development. There is one aspect of management which still has to be addressed: the management of asymptomatic gallstones. Standard surgical teaching based on the results of published studies still applies, that is, that cholecystectomy is not indicated, as the overall morbidity and mortality consequent on this approach would negate any possible benefits [28]. However, it must be recognized that the situation has changed in a number of ways. Thus, for example, treatment with long-acting somatostatin in patients with acromegaly invariably results in gallstone formation, and as this therapy has to be continued indefinitely, all endocrinologists recommend and refer these patients for laparoscopic cholecystectomy; there have been four such instances in the Ninewells series.

A further scenario can be proposed. On the confirmed observation that laparoscopic cholecystectomy causes minimal inconvenience and may indeed be accompanied by a lower operative mortality, should this operation be offered to fit individuals who harbour silent gallstones? This is an important question which carries very substantial cost implications for the Health Service, as the vast majority of gallstones are asymptomatic. The proposal for laparoscopic cholecystectomy in the asymptomatic fit population has to be reconciled with the epidemiological findings that the vast majority of these silent stones do not give rise to symptoms during life [29,30]. None the less, organizations such as the European Society of Endoscopic Surgeons (ESES) and SAGES ought to consider mounting a prospective clinical trial, randomizing patients to laparoscopic cholecystectomy or no treatment. The outcome of this study will require a very long period of follow-up before definite conclusions can be reached. This in itself may limit the practical feasibility of such a study. It should be stressed, however, that laparoscopic cholecystectomy for asymptomatic gallstones is not justified outside such clinical trials.

References

1 Cuschieri A, Dubois F, Mouiel J *et al.* The European experience with laparoscopic cholecystectomy. *Am J Surg* 1991; **161**: 385–387.

2 Dubois F, Berthelot G, Levard H. Cholecystectomy with celioscopy, 330 cases. *Chirurgie* 1990; **116**: 248–250.

3 Perissat J, Collet D, Belliard R. Gallstones: laparoscopic treatment, cholecystectomy and lithotripsy. Our own technique. *Surg Endosc* 1990; **4**: 1–5.

4 Reddick EJ, Olsen D, Alexander W *et al.* Laparoscopic laser cholecystectomy and choledocholithiasis. *Surg Endosc* 1990; **4**: 133–134.

5 The Southern Surgeons Club. A prospective analysis of 1518 laparoscopic cholecystectomies. *New Engl J Med* 1991; **324**: 1073–1078.

6 Spaw AT, Reddick EJ, Olsen DO. Laparoscopic laser cholecystectomy: analysis of 500 procedures. *Surg Laparosc Endosc* 1991; **1**: 2–7.

7 Prospective multi-institutional laparoscopic cholecystectomy study organized by the Society of American Gastrointestinal Endoscopic Surgeons (SAGES). *Surg Endosc* (in press).

8 de Watteville JC, Gailleton R, Gayal F, Testas P. Is routine intravenous cholangiography before laparoscopic cholecystectomy useful? Eurosurgery Congress, June 1992, Brussels.

9 Chamberlain B, Brown JC. *Gynaecological laparoscopy.* The report of a working party on a confidential enquiry of gynaecological laparoscopy 1987. Royal College of Obstetricians and Gynaecologists: London.

10 Hunter JG. Laser or electrocautery for laparoscopic cholecystectomy? *Am J Surg* 1991; **161**: 345–349.

11 Voyles CR, Peto AB, Meena AL *et al.* A practical approach to laparoscopic cholecystectomy. *Am J Surg* 1991; **161**: 365–370.

12 Osborne DH, Imrie CW, Carter DC. Biliary surgery in the same admission for gallstone-associated acute pancreatitis. *Br J Surg* 1981; **68**: 758–761.

13 Aranha GV, Sontag SJ, Greenlee HB. Cholecystectomy in cirrhotic patients: a formidable operation. *Am J Surg* 1982; **143**: 55–60.

14 Neugebauer E, Troidl H, Spangenberger W *et al.* Conventional versus laparoscopic cholecystectomy and the randomized controlled trial. Cholecystectomy study group. *Br J Surg* 1991; **78**: 150–154.

15 Ponsky JL. Complications of laparoscopic cholecystectomy. *Am J Surg* 1991; **161**: 393–395.

16 Frazee RC, Roberts JW, Okeson GC *et al.* Open versus laparoscopic cholecystectomy. A comparison of postoperative pulmonary function. *Ann Surg* 1991; **213**: 651–653.

17 Baadsgaard SE, Bille S, Egeblad K. Major vascular injury during gynaecological laparoscopy. *Acta Obstet Gynecol Scand* 1989; **68**: 283–285.

18 Fitzgibbons RJ, Salerno GM, Filipi CJ. Open laparoscopy. In: Zucker KA (ed), *Surgical Laparoscopy.* Quality Medical Publishing Inc; St Louis 1991; pp. 87–97.

19 Nathanson LK, Easter DW, Cuschieri A. Ligation of the structures of the cystic pedicle during laparoscopic cholecystectomy. *Am J Surg* 1991; **161**: 350–354.

20 Nathanson, LK, Shimi S, Cuschieri A. Laparoscopic cholecystectomy: the Dundee technique. *Br J Surg* 1991; **78**: 155–159.

21 Newman CE, Hamer JD. Non-absorbable cystic duct ligatures and common bile duct calculi. *Br Med J* 1975; **4**: 504–507.

22 Janson JA, Cotton PB. Endoscopic treatment of bile duct stone containing a surgical staple. *HPB Surg* 1990; **3**: 67–71.

23 Easter DW, Moossa AR. Laser and laparoscopic cholecystectomy. A hazardous union? *Arch Surg* 1991; **126**: 423.

24 Moossa AR, Easter DW, Van Sonnenberg EV. Laparoscopic injuries to the bile duct: a cause for concern. *Ann Surg* 1992; **215**: 203–208.

25 Blumgart LH, Kelley CJ, Benjamin IS. Benign bile duct stricture following cholecystectomy: critical factors in management. *Br J Surg* 1984; **71**: 836–841.

26 Davidoff AM, Pappas TN, Murray EA *et al.* Mechanisms of major biliary injury during laparoscopic cholecystectomy. *Ann Surg* 1992; **215**: 196–202.

27 Maki T, Matsushiro T *et al.* The role of sulphated glycoprotein in gallstone formation. *Surg Gynecol Obstet* 1971; **132**: 446–448.

28 Ransohoff DF, Gracie WA, Wolfsen LB, Neuhauser D. Prophylactic cholecystectomy or expectant management for silent stones. *Ann Intern Med* 1983; **99**: 199–204.

29 Barker DJP, Gardner MP, Power C, Hutt MSR. Prevalence of gallstones at necropsy in nine British towns. A collaborative study. *Br Med J* 1979; **2**: 1389–1392.

30 Godfrey PJ, Bates T, Harrison H *et al.* Gallstones and mortality: a study of all gallstone-related deaths in a single health district. *Gut* 1984; **25**: 1029–1033.

8 : Laparoscopic cholecystolithotomy and cholecystostomy

This chapter deals with three forms of therapy for gallstone disease which, though related, are different in terms of their clinical relevance. The first, percutaneous treatment of gallbladder stones, is considered as an alternative to cholecystectomy, at least in some patients. Although this view is not widely held, none the less it has its staunch advocates. The second procedure is laparoscopic removal of gallstones in a small subgroup of patients with functioning gallbladder, in whom cholecystectomy is known to be followed by adverse consequences. The third approach relates to the emergency management of poor-risk patients with severe acute cholecystitis, in whom the postoperative mortality following cholecystectomy is known to be high.

Percutaneous gallstone treatment

The various percutaneous procedures performed under radiological/ultrasound control include local dissolution by use of methyl tert-butyl ether (MTBE) [1,2], and stone extraction through an Amplatz tube system [3–5]. For large stones mechanical, electrohydraulic, ultrasonic, pulsed-dye laser, and more recently, high-speed rotary electromechanical lithotripsy (Kinsey–Nash) have been employed. All these techniques require the establishment of a percutaneous access to the gallbladder, usually through the edge of the right lobe of the liver (Fig. 8.1) but at times directly through the fundus. In the authors' opinion, all these techniques have intrinsic disadvantages which preclude their widespread application. In particular, none of the procedures is uniformly successful and most require prolonged catheter drainage of the gallbladder. Apart from the risks inherent in dislodgement of the catheter, no-one has reported any information on the integrity of the gallbladder mucosa following catheter drainage for 1–2 weeks. Other disadvantages include the complications inherent to the techniques. With MTBE dissolution, the risks are diminished, but not abolished, by the use of microprocessor-controlled pumps to minimize gallbladder distension and leakage of the solvent through the cystic duct into the biliary tract and duodenum. Experience with the percutaneous electromechanical high-speed lithotripsy is limited, but the data presented by some of the centres show a significant morbidity. The limitation of this otherwise ingenious device is the trauma to the gallbladder caused by the high-speed bombardment of the mucosa by the gallstone fragments.

It would be wrong to dismiss these approaches altogether because they do have a place, especially in poor-risk patients after percutaneous drainage for severe acute obstructive cholecystitis (see below).

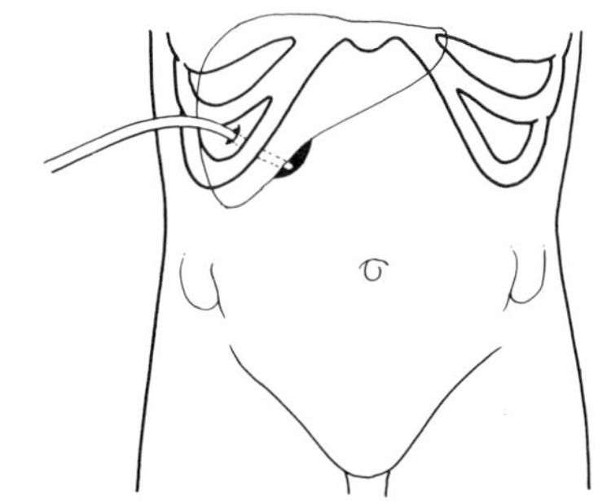

Fig. 8.1 Percutaneous transhepatic cholecystostomy.

Laparoscopic cholecystolithotomy

Although the correct treatment for the vast majority of patients with symptomatic gallstone disease is cholecystectomy, in a few patients this results in undesirable side-effects. There are two patient groups which come into this category: patients who develop symptomatic gallstone disease after previous vagotomy and drainage or partial gastrectomy, and patients with co-existing gastro-oesophageal reflux disease. Cholecystectomy results in significant changes in the enterohepatic circulation of bile salts [6], promotes both enterogastric [7] and gastro-oesophageal reflux [8] and results in impaired function of the antropyloric motor unit [9]. In patients after gastric surgery, the removal of a functioning gallbladder is attended by a high risk of development of explosive diarrhoea [10]. In these patients cholecystolithotomy is a much safer option and is the treatment adopted in the authors' institution [11]. In patients with established gastro-oesophageal reflux disease, there are two alternatives: combined laparoscopic cholecystectomy and antreflux surgery, and cholecystolithotomy. Finally there is a group of young patients with functioning gallbladder who refuse cholecystectomy because of the alleged enhanced risk of colonic carcinoma after gallbladder removal. *Whatever the patient group, laparoscopic cholecystolithotomy is only indicated in the presence of a non-contracted functioning organ.*

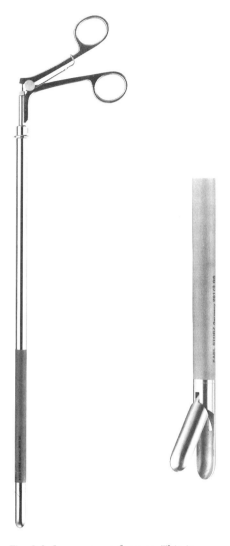

Fig. 8.2 Semm spoon forceps. This is introduced through a 10.0 mm cannula.

Cannula sites and instrumentation

The number of trocar/cannula sites used is identical to those used in laparoscopic cholecystectomy (Chapter 4). In addition to the basic instrument set, the Semm spoon forceps (Fig. 8.2), a flexible choledochoscope and two needle-holders are necessary.

Aspiration of bile

The gallbladder is aspirated of bile using the Veress needle attached to an activated suction line. Although this step may be avoided, it has the merit of minimizing bile leakage.

Cholecystotomy and stone removal

The gallbladder fundus is grasped by the assistant using an atraumatic forceps, and lifted up together with the right lobe to gain the necessary exposure. A 1.0 mm incision is made on the anterior aspect of the fundus, just distal to the grasping forceps (Fig. 8.3). The Semm spoon forceps is then introduced through the 10.0 mm left subcostal cannula and the suction probe through the 5.0 mm right midclavicular cannula. The sucker (non-activated) is used as a probe to squeeze the stones out of the incision by massage of the gallbladder from the neck distally (Fig. 8.4). As the stones escape they are grasped by the spoon forceps and removed (Fig. 8.4). The process is repeated until the gallbladder is emptied of calculi. The sucker is activated intermittently during this process to aspirate any escaping bile. The neck of the collapsed gallbladder is then temporarily occluded by an atraumatic forceps and the gallbladder lumen is irrigated with Hartmann's solution (Fig. 8.5).

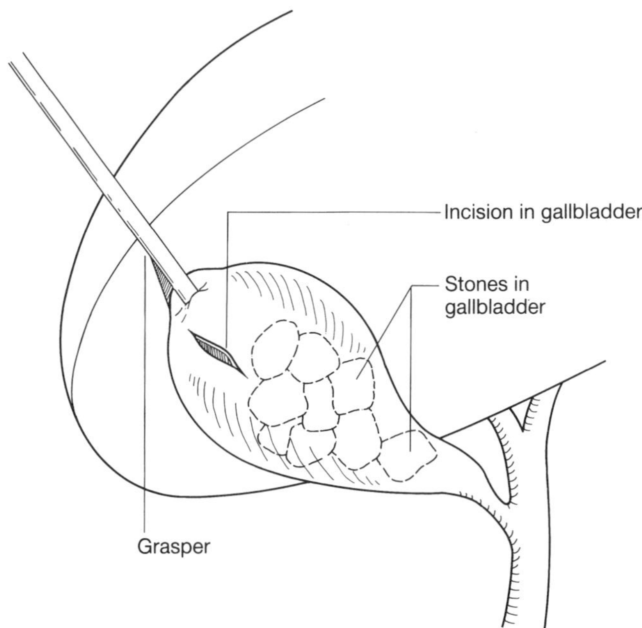

Fig. 8.3 After the gallbladder fundus has been grasped by the assistant using an atraumatic forceps, a 1.0 mm incision is made on the anterior aspect of the fundus just distal to the grasping forceps.

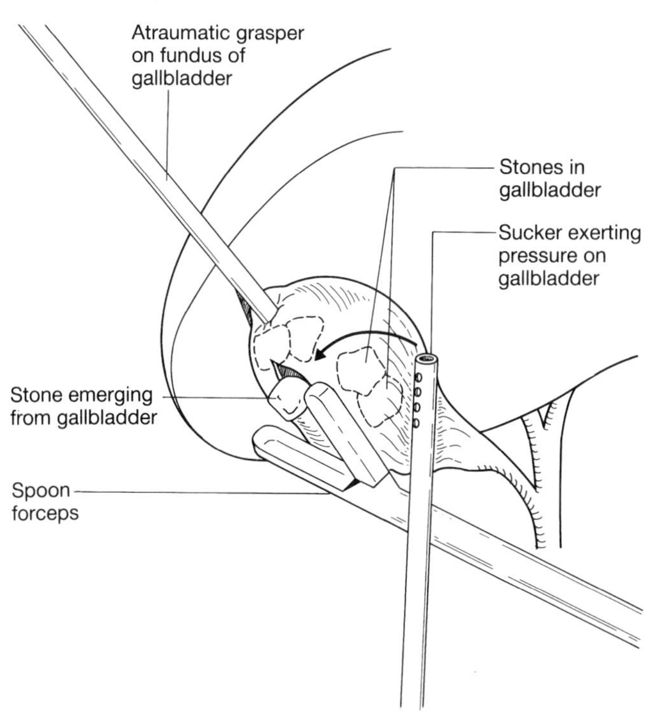

Fig. 8.4 The sucker (non-activated) is used as a probe to squeeze the stones out of the incision by massage of the gallbladder from the neck distally. It is important that this massaging process is maintained in the same direction, i.e. away from the neck of the gallbladder. As stones escape they are grasped by the spoon forceps and removed. The process is repeated until the gallbladder is emptied of calculi.

Endoscopic inspection

The flexible choledochoscope is then introduced into the gallbladder lumen, and the gallbladder wall around the incision is gathered around the flexible scope to prevent leakage of crystalloid solution during the endoscopic

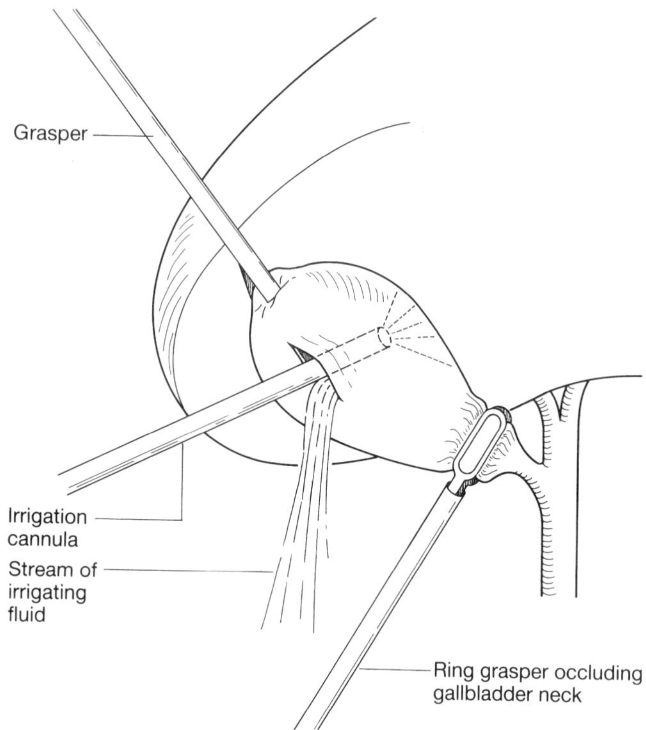

Fig. 8.5 The neck of the collapsed gallbladder is occluded temporarily by an atraumatic forceps and the gallbladder lumen is irrigated with Hartmann's solution.

examination of the interior of the gallbladder (Fig. 8.6). A thorough inspection is made to ensure that there are no residual stones and to exclude other unsuspected pathology. An excellent view of the cystic duct orifice is obtained (Fig. 8.7).

Suture of the cholecystotomy

The endoscope is withdrawn and the incision in the gallbladder closed with a continuous 3/0 absorbable suture mounted on an endoski needle (Fig. 8.8) using the technique outlined in Chapter 10. This requires the use of a preformed jamming loop knot and two needle-holders.

Cholecystocholangiography

A cholecystocholangiogram is essential for two reasons: first to ensure cystic duct patency, and second to establish that the common duct is clear of calculi. The cholecystocholangiogram is performed by direct puncture of the closed gallbladder and the instillation of 30–50 ml of contrast medium. *It is essential that the puncture site is not ligated by an endoloop.* The authors have encountered postoperative bile leakage in a patient following the application of an endoloop to seal the cholangiography puncture site. At relaparoscopy a small circular necrotic perforation at the site of the ligature was found. This

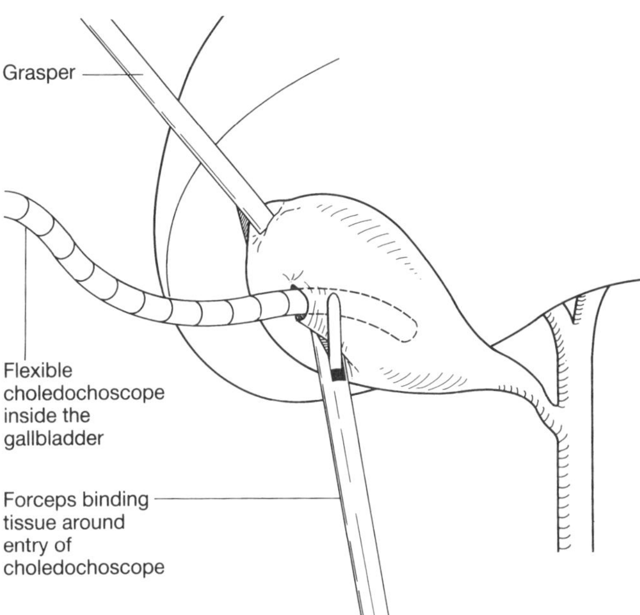

Fig. 8.6 The flexible choledochoscope is introduced into the gallbladder lumen and the gallbladder wall around the incision gathered around the flexible scope to prevent leakage of crystalloid solution during the endoscopic examination of the interior of the gallbladder.

was treated by the insertion of a balloon catheter through the perforation, and thorough peritoneal lavage. The patient made an uneventful recovery. If the cystic duct is patent, the small puncture site seals rapidly due to the elasticity of the gallbladder wall. If leakage persists, then this should be secured by a single interrupted suture.

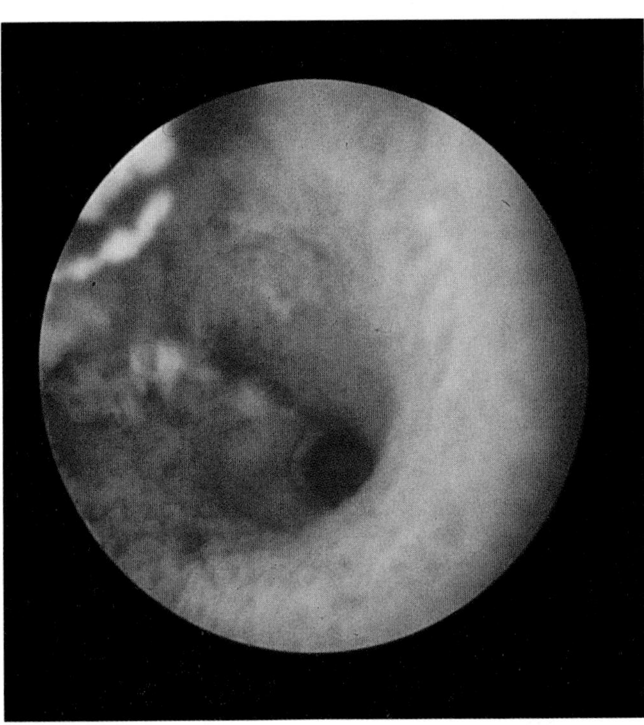

Fig. 8.7 View of the interior of the gallbladder and cystic duct orifice.

Final inspection and irrigation

On completion of the operation, the gallbladder is inspected closely for bile leakage, the peritoneal gutters are irrigated and aspirated, and a small drain is inserted in the subhepatic pouch. This is removed after 48 hours.

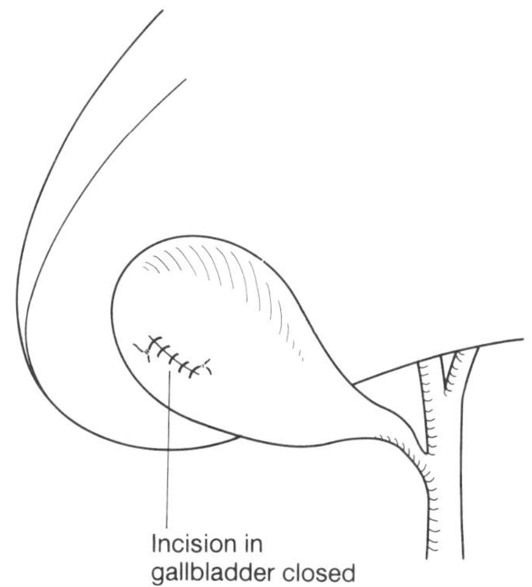

Fig. 8.8 The cholecystotomy is closed with a continuous 3/0 absorbable suture.

Laparoscopic cholecystostomy for severe acute cholecystitis

Percutaneous drainage of the inflamed gallbladder can be performed either under radiological/ultrasound guidance [12–14] or under direct visual control through the laparoscopic approach [15–19]. The other alternative to formal open surgery for poor-risk patients is the minicholecystostomy technique of Burhenne and Stoller [20–22].

Indications for percutaneous cholecystectomy

Although routine elective cholecystectomy in the fit adult is a safe procedure and carries a low mortality, emergency surgery for acute cholecystitis in the elderly carries a reported mortality of 9.8–12.5% from postoperative cardiorespiratory complications [20,23–25]. Furthermore, these patients are at greater risk of developing empyema, which doubles these mortality figures. In addition to being immunocompromised, elderly patients tend to have intercurrent cardiorespiratory disease, which enhances the anaesthetic risk and contributes significantly to the postoperative mortality. Several published reports have documented that cholecystectomy is also a high-risk procedure in cirrhotic patients [26]. Ultrasound-guided percutaneous transhepatic cholecystostomy has been used in patients suffering from acute acalculous cholecystitis [14]. In many of these patients subsequent tube cholangiography showed complete resolution and their clinical progress was uncomplicated, with no late manifestations of gallbladder disease. In all these high-risk groups, a relatively minor percutaneous intervention which can effectively and safely drain the acutely inflamed gallbladder can tide the patient over the critical period. The indications for percutaneous gallbladder drainage for acute disease are shown in Table 8.1.

If local expertise is available, drainage is best achieved by the laparoscopic route. Although the procedure can be performed under local analgesia and sedation, general anaesthesia is preferable. Alternatively, percutaneous drainage of the inflamed gallbladder can be carried out under fluoroscopic/ultrasound control. In either case, drainage, which is usually followed by marked improvement of the patient's condition within 24 hours, is maintained for at least 7 days.

Table 8.1 Indications for percutaneous/laparoscopic cholecystostomy in patients with severe acute cholecystitis

Progressive acute obstructive cholecystitis in poor-risk and elderly patients
Acute acalculous cholecystitis
Severe acute cholecystitis encountered during laparoscopic surgery

Complications of percutaneous drainage of the gallbladder

With experience and the necessary precautions, percutaneous drainage of the gallbladder, whether performed radiologically or through the laparoscopic approach, is safe. The reported complications include catheter dislodgement,

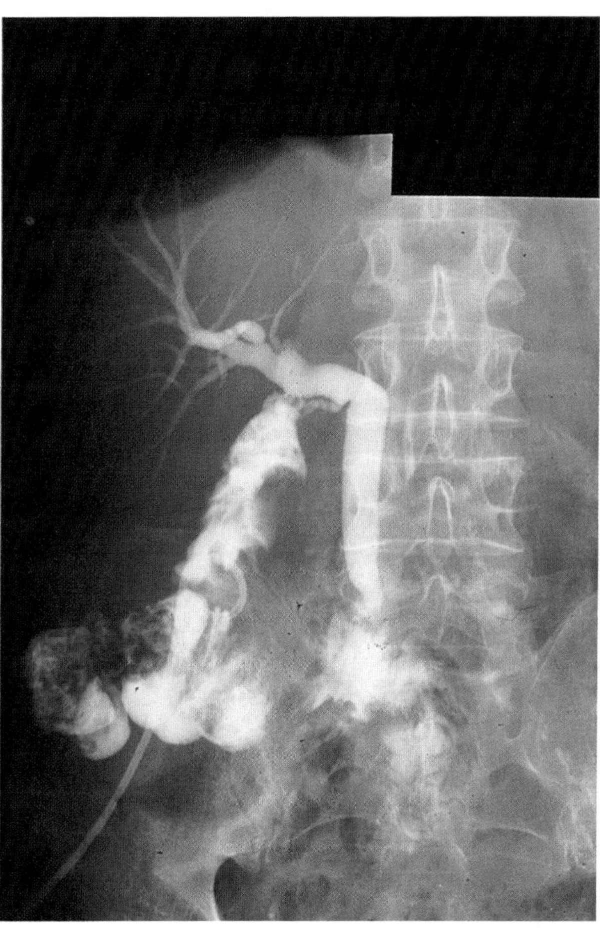

Fig. 8.9 Cholecystocolic fistula after percutaneous ultrasound-guided drainage of empyema in a poor-risk elderly male.

bile leakage into the peritoneal cavity, bleeding when the transhepatic route is used, and damage to the hepatic flexure of the colon. These complications underline the importance of a tube cholecystocholangiogram 24 hours after the procedure is performed. Iatrogenic cholecystocolic fistula (Fig. 8.9) has been reported only after ultrasound-guided percutaneous cholecystostomy, usually with the subcostal direct fundal puncture technique. In a computed tomographic study on the anatomical considerations of this procedure, the right hemicolon was found to lie between the gallbladder fundus and the skin in 13% of patients [27].

Minicholecystostomy

A different combined surgical–radiological approach, the minicholecystostomy, has been practised by Burhenne, Stoller and colleagues [20,21]. The gallbladder and liver edge are located by ultrasound scanning and their position is marked on the skin. Under local anaesthesia, a small oblique abdominal wall incision, approximately 5.0 cm in length, is made over the gallbladder fundus, in which a purse-string suture is inserted. A Fr 24 Foley catheter is then introduced and the purse-string suture tightened and used to anchor the catheter. These authors report no death or significant wound infections in 21 consecutive patients. This minimal-access procedure is a safe and viable alternative to percutaneous drainage in poor-risk patients. Prospective trials comparing it with ultrasound-guided or laparoscopic catheter drainage are needed, as there is currently no reliable information on the comparative efficacy and safety of these procedures.

Technique of laparoscopic cholecystostomy

Anaesthesia

The procedure is best performed under general endotracheal anaesthesia, but if the patient's condition precludes this, local infiltration anaesthesia with 1% lignocaine and intravenous sedation with midazolam may be used instead. Excellent anaesthesia is produced by a lower-right intercostal nerve block (10th–12th). Full monitoring of the cardiovascular and respiratory systems is necessary throughout the operation.

Pneumoperitoneum and confirmation of the diagnosis

The pneumoperitoneum is established as described in Chapter 3, but much less gas is needed. If the procedure is carried out under local anaesthesia and intravenous sedation, insufflation with nitrous oxide causes less discomfort than CO_2. However, nitrous oxide pneumoperitoneum precludes the use of electrocoagulation. In high-risk patients a low-pressure pneumoperitoneum is used (4.0–6.0 mmHg). This is now possible by employing the abdominal wall sling lift (Chapter 3).

The 10.5 mm trocar/cannula for the telescope is situated in the immediate infraumbilical region. Two 5.0 mm accessory cannulae are introduced under vision: left upper paramedian and right midclavicular at the umbilical level. A palpating probe is used to gently tease away omentum from the right upper quadrant. In some patients the hepatic flexure is interposed between the abdominal wall and the inflamed gallbladder. This requires gentle downward displacement with the palpating probe.

The tense inflamed gallbladder is often surrounded by adherent omentum. Not infrequently, green patches of localized gangrene are evident. Visualization of the fundus of the gallbladder is essential for safe laparoscopic cholecystostomy. Some cases are unsuitable and require conversion to open surgery. The indications for immediate laparotomy are shown in Table 8.2.

Table 8.2 Indications for immediate laparotomy in patients with acute cholecystitis

The gallbladder cannot be visualized because of the inflammatory phlegmon
Localized pericholecystic abscess formation
Free perforation with localized or generalized peritonitis
Extensive gangrene of the gallbladder, including emphysematous cholecystitis
Carcinoma of the gallbladder
Carcinoma of the hepatic flexure penetrating the gallbladder

Evacuation of the gallbladder contents

Two techniques can be used: the Mayo–Ochsner suction trocar/cannula or the Veress needle technique.

Mayo–Ochsner cannula. The important features of this cannula (Fig. 8.10) are an integral suction port, complete occlusion of the cannula lumen when the

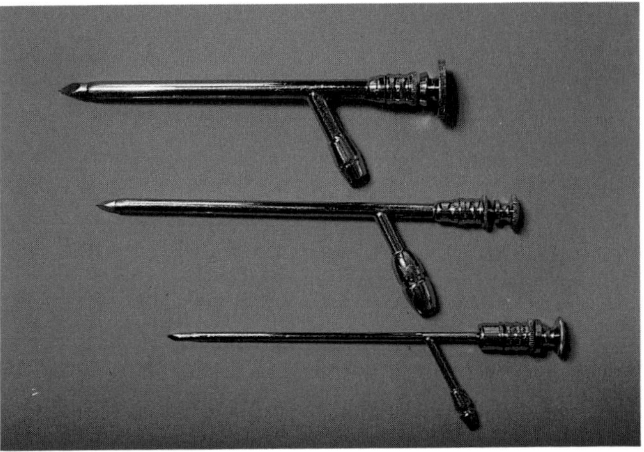

Fig. 8.10 Mayo–Ochsner suction trocar/cannula.

trocar is held in full projection, and the screw-cap seal of the cannula. These features prevent contamination during evacuation of the gallbladder contents. The selected trocar/cannula is connected to a suction line which is activated. The appropriate site on the abdominal wall for insertion of the trocar/cannula is selected by finger depression while viewing the abdominal wall with the telescope. A position directly opposite the intended puncture site in the fundus of the distended gallbladder is selected. A small stab wound is made in the skin and subcutaneous tissue. The trocar/cannula is held such that the palm presses against the plunger, thus ensuring full and fixed projection of the trocar. It is introduced through the abdominal wall under visual guidance. The tip of the trocar is then directed to the fundus and further sustained pressure is exerted until the gallbladder is perforated. Contrary to the non-inflamed organ, fixation by a holding grasper is unnecessary and undesirable, since the walls are softened by the inflammatory oedema and gallbladder mobility is restricted. It is important that the cannula shaft is seen to be well inside the gallbladder lumen before the trocar is withdrawn and the contents are evacuated. The cannula is left in place for introduction of the drainage catheter (see below).

Veress needle. The authors now prefer to use this technique as it is simpler and equally safe and effective. The Veress needle attached to an activated suction line with an intervening trap is introduced under vision, with the trap closed, directly opposite to the fundus and in line with the long axis of the organ. The outer sheath is held retracted until the gallbladder wall is punctured, when the spring-loaded mechanism is released. The position of the needle inside the gallbladder can be easily checked by tilting the needle shaft to gently elevate the wall of the organ. The tap on the Veress needle is then opened and the fluid contents of the gallbladder are evacuated. The Veress needle is then removed and provided decompression is complete, this is not followed by leakage through the small puncture site.

With either technique a specimen of the purulent material is sent for immediate Gram staining and subsequent bacteriological studies.

Tube cholecystostomy

There are three techniques for insertion of a balloon catheter into the inflamed gallbladder: the transperitoneal route, the transcannular method and the guidewire Amplatz technique. The authors now favour the first because it is simpler and puts no restriction on the catheter size used.

Transperitoneal route. A suitably sized balloon silicon or latex Foley catheter is introduced into the peritoneal cavity and the tip directed to the puncture site on the fundus of the gallbladder. After the walls have been gently grasped, the puncture site is enlarged with scissors and the catheter introduced into the lumen of the gallbladder. The balloon is then inflated with saline. Traction is applied to the catheter to ensure an adequate seal. The external part of the catheter is fixed to the abdominal wall in the desired position after reducing the pneumoperitoneum to about 6.0 mmHg.

Transcannular method. The size of the cannula selected for emptying the gallbladder contents determines the maximum size of the balloon catheter which can be inserted into the gallbladder lumen; this is the main limitation of the technique. Following evacuation, the screw cap of the cannula is undone and the trocar removed. The catheter is then introduced down the cannula into the gallbladder lumen and the balloon inflated with saline. This step is performed under vision. The cannula is then exteriorized over the catheter. Another limitation of the technique is that the cannula cannot be removed over the catheter. After disinfection, it is strapped to the abdominal wall distal to the external fixation site of the catheter.

Percutaneous biliary or nephrostomy set. This is a well-validated technique for drainage of the biliary tract and uses a guidewire, a stiffener tube and an outer Amplatz-type sheath. It is more expensive and time-consuming than the above methods.

Peritoneal toilet

The right supracolic compartment is irrigated with Hartmann's solution and aspirated dry. The other peritoneal gutters including the pelvis are then inspected and aspirated of any fluid.

Apart from the removal of small calculi during suction evacuation of the gallbladder contents, no attempt should be made at mechanical stone extraction or lithotripsy at this stage, as the gallbladder wall is friable and easily perforated by the instruments. Syringing of the gallbladder is also unnecessary and may dislodge small calculi into the common bile duct.

Connection and fixation of the drainage catheter

Irrespective of the method used, the final position of the catheter is established after reducing the pneumoperitoneum to about 6.0 mmHg.

Traction is then applied to the catheter. This achieves two objectives: it seals the entry hole in the gallbladder, and shortens and straightens the tract from the gallbladder to the abdominal wall. In most instances the fundus can be made to touch the parietal peritoneum of the right hypochondrium. This approximation, together with a straight course, considerably facilitates subsequent dilatation of the tract and percutaneous stone fragmentation or extraction. The catheter is sutured to the abdominal wall in the desired position and then connected to a closed drainage system. The area is sealed with an occlusive dressing to ensure against accidental dislodgement. If the transcannular technique is used, the cannula is strapped to the abdominal wall further down.

Cholecystocholangiogram

These patients should have a contrast examination 24 hours later. The cholecystocholangiogram establishes that the catheter is *in situ* and also provides useful information regarding the pathological state of the biliary tract, the extent of the stone load and the presence of ductal calculi. Thus apart from being an essential safety check, it indicates the appropriate subsequent therapy when the patient has recovered from the acute episode.

Subsequent therapy

This depends on the condition of the patient, especially the cardiorespiratory state and the findings of the cholecystocholangiogram. In patients with acalculous cholecystitis, no further therapy is necessary. The catheter is removed after 10–14 days, or longer if the patient is immunocompromised or a diabetic. One report from Holland has shown excellent results, with return to normal gallbladder function in these patients [14].

In the case of calculous disease, if the patient's condition improves and he is considered fit for surgery, an elective cholecystectomy is performed, laparoscopically in most cases. The only difficulty encountered is mobilization of the gallbladder from the abdominal wall, omentum and hepatic flexure. Thus although tedious, the laparoscopic procedure is safe, though often prolonged.

If the patient has severe cardiorespiratory disease, percutaneous lithotripsy or stone extraction or MTBE dissolution can be performed. In the future, chemical ablation of the gallbladder mucosa by sclerosants after cystic duct occlusion would constitute the ideal definitive treatment in these patients [28,29]. In view of their limited life expectancy, the long-term potential hazards of chemical cholecystectomy, such as the development of cancer of the gallbladder, would not apply to these patients.

An endoscopic sphincterotomy and stone extraction is performed in those patients who are found to harbour ductal calculi.

References

1 Allen MJ, Borody TJ, Bugliosi TF *et al.* Rapid dissolution of gallstones by methyl tert-butyl ether. Preliminary observations. *New Engl J Med* 1986; **314**: 818–822.
2 van Sonnenberg E. Horizons in gallstone therapy—1988. *AJR* 1988; **150**: 43–46.
3 Kerlan RK, LaBerge JM, Ring EJ. Percutaneous cholecystolithotomy: preliminary experience. *Radiology* 1985; **157**: 653–656.
4 Kellet MJ, Wickham JEA, Russell RCG. Percutaneous cholecystolithotomy. *Br Med J* 1988; **296**: 453–455.
5 Gajetta DJ, Cohen MJ, Crummy AB *et al.* Ultrasonic lithotripsy of gallstones after cholecystostomy. *AJR* 1984; **143**: 1088–1089.
6 Thaysen EH, Pedersen L. Idiopathic bile acid catharsis. *Gut* 1976; **17**: 965–970.
7 Brown TH, Walton G, Cheadle WG, Larson GM. The alkaline shift in the gastric pH after cholecystectomy. *Am J Surg* 1989; **157**: 58–65.
8 Walsh TN, Jazrawi S, Byrne PJ *et al.* Cholecystectomy and oesophageal reflux. *Br J Surg* 1991; **78**: 753.
9 Johnson AG. Pyloric function and gallstone dyspepsia. *Br J Surg* 1972; **59**: 449–454.
10 Taylor TV. Postvagotomy and cholecystectomy syndrome. *Ann Surg* 1981; **194**: 625–629.
11 Cuschieri A. Postvagotomy diarrhoea: is there a place for surgical management? *Gut* 1990; **31**: 245–246.
12 Lindemann SR, Tung G, Silverman SG, Mueller PR. Percutaneous cholecystostomy. *Sem Intervent Radiol* 1988; **5**: 179–185.
13 Pearse DM, Hawkins IF Jr, Shaver R, Vogel S. Percutaneous cholecystostomy in acute cholecystitis and common duct obstruction. *Radiology* 1984; **152**: 365–367.
14 Eggermont AM, Lameris JS, Jeekel J. Ultrasound-guided percutaneous transhepatic cholecystostomy for acute acalculous cholecystitis. *Arch Surg* 1985; **120**: 1354–1356.
15 Cuschieri A. Value of laparoscopy in general surgery and gastroenterology. *J Hosp Med* 1980; **24**: 252–257.
16 El Ghany AB Abd, Holley MP, Cuschieri A. Percutaneous clearance of the gallbladder through an access cholecystostomy: a laparoscopic guided technique. *Surg Endosc* 1989; **3**: 126–130.
17 Berci G, Cuschieri A. *Practical Laparoscopy.* Baillière Tindall, London, 1986.
18 Frimberger E. Operative laparoscopy: cholecystotomy. *Endoscopy* 1989; **21**: 299–384.
19 Buess G, Mentges B, Melzer A *et al.* Laparoscopic microsurgical cholecystostomy in gallstone disease. *Surg Endosc* 1990; **4**: 55 (Abstr).
20 Stoller JL, Burhenne HJ. Empyema of the gallbladder. *Lancet* 1984, **i**: 1187.
21 Burhenne HJ, Stoller JL. Minicholecystostomy and radiologic stone extraction in high-risk cholelithiasis patients. *Am J Surg* 1985; **149**: 632–635.
22 Gibney RG, Fache JS, Becker CD *et al.* Combined surgical and radiologic intervention for complicated cholelithiasis in high-risk patients. *Radiology* 1987; **165**: 715–719.
23 Glenn FW, Hays DM. The age factor in the mortality rate of patients undergoing surgery of the biliary tract. *Surg Gynecol Obstet* 1955: **100**: 11–15.
24 Condon RE, Nyhus LM. Cholecystectomy in the aged. *Am J Surg* 1960; **100**: 544–550.
25 McSherry CK, Glenn F. The incidence of death following surgery for non-malignant biliary tract disease. *Ann Surg* 1980; **191**: 271–275.
26 Aranha GV, Sontag SJ, Greenlee HB. Cholecystectomy in cirrhotic patients: a formidable operation. *Am J Surg* 1982; **143**: 55–60.
27 Warren LP, Saadoon K, Dunnick NR. Percutaneous cholecystostomy: anatomic considerations. *Radiology* 1988; **168**: 615–616.
28 Becker CD, Quenville NF. Burhenne HJ. Gallbladder ablation through radiologic intervention: an experimental alternative to cholecystectomy. *Radiology* 1989; **171**: 235–240.
29 Cuschieri A, El Ghany AB Abd, Holley MP. Successful chemical cholecystectomy: a laparoscopic guided technique. *Gut* 1989; **30**: 1786–1794.

9 : Laparoscopic treatment of common duct stones

Although stones in the common duct may remain asymptomatic for varying periods, they are prone to give rise to serious complications which are attended by a significant morbidity and an appreciable mortality, and for this reason, always require treatment. The majority of ductal calculi originate from the gallbladder by migration through the cystic duct (secondary), but some originate *de novo* in the common duct. These primary ductal pigment stones are aetiologically associated with distal obstruction of the bile duct (functional or organic) and the bacterial colonization of bile. In surgical practice, ductal calculi are encountered in four different clinical settings:

1 Complicated: obstructive jaundice, cholangitis and acute pancreatitis.

2 Subclinical obstructive: minor elevations of some of the parameters of the liver function tests, particularly an elevated alkaline phosphates or an ultrasound-detected dilatation of the common duct.

3 Unsuspected: ductal stones discovered by intraoperative cholangiography (IOC) during cholecystectomy in patients with normal preoperative liver function tests and biliary ultrasound scanning.

4 Postcholecystectomy: symptomatic stones after a previous cholecystectomy.

The postcholecystectomy group are often missed or retained stones (undetected though present at the time of cholecystectomy) but others form subsequent to this operation (recurrent). It is often difficult to determine in the individual patient whether the ductal calculi are retained or recurrent. A cutoff period of 2 years post-cholecystectomy was suggested by Schein as a useful differentiating criterion in deciding whether the stones are missed or recurrent in nature [1].

The unsuspected stones, which account for 2–5% of cases, are important because they can always be detected by good IOC and removed at the time of surgery. This indeed is one of the benefits of routine IOC during cholecystectomy, irrespective of whether this is conducted by the open or the laparoscopic approach. It must be stressed that the routine preoperative work-up (liver function tests and ultrasound) does not reliably exclude ductal calculi, and routine recourse to preoperative ERCP is untenable because of increased morbidity [2] and poor yield, which in one large series was only 16% [3].

Options and practice

The options for management of ductal calculi are:

1 Endoscopic sphincterotomy and stone extraction.

2 Open surgical common duct exploration.

3 Laparoscopic treatment.

4 Percutaneous extraction via the T-tube tract.

The advent of laparoscopic surgery has intensified the controversy regarding the use of these management options. However, many of the arguments for and against a given treatment approach have been advanced without reference to the clinical setting, and for this reason have further clouded the issue. The correct treatment in the individual patient depends on five factors: (i) the clinical setting, (ii) the condition of the patient, (iii) the calibre of the common bile duct and extent of the stone load, (iv) the level of local expertise in endoscopic treatment, and (v) the experience of the surgeon in laparoscopic biliary surgery.

Ductal calculi discovered before surgery

The overriding factor in deciding the appropriate management here is the condition of the patient. There is no doubt that patients who are deeply jaundiced, those with cholangitis and poor-risk patients are best treated by endoscopic sphincterotomy and stone extraction. Laparoscopic cholecystectomy is undertaken once the condition of the patient has improved.

By contrast, good-risk patients with or without mild jaundice and no clinical features of cholangitis are better managed with laparoscopic stone extraction if the necessary surgical expertise is available. This approach is likely to carry a lower morbidity than preoperative endoscopic stone extraction followed by cholecystectomy. In one prospective study, the morbidity of this combined endoscopic-surgical approach was found to be higher than cholecystectomy with common bile duct exploration by the open route [2]. There is one important contraindication to elective laparoscopic stone extraction which is being overlooked. This concerns patients with gross dilatation of the bile duct (>2.0 cm) and multiple ductal calculi. These patients need a drainage procedure and the correct treatment is either open cholecystectomy with choledochoduodenostomy, preferably by the transection technique [4] or adequate endoscopic sphincterotomy.

Ductal calculi discovered during surgery

The experience to date suggests that the best treatment for these unsuspected ductal calculi is laparoscopic stone extraction, either through the cystic duct or via limited supraduodenal choledocholithotomy. For small calculi, the success of cystic duct extraction now approaches 80% [5–8]. Although these procedures add an extra 1–1.5 hours to the operating time, the benefits include the completing of treatment in one procedure and negligible morbidity. For this subgroup, laparoscopic stone extraction may be safer and more cost-effective than postoperative endoscopic stone extraction. Furthermore, it avoids the necessity for a sphincterotomy, which is an important consideration in young and middle-aged patients.

However, laparoscopic extraction for unsuspected calculi at the time of cholecystectomy may be inadvisable in patients with a narrow common bile duct. The risk of complications, particularly ductal stricture following any bile duct exploration (laparoscopic or open), cannot be ignored, and for this reason this subgroup may be better treated by postoperative endoscopic extraction, or simply followed up and treated if symptoms develop.

Ductal calculi discovered after surgery

In those patients with retained stones who have access to the biliary tree (T-tube), endoscopically guided percutaneous stone extraction via the T-tube tract is the preferred option [9]. A few weeks is allowed for maturation of the tract before the procedure is undertaken. After the insertion of a guidewire, the T-tube is removed and the tract dilated. An Amplatz sheath is then inserted before passage of the flexible choledochoscope over the guidewire into the common bile duct. Good fluoroscopy is also needed for this procedure.

In patients without a T-tube, endoscopic sphincterotomy and stone extraction remains the treatment of choice. In experienced hands this has a success rate of 90–95%. This technique fails and special measures are needed in patients with the duodenal diverticulum, the anatomically difficult papilla, in the presence of occluding stones, and in patients after Polya gastrectomy. These special techniques includes precutting, transpapillary guided endoscopic sphincterotomy, and, as a last resort, transhepatic guided endoscopic division of the sphincter.

Laparoscopic extraction of calculi through cystic duct

This is applicable to calculi in the distal common duct, which fortunately account for the vast majority. It can be performed under radiological control or by direct visual guidance, and is applicable to small calculi (up to 0.5 cm). It is unsuitable for proximal stones and multiple large occluding calculi, where laparoscopic supraduodenal bile-duct exploration is indicated (see below).

Radiologically controlled technique

This has been popularized by Hunter [8]. Its advantages include the avoidance of the need to dilate the cystic duct, and multiple stone evacuation per single basket passage. It necessitates good real-time fluoroscopy. In this respect the authors have found the 'road mapping' mode of the OEC Diasonics C-arm particularly useful, as it shows, in relief and with remarkable clarity, the basket against the contrast background and filling defects caused by the calculi.

The procedure is performed with the patient in the reversed Trendelenburg position. The cholangiogram catheter is replaced by a Fr 4 ureteral stone basket with filiform tip. Under screening control (preferably in the roadmapping mode) the basket is passed down the cystic duct into the distal common bile duct so that its floppy tip lies in the duodenum. When this position is ascertained, the 8.0 mm helical Dormia or Segura basket is opened just above the lower choledochal sphincter (Fig. 9.1) and pulled back into the cystic duct, where the basket is closed on to the stones caught in the troll. Careful closure of the basket to the appropriate extent—i.e. sufficient to ensnare without crushing the stones—is the desired objective. However, if the stones are larger than the cystic duct orifice, further closure of the basket

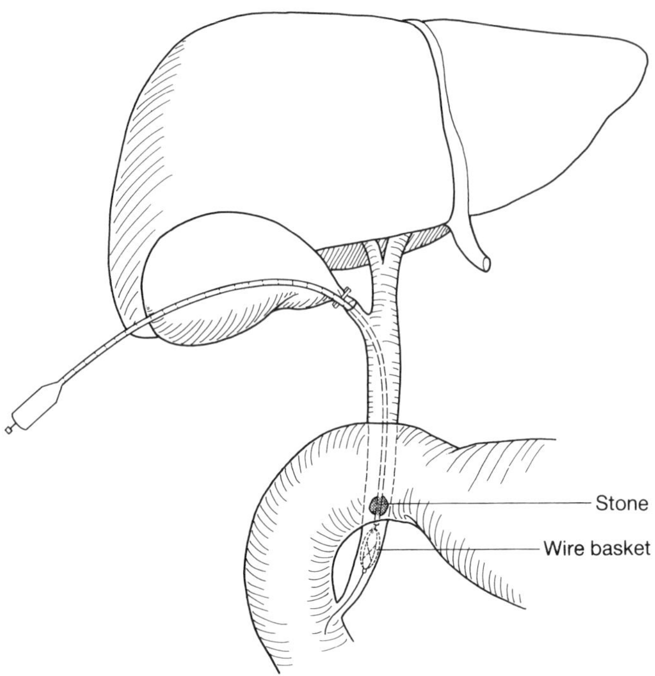

Fig. 9.1 Under screening control the basket is passed down the cystic duct into the distal common bile duct, so that its floppy tip lies in the duodenum. When this position is ascertained, the 8.0 mm helical Dormia basket is opened just above the lower choledochal sphincter and pulled back into the cystic duct, where the basket is closed on to the stones caught in the troll.

is necessary to achieve crushing. The process is repeated until ductal clearance of all discernible fragment is obtained. At this stage the cholangiocatheter is reintroduced and the biliary tract flushed and filled with saline. This washes out any debris and removes air bubbles. The cholangiogram is then repeated, and if ductal clearance is confirmed, the cholangiocatheter is removed and the cystic duct is ligated in continuity with catgut (Chapter 4), or cut and then secured with a preformed endoloop.

An alternative technique which the authors have used on several

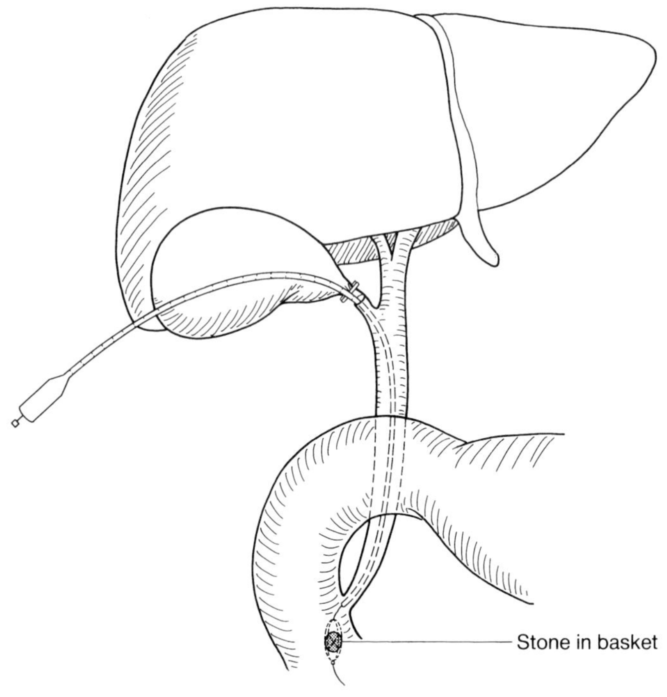

Fig. 9.2 Alternatively the basket is passed with its load into the duodenum, where the stones are released or crushed. This is quick and effective but must be limited to one, or at most two, passages, otherwise the risk of postoperative pancreatitis is increased.

occasions is to trap the stone in the basket and then pass this with its load into the duodenum, where the stones are released or crushed by full closure of the basket so that the fragments drop into the duodenal lumen (Fig. 9.2). This is quick and effective, but must be limited to one or at most two passages, otherwise the risk of postoperative pancreatitis is increased. The other possible complication of this technique is impaction of the basket in the sphincter.

Visually guided technique

This technique was pioneered by Dubois in France and Phillips *et al.* in Los Angeles [5,6]. It necessitates the dilatation of the cystic duct, followed by the introduction of a small-calibre flexible endoscope attached to a CCD camera for visually guided transcystic extraction of the ductal calculi. The technique should not be attempted in patients with a narrow cystic duct as the risk of splitting of this duct is substantial.

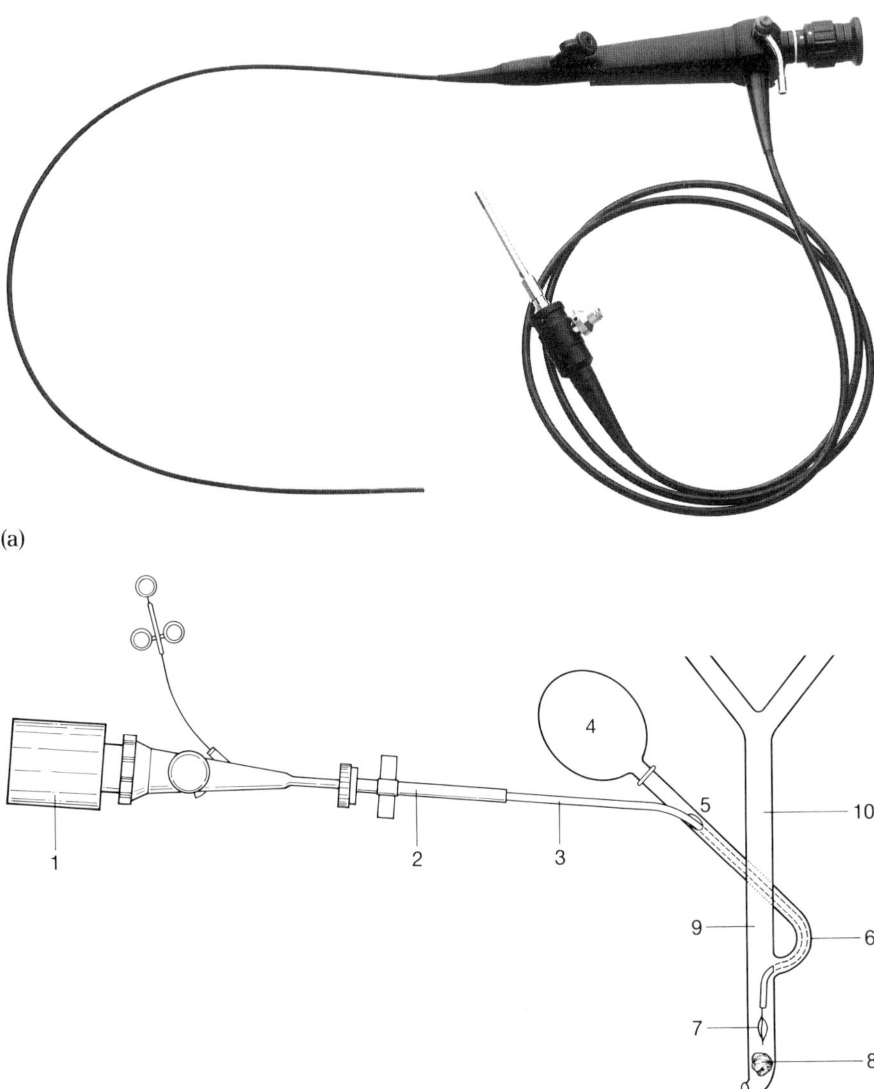

Fig. 9.3 (a) Flexible ureteroscope used for extraction of ductal calculi through the cystic duct. (b) Principle of visually guided extraction through the cystic duct using a Dormia basket through the operating channel of the ureteroscope.

The most useful flexible endoscope for this purpose is the urethroscope (Fig. 9.3). This has a functional length of 30 cm, an outer diameter of 3.4–3.6 mm and an instrument channel of 1.2 mm. Finer endoscopes are available and can be used, but these must have an instrument channel of at least 1.0 mm, otherwise irrigation is impossible once the basket is introduced. The other items of equipment needed are angioplasty balloon dilators and guidewires. The balloon dilators should be Fr 6–7 gauge with a balloon length of 40 mm and achieve maximal dilatation of 5.0 mm. They are insufflated with saline through a customized pressure gauge using a special syringe. Torque guidewires with soft pliable tips, or J-wires which fit the balloon catheters, are used.

When the operative cholangiogram demonstrates calculi (Fig. 9.4), the guidewire is inserted under fluoroscopic control through the cholangiocatheter into the common bile duct and, if possible, into the duodenum. The cholangiocatheter is then removed and replaced by the balloon catheter over the guidewire. If the common bile duct is dilated, the balloon is positioned under fluoroscopic control across the choledochal sphincter and then inflated. Following dilatation of the sphincter, the balloon is deflated and the catheter withdrawn until the balloon lies in the cystic duct, where it is reinflated to dilate this structure. The dilatation of the choledochal sphincter is omitted if the common bile duct is not dilated. At this stage an antispasmodic which relaxes the sphincter of Oddi is administered intravenously (secretin, glucagon or ceruletide). This is followed by irrigation of warm saline through the deflated balloon catheter in an attempt to flush small calculi into the duodenum. The effect of this manoeuvre is ascertained by fluoroscopy and the injection of contrast medium. If unsuccessful, the guidewire is inserted inside the balloon catheter through into the common bile duct and the catheter, then withdrawn. The flexible ureteroscope

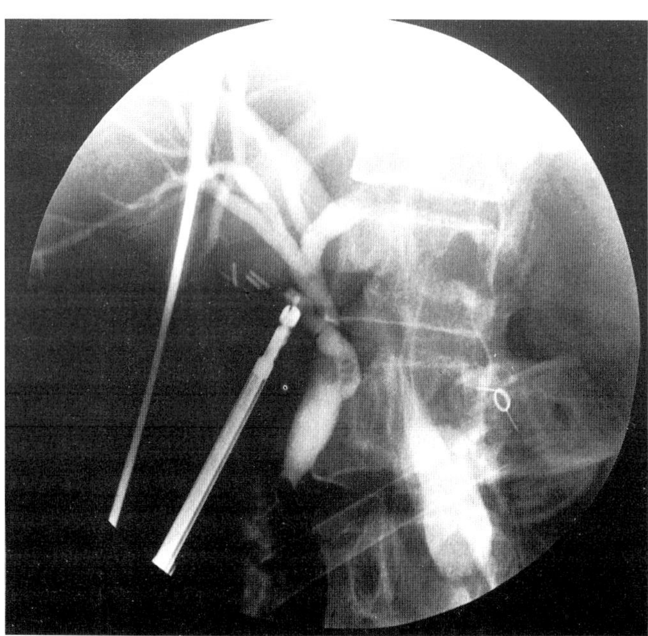

Fig. 9.4 Operative cholangiogram shows stones in the lower end of the cystic and bile ducts. Complete ductal clearance was achieved by visually guided extraction through the cystic duct.

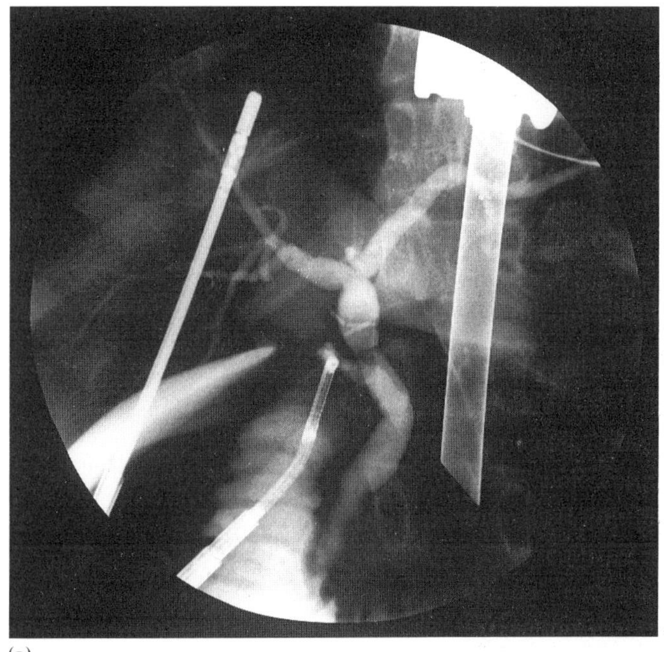
(a)

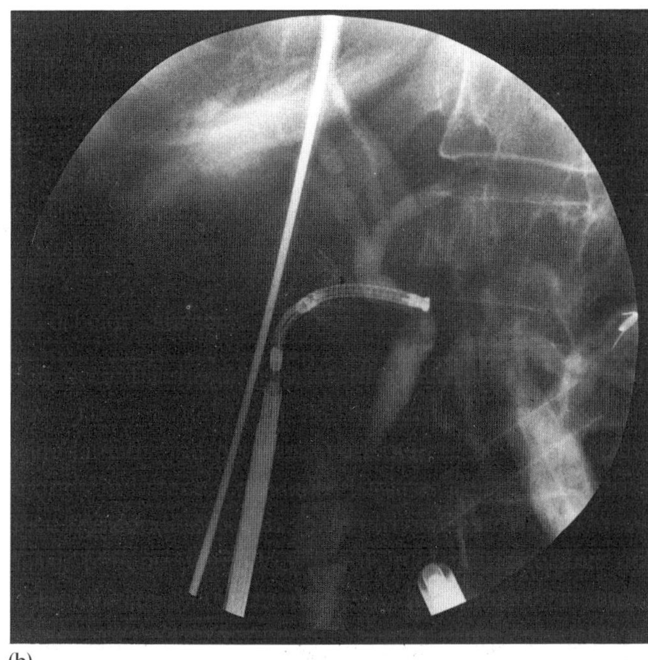
(b)

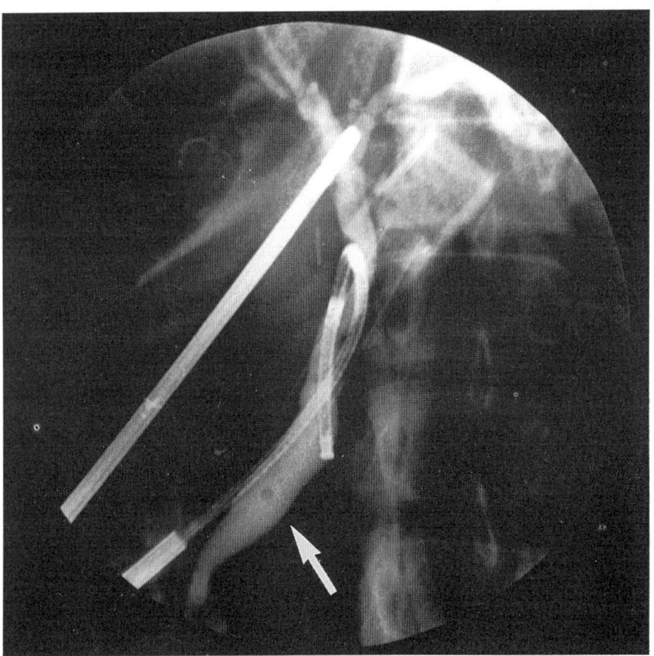
(c)

Fig. 9.5 Insertion of ureteroscope through the cystic duct into the common duct (b). (c) The scope is then manoeuvred towards the stone (arrow) in the lower end of the common bile duct.

connected to the irrigation system (Fenwall pressure cuff) and the CCD camera is inserted through the midclavicular cannula and threaded over the guidewire into the common duct (Fig. 9.5). The guidewire is then replaced by the Dormia basket, which is used to trap and remove the stones under direct vision (Fig. 9.6), either through the cystic duct or into the duodenum.

Special measures are needed if the stone is impacted in the lower choledochal sphincter. The most careful is stone fragmentation by electro-hydraulic lithotripsy (Fig. 9.7) using a Fr 2.7 probe. This requires accurate

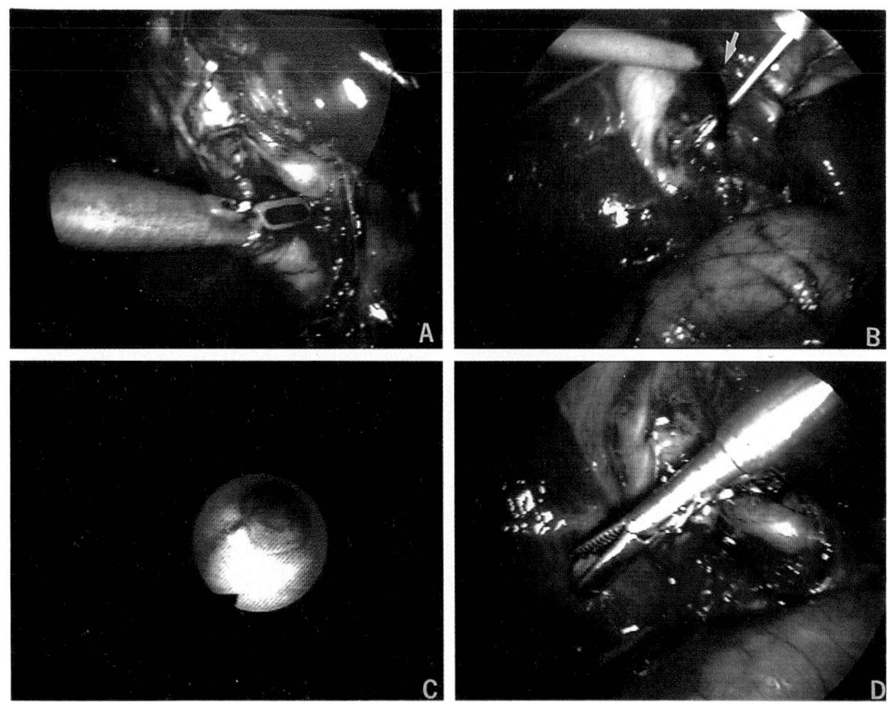

Fig. 9.6 (A) Cholangiocatheter *in situ* held by the cholangiograsper. (B) Flexible ureteroscope is connected to the irrigation system and the CCD camera is inserted through the midclavicular cannula and threaded over the guidewire into the common duct. The guidewire is then replaced by the Dormia basket, which is used to trap and remove the stones under direct vision either through the cystic duct or into the duodenum. (C) Stone in the distal common duct visualized by the ureteroscope. (D) Extracted stone transferred to forceps.

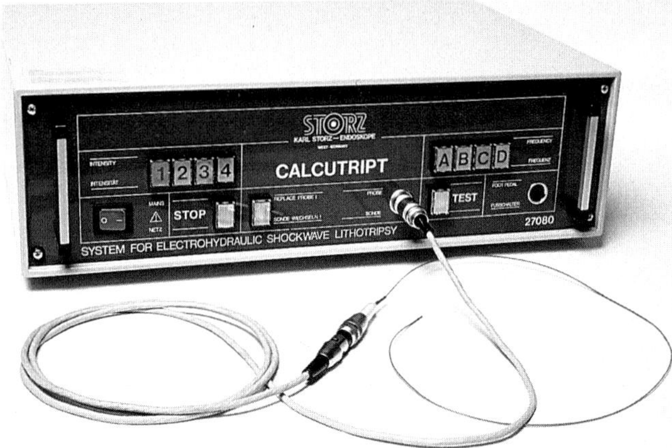

Fig. 9.7 Electrohydraulic lithotriptor.

placement of the tip of the probe on the stone away from the duct wall, otherwise a small perforation may be induced when the electric spark is generated. Other methods of fragmentation, such as pulsed-dye laser (504 nm) transmitted through a thin quartz fibre (300–400 μm) can be used [10,11]. The laser operates at 60 mJ/pulse at 10 Hz and achieves stone fragmentation within 1–2 min. The resulting fragments are extracted if large, or flushed through the ampulla if small (<2.0 mm). A completion cholangiogram is performed to confirm stone clearance. The cystic duct is then ligated in continuity by means of a preformed endoloop. If there is any suspicion of incomplete clearance, a soft infant feeding tube (Fr 5–8) is placed and secured by two catgut ligatures to the cystic duct stump (see below). This provides ductal drainage and access for postoperative cholangiography. If the cholangiogram is normal, the patient is discharged home with the sealed cannula *in situ* and returns for removal of the cannula on the 7th-10th day.

Laparoscopic supraduodenal bile duct exploration

At Ninewells this is now the preferred technique if the common duct diameter is larger than 1.0 cm. It is essential in all patients with proximal stones. Initially, the authors, like others [12], used to insert a T-tube after completion of the supraduodenal bile duct exploration, but increasingly we now prefer to drain the biliary tract through the cystic duct. The equipment needed for supraduodenal bile duct exploration includes the flexible choledochoscope, the dipping endoretractor, sharp microscissors or retractable diamond knife, Dormia basket, two needle-holders and 4/0 absorbable atraumatic sutures mounted on an endoski needle. The dipping endoretractor (Chapter 3) is very useful for elevation of the quadrate lobe ahead of the optic, and thereby provides excellent exposure of the common bile duct. If not available, an additional cannula is needed to insert a retractor to lift the quadrate lobe. This is best placed below and to the left of the xiphoid. The retracting rod is passed beneath the round ligament, which is lifted together with the liver. The abdominal wall sling (Chapter 3) provides added exposure.

Supraduodenal exploration and stone extraction

The catheter used for the cholangiogram is left *in situ*. Minimal dissection of the common duct is needed as only the anterior wall needs to be exposed. Stay sutures are unnecessary and counterproductive, as they use up ports. The incision on the common bile duct is normally 1.0 cm. It is made on the anterior wall in a vertical-oblique fashion (Fig. 9.8), preferably with a diamond knife. At this stage saline is injected forcibly through the cystic duct cannula. This may result in the escape of the stone, which is then picked up

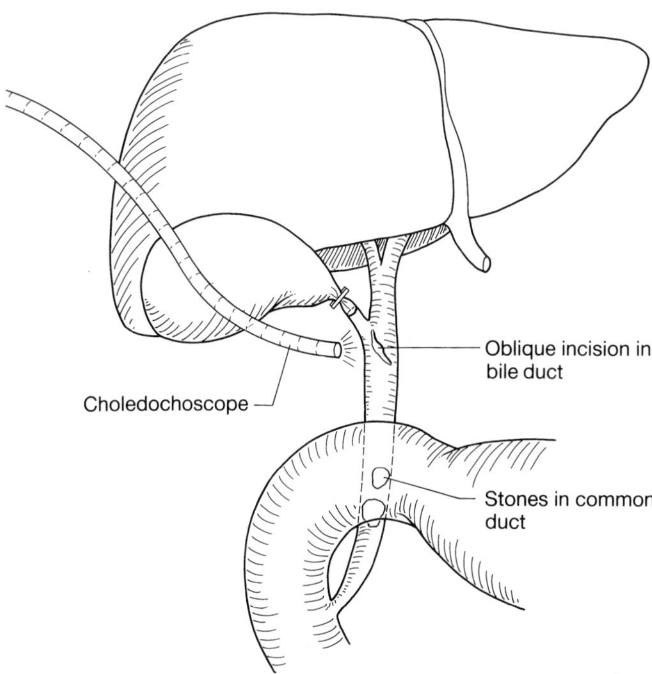

Fig. 9.8 Vertical-oblique incision on the anterior wall of the common bile duct for supraduodenal exploration.

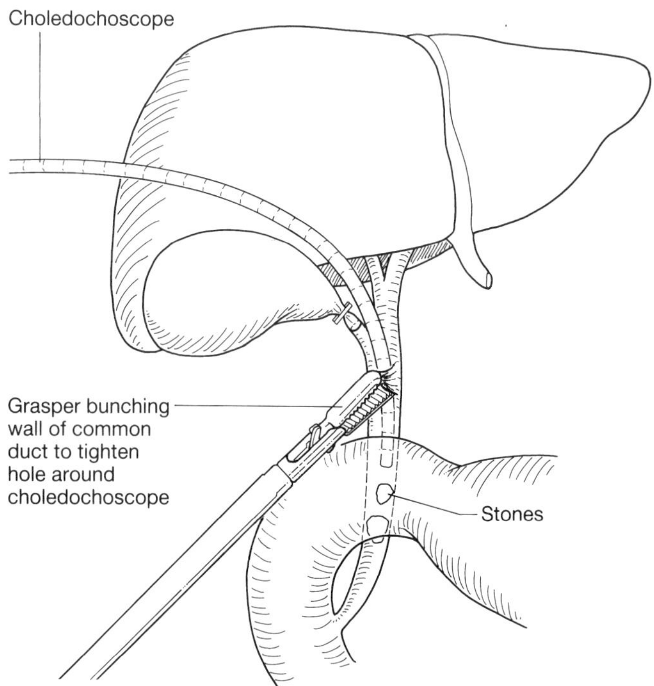

Fig. 9.9 The walls of common bile duct are gathered around the flexible endoscope by an atraumatic forceps to minimize leakage during irrigation, which is necessary for adequate choledochoscopic examination.

by the spoon forceps and retrieved. If not, the flexible choledochoscope connected to the irrigation system (Fenwall) and the CCD camera is introduced through the right midclavicular cannula and inserted into the common bile duct through the choledochotomy. The walls of the common bile duct are gathered around the flexible endoscope by an atraumatic forceps to minimize leakage during irrigation (Fig. 9.9). The entire biliary tract is inspected proximally and distally, and any stones are trapped and removed under vision through the choledochotomy by means of a Dormia basket. Once outside the bile duct, the stones are transferred on each occasion to a spoon forceps and retrieved. Once clearance is achieved, repeat choledochoscopic inspection of the biliary tract is performed.

Bile duct drainage

Drainage of the bile duct is essential after supraduodenal bile duct exploration, as hold-up due to oedema is encountered for several days after this procedure [13]. In addition, the drainage tube provides a ready access for postoperative cholangiography as a final check against retained stones. There are two techniques which can be used to provide biliary drainage: insertion of a T-tube and cystic duct decompression.

T-tube method. This is the standard technique. The horizontal limb of a Fr 12–14 latex tube is trimmed to a total length no longer than 1.5 cm and is filleted. These modifications greatly facilitate the insertion of the horizontal part into the common bile duct. The tube is inserted into the peritoneal cavity through a stab wound in the right flank, so that the long limb runs a straight course

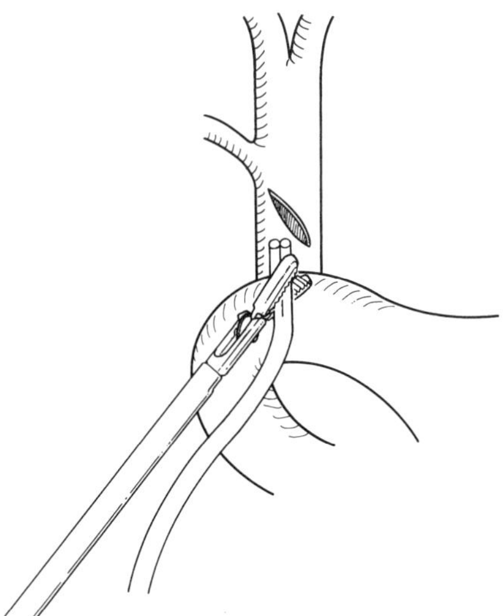

Fig. 9.10 Insertion of T-tube through the choledochotomy.

to the choledochotomy. This straight alignment of the long limb of the T-tube is important should any residual stones be discovered by the postoperative cholangiogram, as a straight tube tract renders percutaneous stone extraction by this route much less difficult than when the T-tube pursues a tortuous course. In this respect it is a mistake to use one of the cannula sites for the insertion of the T-tube, as more often than not these do not provide the ideal location. Once the tube is in the peritoneal cavity, its short horizontal limbs are compressed together by means of an atraumatic forceps and then fed into the common bile duct, when the forceps is released. When the T-tube is in place, saline is instilled through it into the biliary tract (Fig. 9.10).

Cystic duct drainage. At Ninewells the authors now prefer this technique because it results in the quicker recovery of the patient. Furthermore, our experience has confirmed that a Fr 5–8 soft polyethylene cannula provides adequate drainage (average 300 ml/day) and excellent access for postoperative cholangiography. We have been familiar with the technique of cystic duct drainage in open surgery for several years [14], and this experience led us to use it in patients undergoing laparoscopic supraduodenal exploration [15], with no complications to date.

Following completion of the ductal exploration, the cholangiocatheter is replaced by an infant feeding tube (Fr 5–8). This is introduced into the right flank via a large Medicut cannula (Fig. 9.11) and then inserted through the cystic duct well into the common bile duct. The cystic duct is then tied over the tube in continuity using a Roeder slip knot of 0 chromic catgut. A second Roeder slip knot is applied a few millimetres further laterally, but medial to the clip on the gallbladder end of the cystic duct. The cystic duct is then

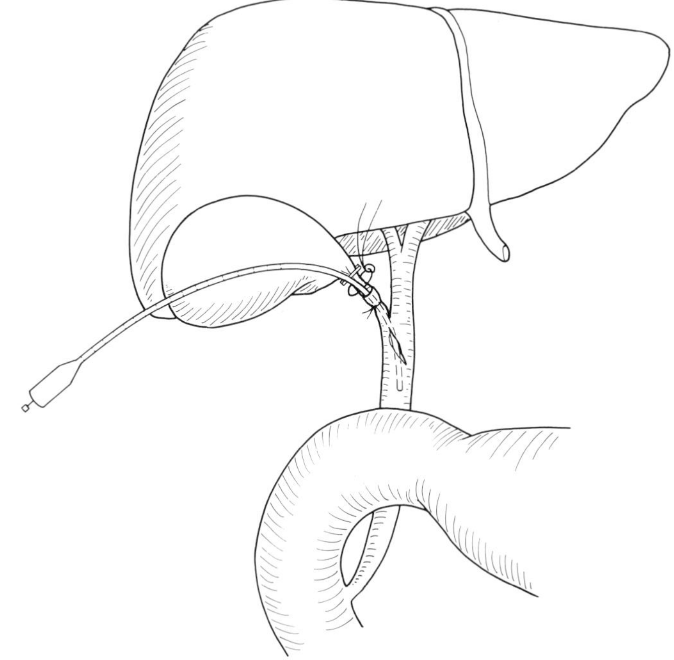

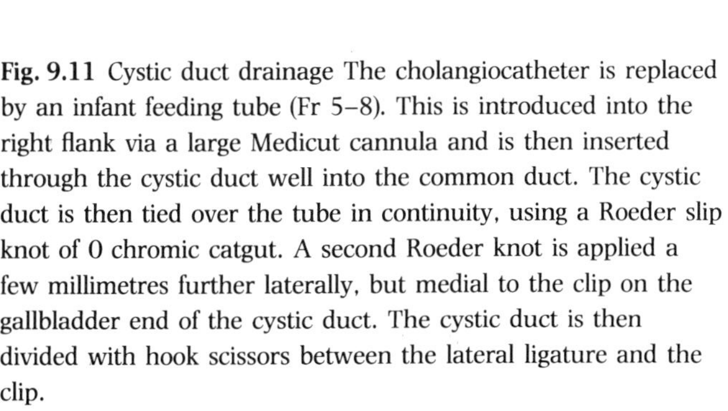

Fig. 9.11 Cystic duct drainage The cholangiocatheter is replaced by an infant feeding tube (Fr 5–8). This is introduced into the right flank via a large Medicut cannula and is then inserted through the cystic duct well into the common duct. The cystic duct is then tied over the tube in continuity, using a Roeder slip knot of 0 chromic catgut. A second Roeder knot is applied a few millimetres further laterally, but medial to the clip on the gallbladder end of the cystic duct. The cystic duct is then divided with hook scissors between the lateral ligature and the clip.

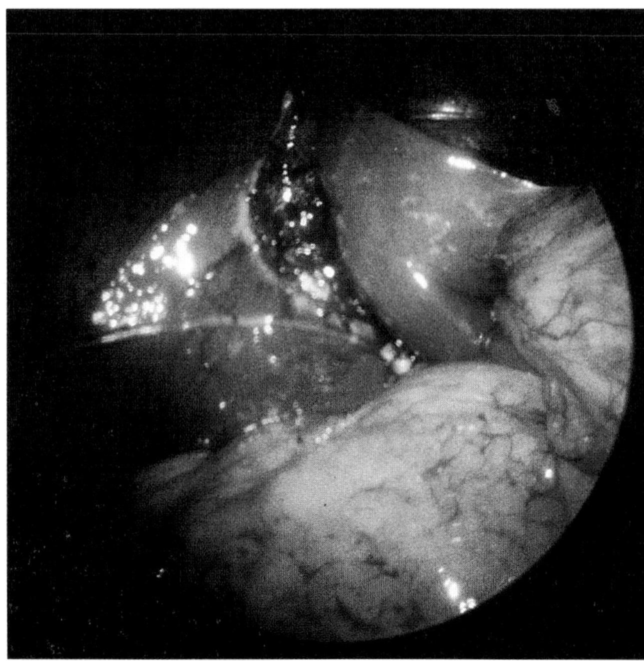

Fig. 9.12 Saline is infused through the cystic duct cannula to ensure patency.

divided with hook scissors between the lateral ligature and the clip. Saline is infused through the cystic duct cannula to ensure patency (Fig. 9.12).

Closure of the choledochotomy

The incision in the common bile duct is then closed by 2 or 3 interrupted 4/0 absorbable sutures. If a T-tube is placed, the choledochotomy is closed above the long limb, which then comes to lie at the bottom of the closed incision (Fig. 9.13). The interrupted knots may consist of the standard surgeon's knot or the tumbled square knot or the Dundee jamming loop knot with a locking hitch. When closure of the duct is complete, saline is injected through the cystic duct cannula or T-tube to ensure a watertight seal.

Fig. 9.13 (a) If a T-tube is placed, the choledochotomy is closed above the long limb which then comes to lie at the bottom of the closed incision. (b) The incision is closed completely when cystic duct drainage is used. (c) T-tube in common bile duct after supraduodenal exploration.

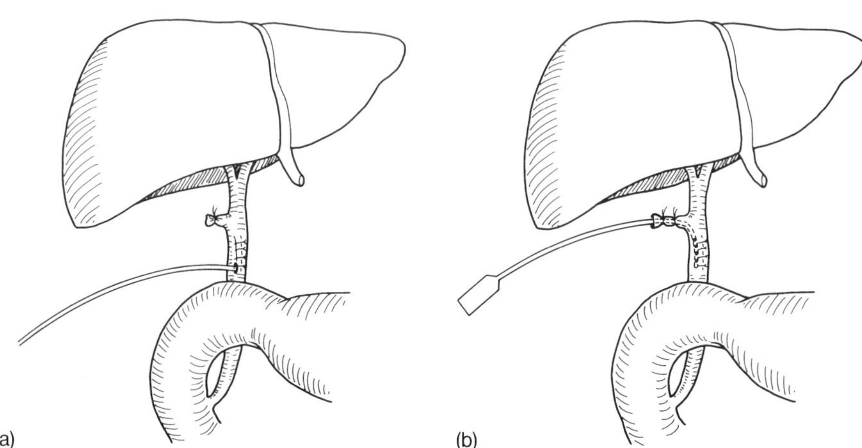

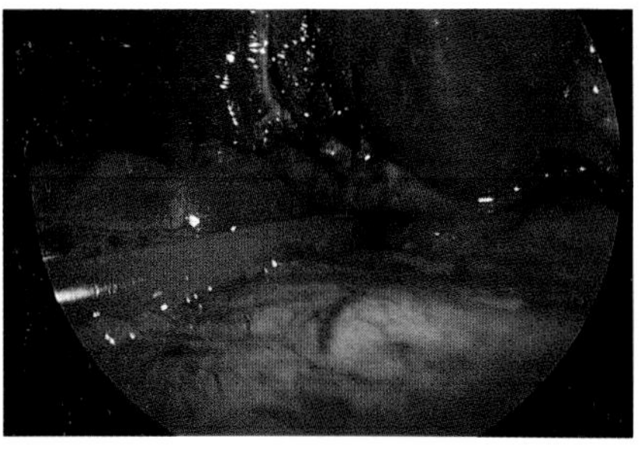

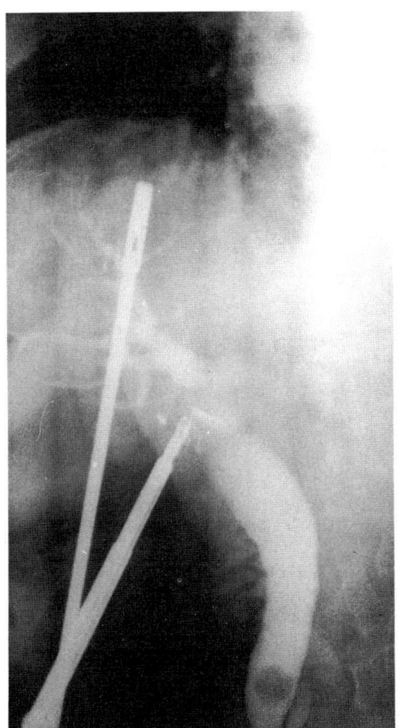

(a)

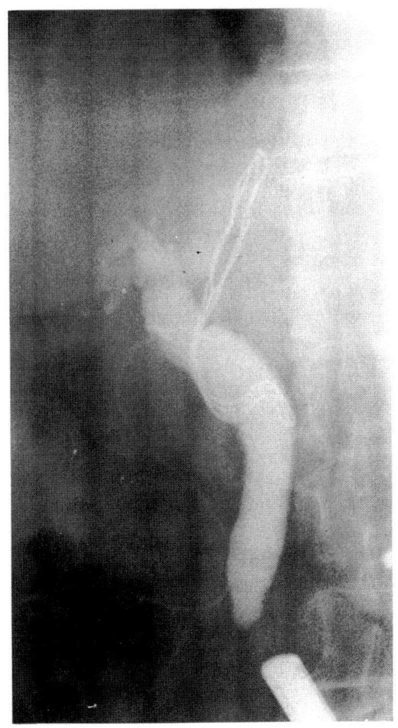

(b)

Fig. 9.14 (a) Intraoperative cholangiogram showing a large stone in the lower end of the common bile duct. (b) Completion cholangiogram after supraduodenal exploration with closure of the duct and cystic duct drainage.

Occluding calculi

We have had to treat a number of patients with large occluding calculi (2–3 cm) impacted at the lower end of the common bile duct after unsuccessful attempts at endoscopic stone extraction. In these patients the following laparoscopic procedure has been employed with successful completion and no complications. A low large vertical choledochotomy is made (commensurate with the size of the stone). On opening the bile duct in these patients we have been surprised with the excessive amount of air (causing frothing of the bile) and mucus emerging from the proximal dilated duct. A biliary balloon catheter (Fr 4–5) is introduced through a large Medicut cannula in the right subxiphoid region and inserted into the bile duct until the tip has negotiated the stone. The balloon is then inflated and traction applied until the stone is dislodged. Several attempts may be required to achieve this. Once the stone is dislodged, its convexity appears at the lower limit of the choledochotomy. Thereafter, the stone is engaged between the closed Semm's spoon biopsy forceps placed on the lateral aspect of the bile duct and the suction probe on its medial side. In this fashion, the stone is milked out of the duct where it is caught by the Semm's spoon forceps and removed. Completion choledochoscopy of the entire biliary tree is then performed. Because of the large choledochotomy and the cholangitis, we have always inserted a Fr 14 T-tube in these cases. Closure of the choledochotomy with interrupted 4/0 Polysorb sutures has to be meticulous to achieve a water-tight anastomosis.

Completion cholangiogram and insertion of drain

A completion contrast study is performed in all cases to confirm ductal clearance (Fig. 9.14). A subhepatic drain is advisable in all these patients. This is introduced through the midclavicular cannula, placed in the subhepatic pouch close to the choledochotomy, and connected to a closed drainage system. Thereafter, the peritoneum is desufflated and the drain and T-tube or cystic duct cannula are sutured to the skin.

Postoperative management

Cystic duct cannula. This is kept on free closed drainage for 48 hours (Fig. 9.15) and then sealed, provided the output from the subhepatic drain is negligible. The patient is observed during the next 12 hours and if the interruption of the external biliary drainage does not result in any increased output from the subhepatic drain, this is removed and the patient discharged home with the sealed cannula protected by an occlusive dressing. The patient returns for a postoperative cholangiogram (Fig. 9.16) 7–10 days later, and if this is satisfactory, the cannula is withdrawn under intravenous sedation.

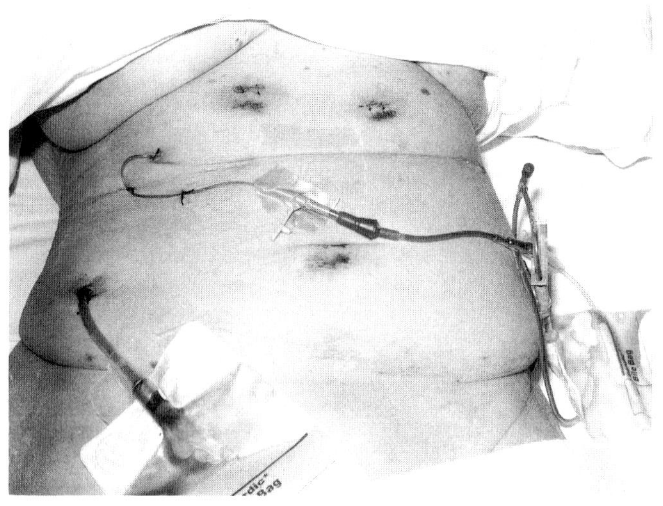

Fig. 9.15 The cystic duct drainage cannula is kept on free closed drainage for 48 hours and then sealed, provided the output from the subhepatic drain is negligible.

Table 9.1 Treatment of ductal calculi encountered during laparoscopic cholecystectomy. Results from seven centres: courtesy of Drs M Arian and S T Ko (Chicago), Dr M Franklin (San Antonio), Dr J Hunter (Salt Lake City), Dr J Petelin (Kansas City), Dr E Phillips (Los Angeles), Dr S Shapiro (Los Angeles) and Dr A. Cuschieri (Dundee)

Surgeon	Total	Cystic duct extraction	CBD exploration	Conversion to open surgery	E.S.*
Arian, Ko	25	16	4	3	2
Cuschieri	35	12	16	1	6
Franklin	27	0	27	0	0
Hunter	26	18	4	4	0
Petelin	65	60	2	1	2
Phillips	66	56	3	4	3
Shapiro	30	24	1	5	0
	274	186(68%)	57(21%)	18(6%)	13(5%)

*Endoscopic sphincterotomy.
CBD = Common bile duct.

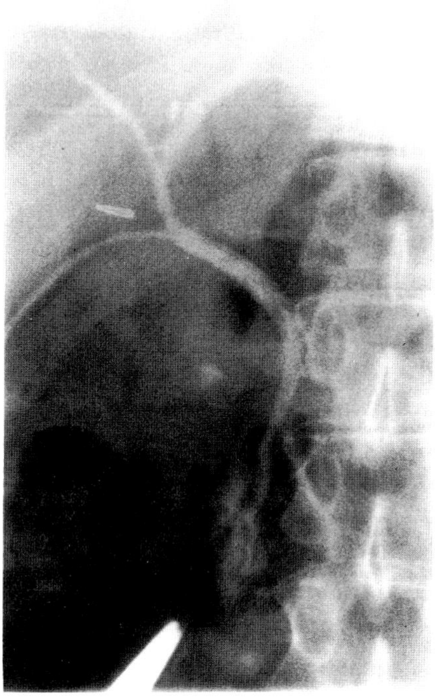

Fig. 9.16 Normal postoperative cholangiogram performed through the cystic duct cannula.

T-tube. The patients with this type of drainage are slower to recover and usually have some ileus, which resolves within 48 hours. They are ready for discharge on the 6th–8th day with the T-tube in place but spigoted. The postoperative cholangiogram may be performed either before discharge or when they return for its removal on the 10th–14th day.

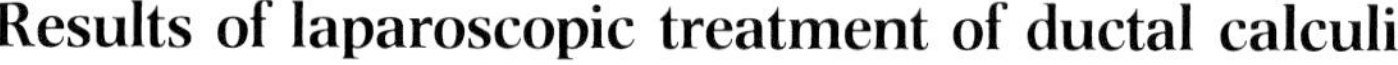

Results of laparoscopic treatment of ductal calculi

The results from seven centres are shown in Table 9.1. In the majority ductal clearance has been achieved via the cystic duct route, which is ideal for small ductal calculi and avoids opening the common duct. Experience with laparoscopic supraduodenal bile duct exploration is more limited and is usually reserved for large stones. There is significant variation in the

Table 9.2 Morbidity and mortality of laparoscopic treatment of ductal calculi ($n = 243$)

Postoperative complication	n (%)
Bile leakage	8(3.2%)
Retained stone	4(1.6%)
Death	3(1.2%)

conversion rate and in the percentage use of postoperative endoscopic sphincterotomy. The Dundee figures reflect the authors' policy of internal drainage in all patients with multiple ductal calculi and significant dilatation of the common bile duct. We also favour endoscopic sphincterotomy in patients with narrow ducts.

Complications of laparoscopic stone removal

Although the reported experience is small, the results to date have been most encouraging, with a low postoperative morbidity and retained stone rate (Table 9.2). Splitting of the cystic duct may result from balloon dilatation. This complication is recognized immediately at operation and is best treated by laparoscopic suture closure of the cystic duct stump. Hyperamylasaemia is common after transcystic removal (20%) but clinically significant pancreatitis is rare. The other complication is bile leakage. This is encountered in 10% of patients after supraduodenal common bile duct exploration, and always resolves provided a subhepatic drain is left in at the time of surgery.

References

1 Schein CJ. *Postcholecystectomy Syndromes.* Harper and Row, Hagerstown, 1978.

2 Neoptolomos JP, Carr-Locke DL, Fossard DL. Prospective randomized study of preoperative endoscopic sphincterotomy versus surgery alone for common bile duct stones. *Br Med J* 1987; **294**: 470–474.

3 Southern Surgeons Club. A prospective analysis of 1518 laparoscopic cholecystectomies. *New Engl J Med* 1991; **324**: 1073–1078.

4 Cuschieri A, Wood RAB, Metcalf MJ, Cumming JGR. Long-term experience with transection choledochoduodenostomy. *World J Surg* 1983; **7**: 502–504.

5 Sackier M. Berci G, Paz-Partlow M. Laparoscopic transcystic choledocholithotomy as an adjunct to laparoscopic cholecystectomy *Am Surg* 1991; **57**: 323–326.

6 Sackier J, Berci G, Phillips E *et al.* The role of cholangiography in laparoscopic cholecystectomy. *Arch Surg* 1991; **126**: 1021–1026.

7 Petelin JB. Laparoscopic approach to common duct pathology. *Surg Laparosc Endosc* 1991; **1**: 33–41.

8 Hunter JG. Laparoscopic transcystic common duct exploration. *Am J Surg* 1992; **163**: 53–58.

9 Berci G, Hamlin AJ. Postoperative removal of retained stones through the T-tube tract. In: Cuschieri A, Berci G (eds) *Common Bile Duct Exploration.* Martinus Nijhoff, Boston, 1984; pp. 89–99.

10 Berci G, Hamlin JA, Daykhovsky L, Sackier J, Paz-Partlow M. Common bile duct lithotripsy. *GI Endosc* 1990; **36**: 137–139.

11 Shapiro SJ, Gordon LA, Daykhovsky L, Grundfest W. Laparoscopic exploration of the common bile duct. *J Laparosc Endosc* 1991; **1**: 333–341.

12 Jacobs M, Verdeja J-C, Goldstein HS. Laparoscopic choledocholithotomy. *J Laparosc Endosc Surg* 1991; **1**: 79–82.

13 Cuschieri A, Berci G. *Common Bile Duct Exploration.* Martinus Nijhoff, Boston, 1984.

14 Shimi S, Banting S, Cuschieri A. Cystic duct drainage after laparoscopic exploration of the common bile duct. *Min Invas Ther* (in press).

15 Holdsworth RJ, Sadek SA, Ambikar S, Baker PR, Cuschieri A. Dynamics of bile flow through the human choledochal sphincter following exploration of the common bile duct. *World J Surg* 1989; **13**: 300–306.

10 : Laparoscopic management of pancreatic cancer

Experience has demonstrated the value of laparoscopy in the diagnosis of hepatobiliary disease, obstructive jaundice [1–5], and in the staging of intra-abdominal malignancy, particularly pancreatic cancer [6–13]. Laparoscopy has been shown to be superior to ultrasound and CT scanning in the detection of small hepatic deposits and peritoneal involvement in these patients. Staging laparoscopy, which has been in long usage in the authors' institution, confers undoubted benefit to patients with pancreatic cancer, since it avoids unnecessary laparotomy in advanced disease while permitting visualization of the tumour by either the supragastric or the infragastric approach [9,14,15], with procurement of biopsy material for histological confirmation of the diagnosis.

Laparoscopic bilioenteric anastomosis is a logical extension of the use of staging laparoscopy in this condition, providing good and efficient palliation of biliary obstruction in advanced pancreatic malignancy, thereby avoiding the need for readmissions necessitated by endoprosthesis-related complications.

Staging laparoscopy

The laparoscopic staging of pancreatic cancer has three components: the detection of hepatic and peritoneal spread (Fig. 10.1), inspection of the tumour, and biopsy confirmation. It requires three access ports: umbilical for the telescope, left paramedian, and right midclavicular at the level of the umbilicus (for graspers, palpating probe and scissors).

The technique of laparoscopic examination of the liver and peritoneal contents for metastatic deposits, and methods available for tissue diagnosis are outlined in Chapter 11. Any free fluid is aspirated in a suction trap and sent for cytological examination. The local assessment of the tumour and visualization of the pancreas is carried out in an orderly fashion as follows:

1 *Inspection of the duodenal loop and head of the pancreas.* This entails lifting the right lobe of the liver and palpating the head of the pancreas and the duodenum. The supraduodenal extension and fixity of the mass are ascertained and the involvement of the duodenum is assessed by lifting the anterior wall with an atraumatic forceps (Fig. 10.2). If hepatic or peritoneal deposits are not evident, a transduodenal biopsy of the mass lesion is performed at this stage, preferably with the spring-loaded Trucut Biopty device. The biopsy needle is introduced percutaneously under visual guidance. The small perforation on the anterior wall of the duodenum is then closed with a single interrupted 3/0 suture.

2 *Inspection of the lesser sac.* The supragastric technique is tried first, especially in thin patients. With the patient in the head-up position, the liver is elevated using a closed forceps or palpating probe to expose the gastrohepatic omentum. A window is cut through an avascular area of the lesser omentum and the closed forceps or palpating probe is advanced into the lesser sac and used to elevate the liver. The 30° forward oblique 10.0 mm

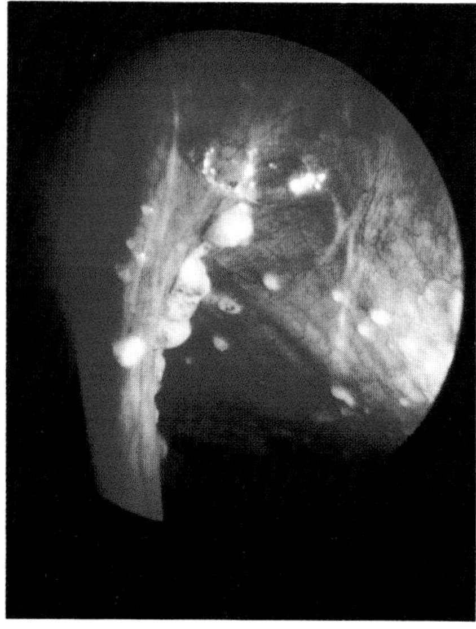

Fig. 10.1 Seedling deposits in the falciform ligament from a primary pancreatic cancer. These small metastatic lesions are not visualized by computed tomography.

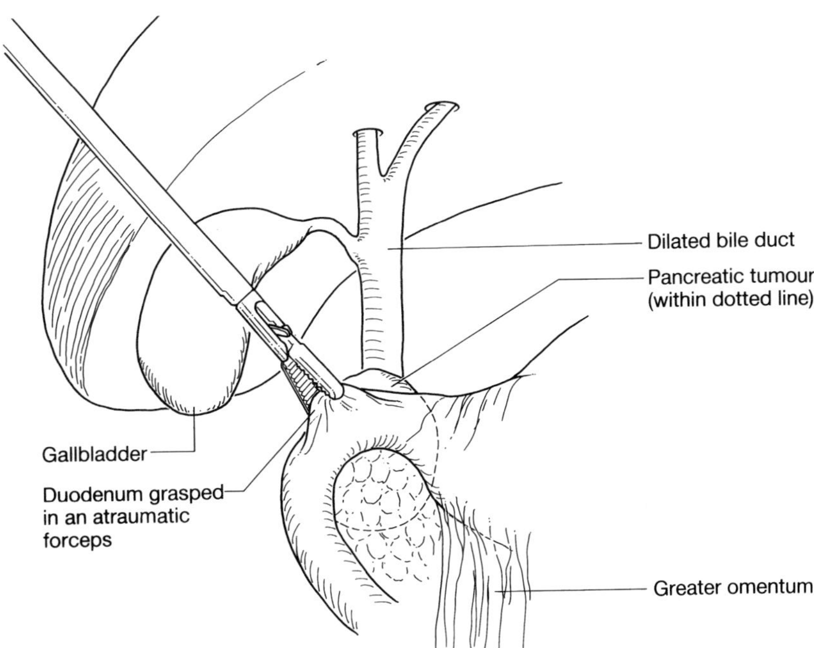

Fig.10.2 Involvement of the duodenum by direct extension of the tumour is assessed by lifting the anterior wall with an atraumatic forceps.

telescope is then advanced for inspection of the neck, body and tail of the pancreas. In some patients, traction of the stomach downwards and anteriorly may be necessary to achieve full inspection of the pancreas.

The infragastric technique gives better visualization of the lesser sac and pancreas but is more technically demanding. Entry into the lesser sac is through an avascular window in the gastrocolic omentum. The probe or closed forceps introduced through the opening into the lesser sac is used to lift up the stomach for inspection of the pancreas by the forward oblique telescope.

Laparoscopic palliation for advanced inoperable cancer of the head of the pancreas

The technique used is based on chronic experiments in pigs, which have enabled the development of safe sutured gastrointestinal and bilioenteric anastomoses undertaken by the laparoscopic route [16]. The method involves the construction of a preformed external jamming loop knot and continuous suturing, using a specially developed endoski needle. In patients with large bile duct obstruction due to advanced incurable cancer of the head of the pancreas, these laparoscopic bypass procedures have the potential for complete palliation, with a short hospital stay, and avoid repeated hospital admissions to deal with the complications of endoscopic stenting, such as encrustation and cholangitis [17].

Indication and timing

The laparoscopic bypass may be conducted during the same session as the staging if the disease is demonstrated to be incurable (presence of hepatic or peritoneal metastases) and the diagnosis is confirmed histologically by frozen section. If the latter is equivocal, it is wise to postpone the endoscopic bilio-enteric bypass until fixed paraffin histology of the lesion or the secondaries has been carried out.

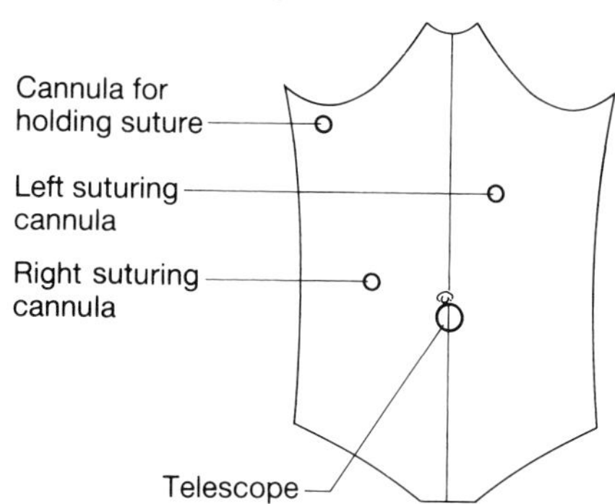

Fig. 10.3 The sites for the trocar/cannulae used for the performance of laparoscopic cholecystojejunostomy. The telescope cannula (11.0 mm) is inserted in the immediate subumbilical region. The right suturing cannula (5.0 mm) is placed along the linea semilunaris well down at the umbilical level, the left one (5.0 mm) half-way up the left paramedian plane. The fourth cannula (5.0 mm) is sited in the right hypochondrium close to the costal margin. It is used by the assistant to hold the tension on the anastomotic line during suturing.

Technique of laparoscopic cholecystojejunostomy

The procedure is conducted with the patient in the supine position and the surgeon operating from the left side. Antibiotic prophylaxis is administered (cephalosporin and metronidazole) after the induction of the pneumoperitoneum. In addition to the trocar/cannulae, the essential instruments are two needle-holders, suture applicator or reducer tube, forward oblique 30° telescope, rubber-shod suture holder, twin-action scissors, suction/aspiration device and electrosurgical hook knife. The Storz dipping endoretractor is a useful accessory for the performance of a choledochojejunostomy.

Access

The sites for the trocar/cannulae used are shown in Fig. 10.3. The telescope cannula (11.0 mm) is inserted in the immediate subumbilical region. The right suturing cannula (5.0 mm) is placed along the linea semilunaris, well down at the umbilical level, and the left one (5.0 mm) half-way up the left paramedian plane. The fourth cannula (5.0 mm) is sited in the right hypochondrium close to the costal margin. This cannula is used by the assistant to hold the suture under tension while suturing is in progress. For this purpose a rubber-shod suture holder (Fig. 10.4) is necessary to avoid damage and fraying of the suture by the grasp of the metal jaws.

Cholecystocholangiogram

The patency of the cystic duct is initially confirmed by a cholecystocholangiogram performed using a Veress needle introduced through the fundus (Chapter 6). After aspiration of the gallbladder bile, 50–70 ml of 20% sodium diatrizoate are injected to outline the biliary tract. This contrast examination is needed to confirm the patency of the cystic duct and the clearance of its insertion from the upper limit of the tumour by at least 1.5 cm (Fig. 10.5). As in open surgery, laparoscopic cholecystojejunostomy is indicated when the junction of the cystic and common hepatic ducts is well clear of the tumour. Otherwise a choledochojejunostomy is performed.

Selection of jejunal loop

A loop of jejunum some 50 cm from the ligament of Treitz is selected for anastomosis to the gallbladder. This is an important step of the procedure. The transverse colon and mesocolon are elevated to reveal the upper jejunum, which is then traced upwards by two graspers until the ligament of Treitz and the duodenojejunal junction are identified. The apex of the selected loop is then grasped and brought up antecolically to the gallbladder to ensure sufficient reach, which will enable the performance of an anastomosis between the two organs without tension.

Type of anastomosis

The bilioenteric anastomosis is performed using a single-layer technique with deep seromuscular absorbable 3/0 sutures (Polysorb or coated polyglactin) mounted on endoski needles. Two sutures are used, one for the posterior and the other for the anterior part of the anastomosis.

An alternative technique consists of using the EndoGIA (US Surgical Corporation) to effect a stapled anastomosis, with closure of the residual defect at the site of insertion of the stapler heads by hand suturing.

Technique of hand-sutured anastomosis

The ideal length of suture is 30 cm. A preformed jamming loop knot is fashioned externally with the knot slipping from the tail (Fig. 10.6). This requires 10.0 cm of length from the tail to fashion and draw easily. The suture is then grasped by a 3.0 mm needle-holder and loaded inside a suture applicator for introduction into the peritoneal cavity. The needle is then

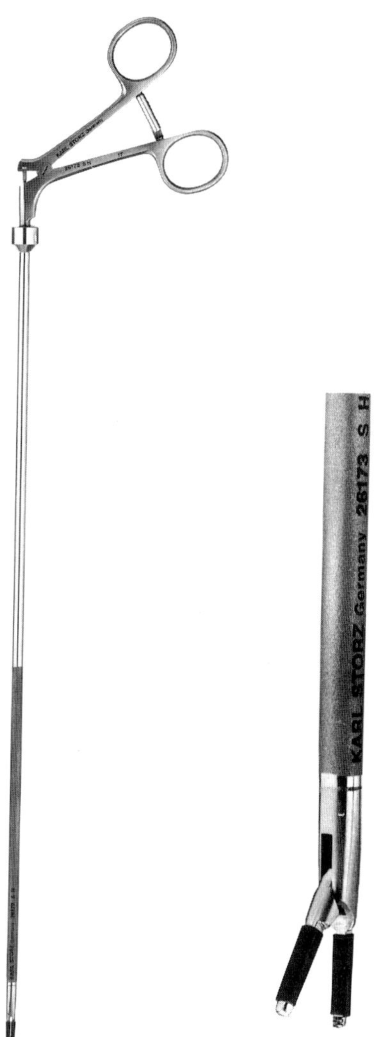

Fig. 10.4 Rubber-shod suture holder.

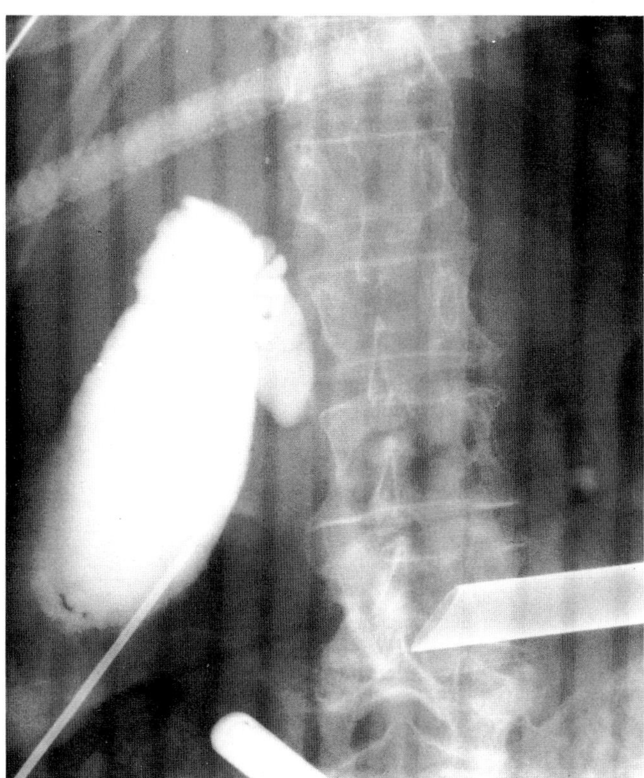

Fig. 10.5 Laparoscopic cholecystocholangiogram showing a patent cystic duct with its insertion well proximal to the upper limit of the tumour.

grasped by the 5.0 mm needle-holder, and after passage through the seromuscular layer of the jejunum and the gallbladder, the suture is pulled until the jamming loop knot impinges on the jejunum. The two organs are approximated with further traction on the suture (Fig. 10.7), and while tension on this is maintained, one of the needle-holders is introduced through the loop (Fig. 10.8) and used to grasp the standing part of the suture which is then pulled through the jamming loop (Fig. 10.9). The loop is then slipped (closed) on the suture from the tail and the knot locked by pulling first the suture and then the tail against counter-traction on the knot by the open jaws of the needle-holder (Fig. 10.10). A continuous posterior seromuscular approximation over a distance of 3.0 cm is next carried out with the assistant holding tension on the suture line (Fig. 10.11). The suturing technique involves the use of the 5.0 mm needle-holder as the active driver with the other needle-holder being used to apply counter-traction on the tissue to facilitate needle passage and to pick up the needle after it emerges through the tissues before transfer to the active needle-holder. The individual suture bites have to be inserted in a deep seromuscular fashion and be evenly spaced. The last but one suture bite is locked, and following a further passage of the needle through the two organs, the suture is tied using the Aberdeen knot (Fig. 10.12). Although the needle can be cut off at this stage leaving a long tail, it is advantageous to leave the needle *in situ*, in case the anterior suture is too short or breaks during the performance of the final part of the anastomosis. If braided polyglactin is used, the terminal Aberdeen knot may be replaced by two locking bites (Fig. 10.13). If this alternative

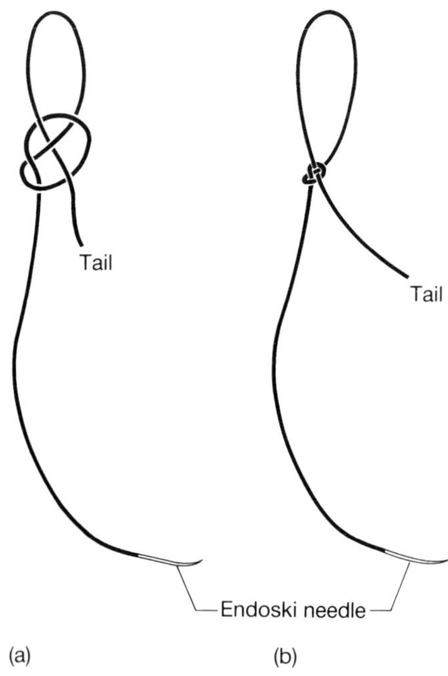

Fig. 10.6 Dundee jamming loop knot fashioned near the tail of the suture: (a) loose, (b) drawn.

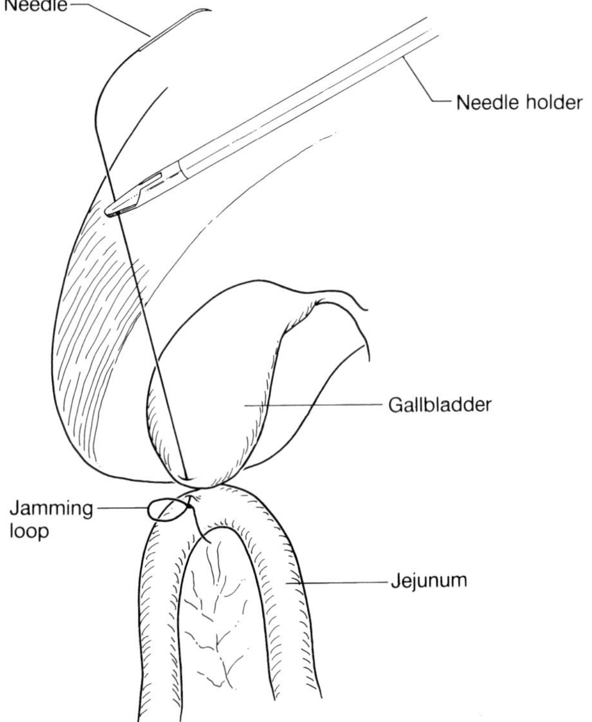

Fig. 10.7 After passage of the needle through the seromuscular layers, the two organs are approximated by traction on the suture.

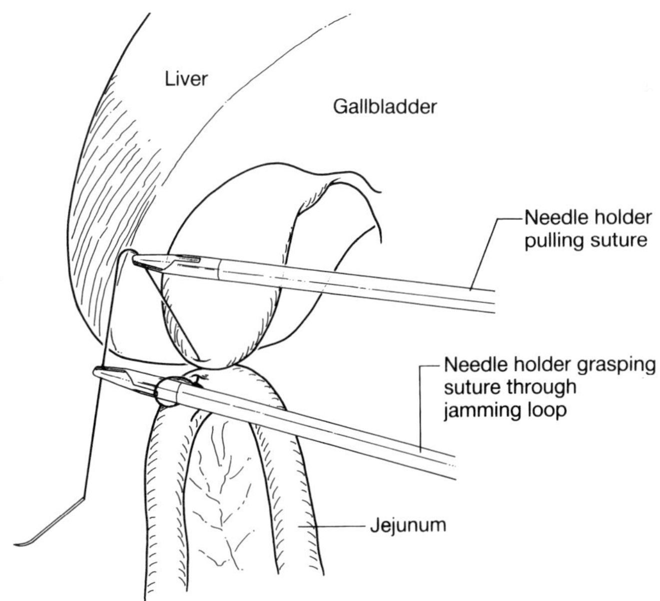

Fig. 10.8 While tension on the suture is maintained, the lower needle-holder is introduced through the loop and used to grasp the standing part of the suture.

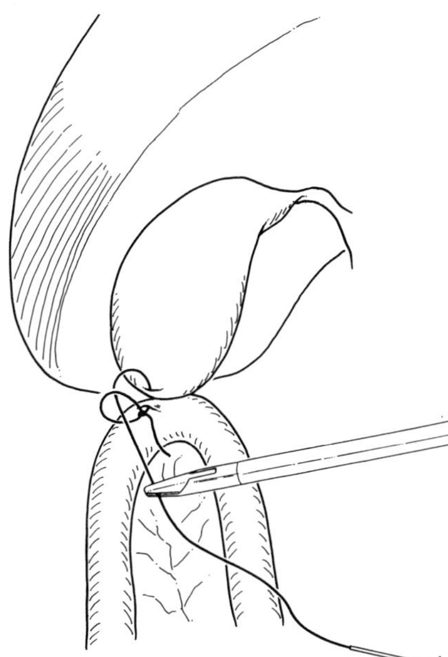

Fig. 10.9 The suture and needle trailing behind it are then pulled through the jamming loop.

is employed, it is important that the posterior suture line is checked for slippage and tightened accordingly, before the final knot joining the two sutures (anterior and posterior) is completed. *The authors do not recommend the practice of applying clips to hold the suture as in order to secure a good grip, the clip has to deform and damage the suture.*

The seromuscular layer of the gallbladder is then incised over a distance of 2.5 cm with the electrosurgical hook knife using a blender monopolar current 0.5 cm anterior and parallel to the completed suture line. With the sucker in place, a small cut is made with the twin-action scissors in the mucosa, the sucker tip is introduced into the gallbladder lumen and the bile is aspirated. The mucosal cut is then extended and the interior wall of the gallbladder inspected and thoroughly irrigated with Hartmann's solution to ensure the removal of all debris and blood clots. Any bleeding from the cut gallbladder wall has to be secured by soft electrocoagulation. The enterotomy is fashioned to an equivalent length and with the same technique, but the intraluminal irrigation step is avoided. With the jejunum attached to the gallbladder, which keeps it tented high up, leakage from the enterotomy does not occur. The anterior wall of the anastomosis is performed using a similar technique. The first suture and jamming loop knot are inserted lateral to the start of the posterior suture line (Fig. 10.14). Once the end of the anterior approximation has been reached (Fig. 10.15), the suture is tied to the tail of the posterior suture using a standard microsurgical knot (Fig. 10.16). The laparoscopic appearances of the various stages of the anastomosis are illustrated in Fig. 10.17 a–f. The completed anastomosis (Fig. 10.18) is inspected closely for defects and the subhepatic pouch and peritoneal gutters are then aspirated and irrigated with Hartmann's solution.

Technique of stapled–sutured anastomosis

A different technique is used to perform a stapled/sutured anastomosis. Two stay sutures introduced through the anterior abdominal wall are inserted at the proposed limits of the anastomosis between the two organs (Fig. 10.19). A small opening is then made on each organ and the EndoGIA (United States Surgical Corporation) inserted, the staple heads are approximated and the instrument is fired (Fig. 10.20). After checking the stapled anastomotic line, the anterior defect is closed with a running suture as described above.

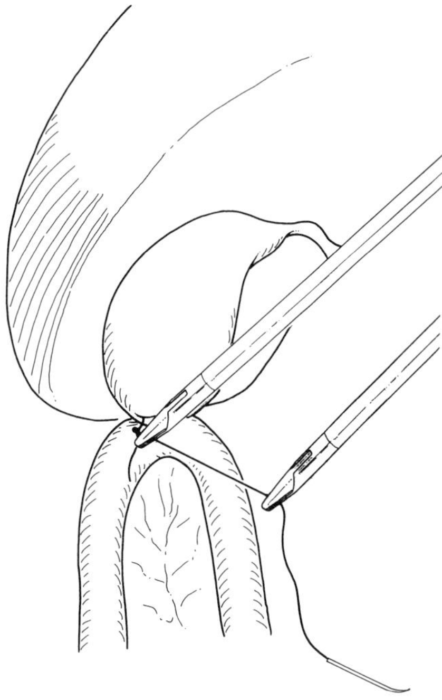

Fig. 10.10 The loop is then slipped (closed) on the suture from the tail and the knot locked by pulling first the suture and then the tail against counter-traction on the knot by the open jaws of the needle-holder.

Choledochojejunostomy

A choledochojejunostomy is undertaken if the drainage of the cystic duct is close to the upper limit of the tumour as demonstrated by the cholecystocholangiogram. The position of the patient is identical to that used for cholecystojejunostomy, and, likewise, the surgeon stands on the left side of the patient. However, an extra cannula (right subxiphoid) is needed for upward retraction of the quadrate lobe (Fig. 10.21) to expose the porta hepatis. The view of the operative field is further enhanced if the abdominal wall–round ligament sling-lift is employed (Chapter 4). The use of the Storz dipping endoretractor is also helpful in this situation.

The suturing technique is otherwise the same as outlined above. As the common hepatic duct is enlarged and prominent (Fig. 10.22), no dissection is necessary and the incision on its anterior wall is made in a transverse direction, using either the retractable diamond knife or curved microscissors (Fig. 10.23). The continuous flow of bile may obscure the field; this problem

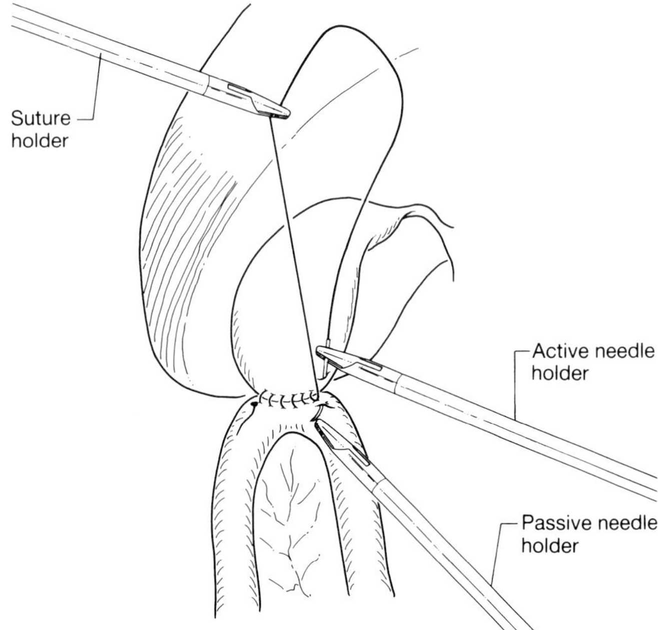

Fig. 10.11 A continuous posterior seromuscular approximation over a distance of 3.0 cm is next carried out with the assistant holding tension on the suture line.

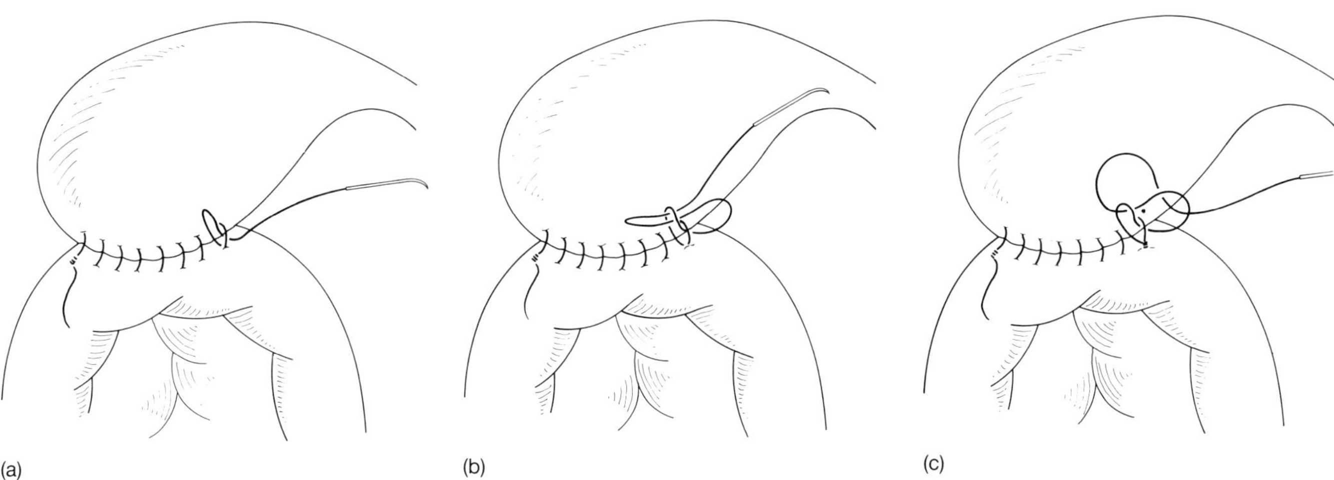

Fig. 10.12 Terminal Aberdeen knot. (a) First locking loop. (b) Second locking loop. This is created after the first loop has been tightened. (c) Third locking loop with the suture pulled through the loop. The knot is tightened against counter-traction by the needle-holder.

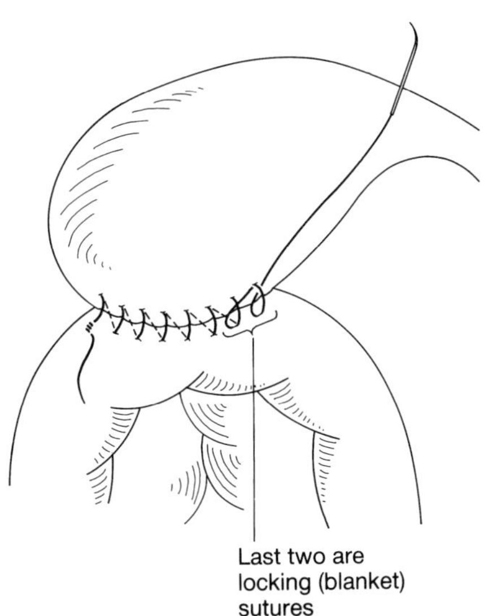

Fig. 10.13 If braided polyglactin is used, the terminal Aberdeen knot may be replaced by two locking bites. If this alternative is employed, it is important that the posterior suture line is checked for slippage and tightened accordingly, before the final knot joining the two sutures (anterior and posterior) is completed.

is resolved by inserting a biliary balloon catheter high up and inflating the balloon with air. This occlusion of the proximal common hepatic duct just below the bifurcation (Fig. 10.24) is maintained until the posterior suture line is nearing completion, when the balloon is deflated and the catheter removed.

Anterior gastrojejunostomy

If a double bypass is needed, the cholecystojejunostomy is performed first and the gastrojejunostomy second. In this fashion the first anastomosis results in automatic approximation of the jejunal loop to the anterior wall of the stomach. The selected loop has to be of sufficient length, usually with its apex some 50–60 cm from the ligament of Treitz. Although the authors have conducted this technique in animals, none of our patients has had duodenal obstruction at the time of the creation of the bilioenteric anastomosis, or developed this complication of the disease subsequently but we have performed this anastomosis in patients with inoperable distal gastric cancer. The escape of CO_2 and loss of the pneumoperitoneum when the stomach is opened is obviated by the use of the Sengstaken or Minnesota trilumen tube. Once in place, the gastric balloon is inflated (preferably with saline) and traction is then applied and maintained to seal the gastro-oesophageal junction (Fig. 10.25) until the anastomosis is completed. Suction is applied through the gastric port to empty the stomach before it is opened.

The antecolic anastomosis between the jejunum and the stomach is performed at least 3.0 cm proximal to the duodenal occlusion. The anastomosis can be stapled (EndoGIA) or sutured using techniques similar to those outlined above. If bleeding is encountered from the stapled line, this is controlled by interrupted sutures. *On no account must electrocoagulation be applied to the stapled anastomotic line.*

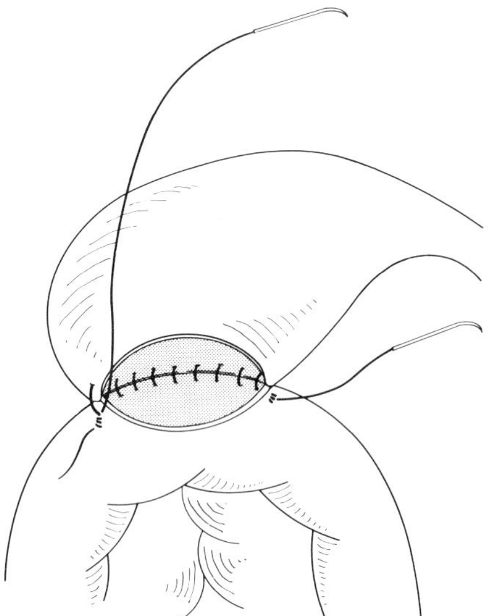

Fig. 10.14 Anterior suture line. The first suture and jamming loop knot are inserted lateral to the start of the posterior suture line.

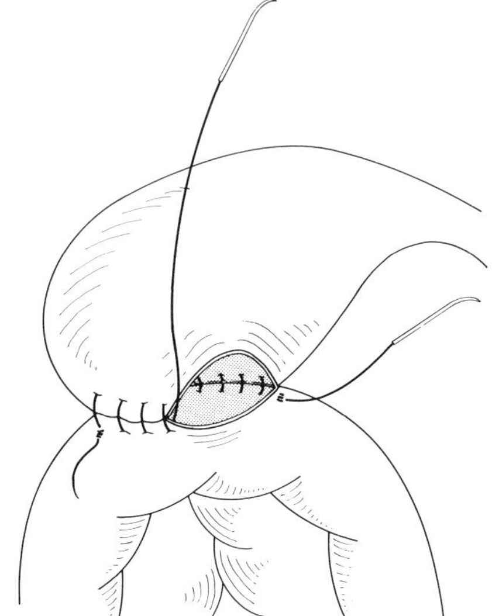

Fig. 10.15 The approximation of the anterior walls of the gallbladder and jejunum is effected using a similar deep seromuscular suturing technique.

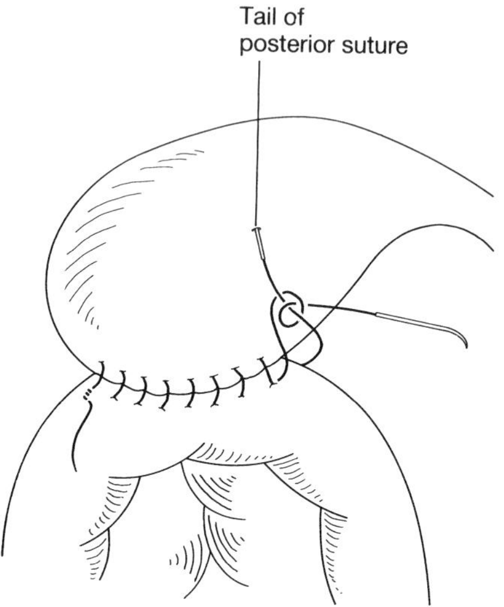

Fig. 10.16 Once the anterior suture line has been completed, the suture is tied to the posterior tail using a standard microsurgical knot.

Postoperative course and outcome

The authors' clinical experience with bilioenteric bypass is limited to six patients, none of whom had duodenal obstruction. The postoperative period was uncomplicated in five patients, who progressed rapidly with minimal ileus and early discharge. The functional patency of the anastomosis was confirmed by biliary scintiscanning (Fig. 10.26) performed in the post-operative period. In one patient, after an initial fall, the bilirubin remained elevated. Both a percutaneous transhepatic cholangiogram and a biliary scintiscan confirmed a non-functioning anastomosis. At reintervention, the otherwise intact anastomosis was found to be obstructed by a bolus of debris and blood clot. This was aspirated and the incision in the gallbladder closed. The patient made a speedy recovery with complete resolution of the jaundice after this minimal procedure. This patient demonstrates the importance of adequate irrigation of the lumen of the gallbladder and meticulous haemostasis during the creation of laparoscopic bilioenteric bypass.

One patient subsequently received supervoltage radiotherapy and three have required a percutaneous coeliac-axis phenol nerve block for pain. All the patients have remained anicteric and none of them has required readmission for cholangitis subsequent to their discharge.

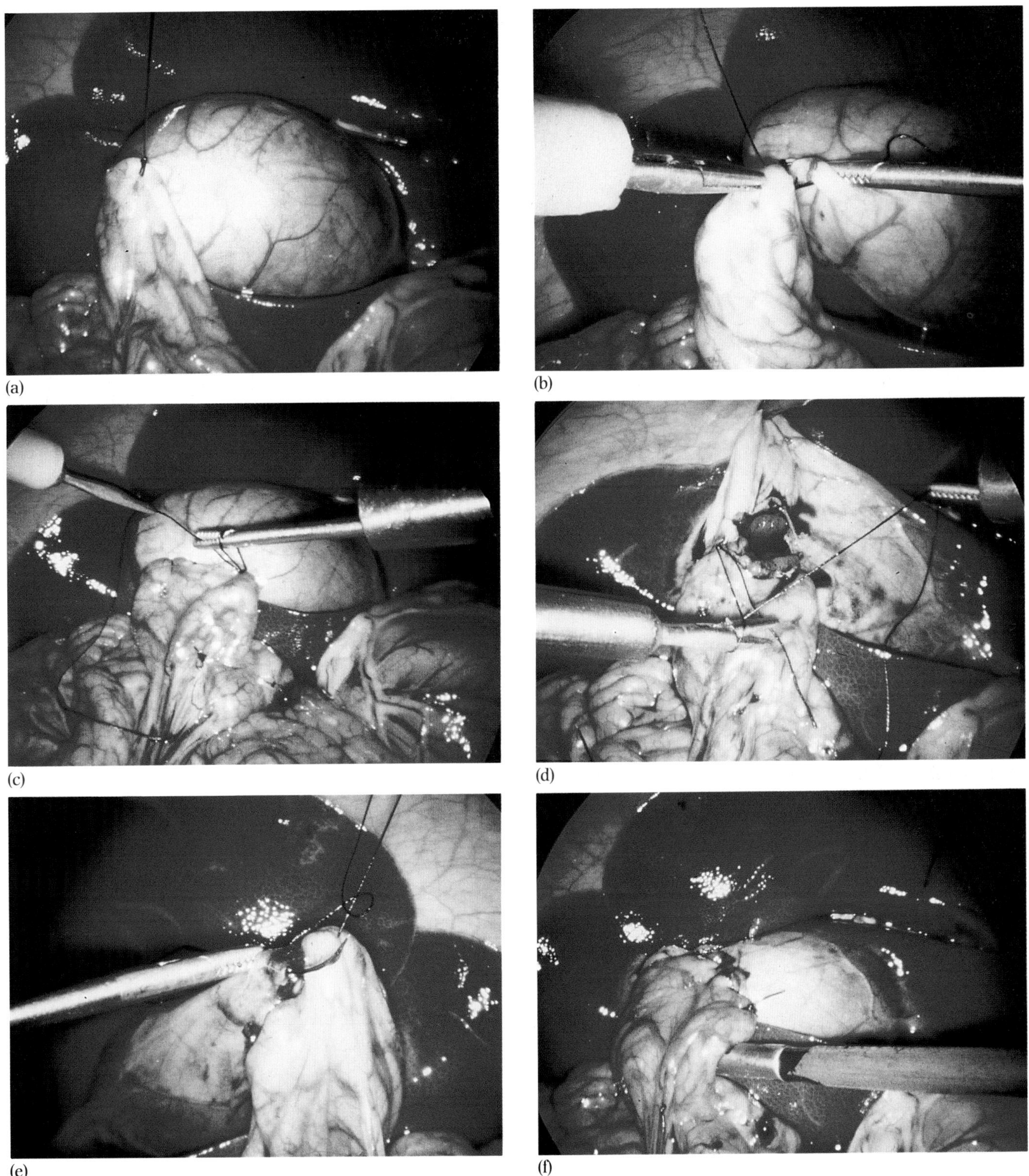

Fig. 10.17 The laparoscopic appearances of the various stages of the anastomosis in the pig. (a) Initial starter knot. (b) Posterior suture line. (c) Aberdeen terminal knot. (d) Opened lumen of the gallbladder and jejunum. (e) Anterior suture line and completed anastomosis.

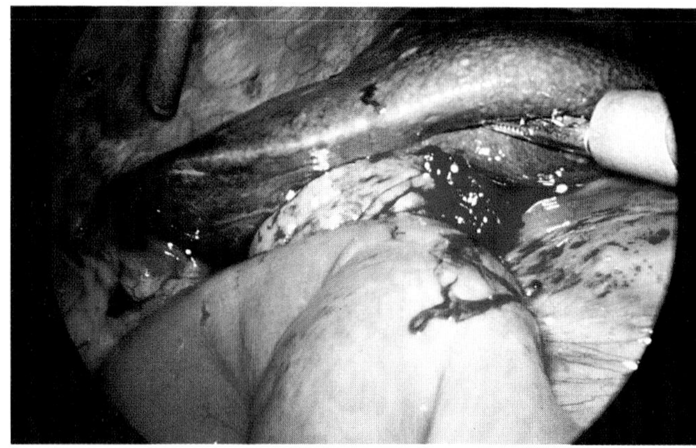

Fig. 10.18 Completed cholecystojejunostomy in a patient with advanced cancer of the head of the pancreas.

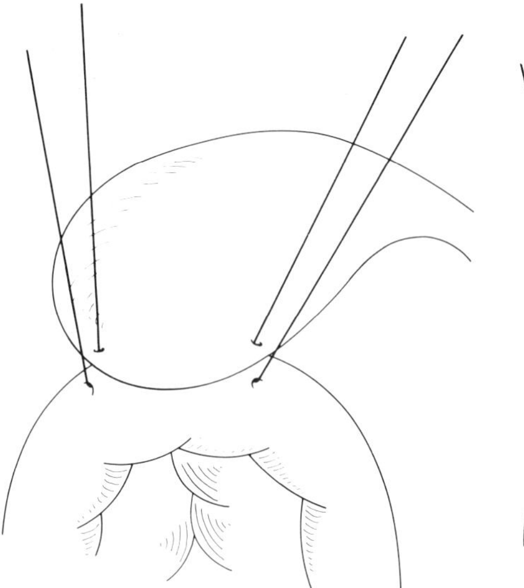

Fig. 10.19 Stapled sutured cholecystojejunostomy. Two stay sutures introduced through the anterior abdominal wall are inserted at the proposed limits of the anastomosis between the two organs.

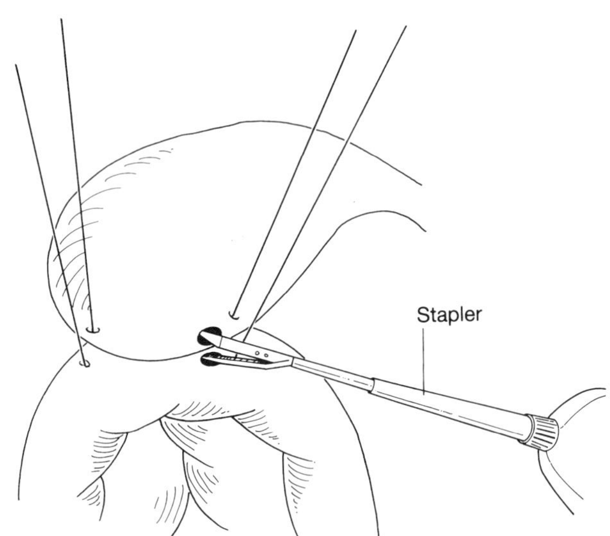

Fig. 10.20 A small opening is then made in each organ and the EndoGIA (United States Surgical Corporation) inserted, the staple heads are approximated and the instrument is fired.

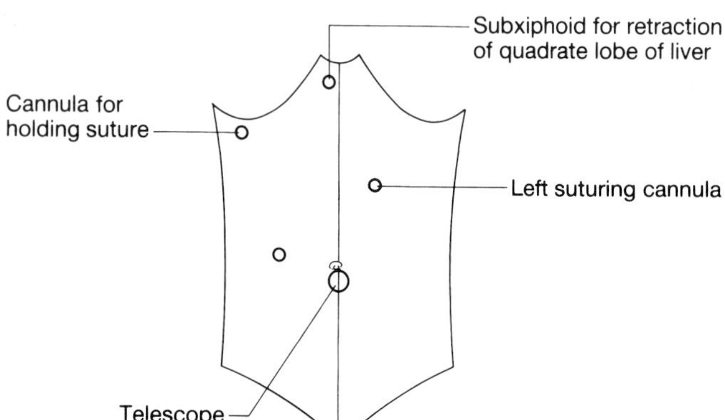

Fig. 10.21 Cannula sites for choledochojejunostomy. The extra right subxiphoid port is needed for retraction of the quadrate lobe of the liver.

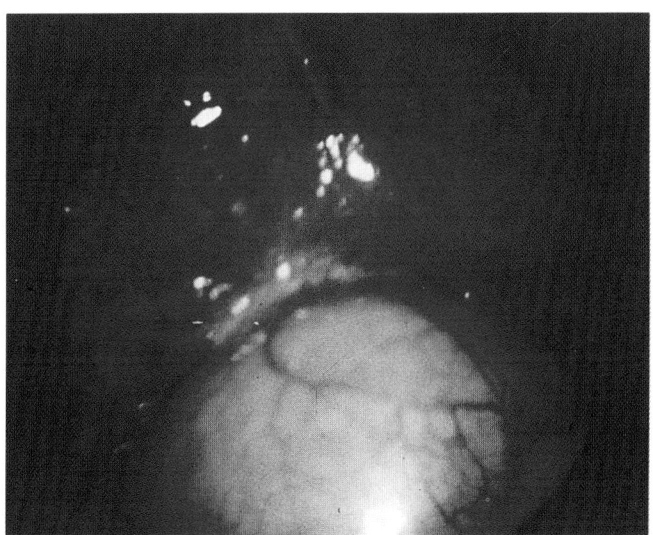

Fig. 10.22 Grossly dilated and prominent common hepatic duct in a patient with advanced cancer of the pancreas.

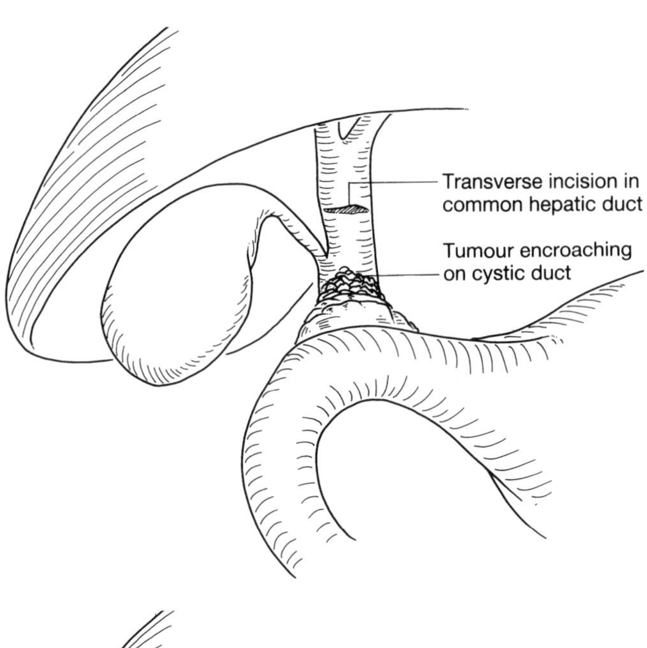

Fig. 10.23 The incision on its anterior wall is made in a transverse direction, using either the retractable diamond knife or curved microscissors.

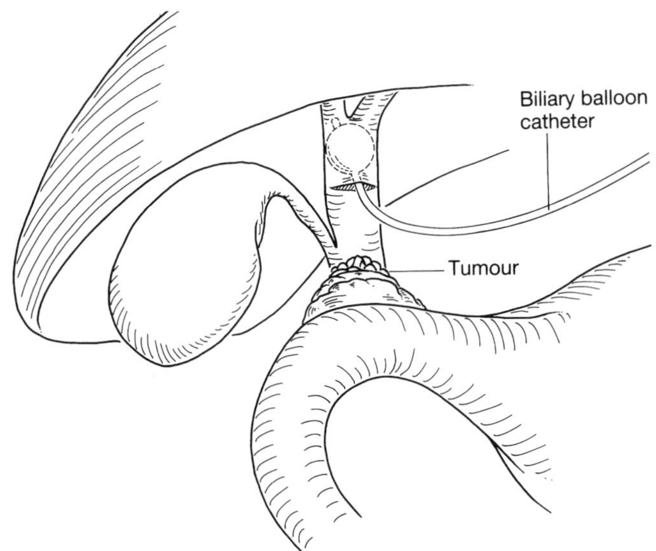

Fig. 10.24 Occlusion of the proximal common hepatic duct just below the bifurcation by a biliary balloon catheter is maintained until the posterior suture line is nearing completion, when the balloon is deflated and the catheter removed.

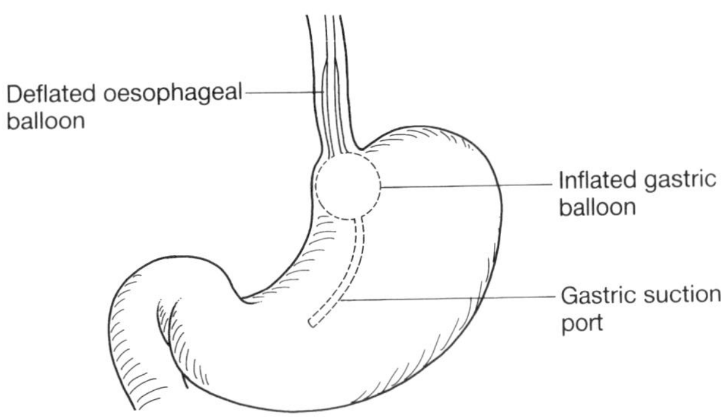

Fig. 10.25 Use of the trilumen tube for laparoscopic gastrojejunostomy to prevent loss of pneumoperitoneum after the stomach is opened. Once in place, the gastric balloon is inflated (preferably with saline) and traction is then applied and maintained to seal the gastro-oesophageal junction until the anastomosis is completed. Suction is applied through the gastric port to empty the stomach before it is opened.

References

1 Berci G, Morgenstern L, Shore JM, Shapiro S. A direct approach to the differential diagnosis of jaundice. Laparoscopy with transhepatic cholecystocholangiography. *Am J Surg* 1973; **126**: 372–378.

2 Cuschieri A. Value of laparoscopy in hepatobiliary disease. *Ann Roy Coll Surg Eng* 1975; **57**: 33–38.

3 Irving AD, Cuschieri A. Laparoscopic assessment of the jaundiced patient. *Br J Surg* 1978; **65**: 678–680.

4 Cuschieri A. Laparoscopy in general surgery and gastroenterology. *Br J Hosp Med* 1980; **24**: 252–258.

5 Berci G, Jensen D. Laparoscopy for the hepatologist and general surgeon. *Acta Endoscopica* 1982; **12**: 3–12.

6 Lightdale CJ. Clinical application of laparoscopy in patients with malignant neoplasms. *Gastrointest Endosc* 1982; **28**: 99–102.

7 Shandall A, Johnson C. Laparoscopy or scanning in oesophageal and gastric carcinoma? *Br J Surg* 1985; **22**: 449–451.

8 Possik RA, Fraco EL, Pires DR *et al.* Sensitivity, specificity and predictive value of laparoscopy for the staging of gastric cancer and for the detection of liver metastases. *Cancer* 1986; **58**: 1–6.

9 Cuschieri A, Hall AW, Clark J. Value of laparoscopy in the diagnosis and management of pancreatic cancer. *Gut* 1978; **19**: 672–677.

10 Ishida H, Furukawa Y, Kuroda H *et al.* Laparoscopic observation and biopsy of the pancreas. *Endoscopy* 1981; **13**: 68–73.

11 Ishida H. Peritoneoscopy and pancreas biopsy in the diagnosis of pancreatic disease. *Gastrointest Endosc* 1983; **29**: 211–218.

12 Warshaw AL, Tepper JE, Shipley WU. Laparoscopy in the staging and planning of therapy for pancreatic cancer. *Am J Surg* 1986; **158**: 76–80.

13 Cuschieri A. Laparoscopy for pancreatic cancer: does it benefit the patient? *Eur J Surg Oncol* 1988; **14**: 41–44.

14 Meyer-Burg J, Ziegler U, Palma C. Zur supragastralen Pankreaskopie. Ergebnisse aus 125 Laparoskopien. *Deutsch Med Wochenschr* 1969; **97**: 1969–1971.

15 Strauch M, Lux G, Ottenjann R. Infragastric pancreascopy. *Endoscopy* 1973; **5**: 30–32.

16 Nathanson LK, Shimi S, Cuschieri A. Sutured laparoscopic cholecystojejunostomy evolved in an animal model. *J Surg Res* (in press).

17 Shimi S, Banting S, Cuschieri A. Laparoscopy in the management of pancreatic cancer: endoscopic cholecystojejunostomy for advanced disease. *Br J Surg* 1992; **79**: 317–319.

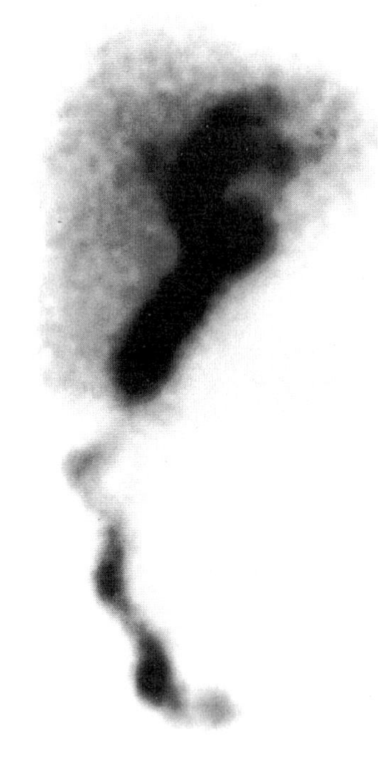

Fig. 10.26 Biliary scintiscan after a laparoscopic cholecystojejunostomy showing a functioning anastomosis.

11 : Diagnostic laparoscopy, tissue diagnosis and other procedures

There are few diagnostic modalities which provide as much useful information on the liver, biliary tract, pancreas and peritoneal cavity as laparoscopy. It is of particular benefit in oncology [1–3] and it is indeed surprising that laparoscopy is not used routinely in the management of patients with intra-abdominal malignancy. The current prevalent practice in these patients is the use of computed tomographic (CT) scanning followed by percutaneous guided-needle biopsy if a localized lesion is encountered in the liver, porta hepatis or pancreas. This requires a second CT examination and in approximately 50% of cases, the needle aspiration is non-informative due to inadequate cell yield. Instead of this costly repeat process, a laparoscopic examination will provide direct visualization of the lesion, permit a more reliable tissue sample and often provide information which is valuable in staging the disease and in establishing dissemination and inoperability. There is no radiological imaging technique that can detect peritoneal seedlings or small metastatic deposits in the liver with the same reliability as laparoscopy [4,5].

Diagnostic laparoscopy should be an integral part of general surgical practice [6]. Over many years the authors have found it particularly useful in influencing patient management in several clinical situations. These are shown in Table 11.1.

Table 11.1 Conditions in which management is often influenced by diagnostic laparoscopy

Acute
Trauma
Acute right iliac fossa pain, particularly in females of childbearing age
Suspicion of mesenteric infarction
Undiagnosed peritonism
Cold
Hepatobiliary disease
Primary and secondary liver tumours
Staging of intra-abdominal cancers: pancreatic, gastric, oesophageal and colorectal
Palpable abdominal mass
Ascites of unknown origin
Unexplained weight loss
Chronic abdominal pain
Second-look assessment (treated malignancy)

Laparoscopic evaluation of liver disease

There are many reports [7–9] and classic atlases [10] which document the usefulness of diagnostic laparoscopy in the evaluation of both benign and malignant liver disease.

Chronic liver disease

The benefits of laparoscopy in the assessment of chronic liver disease include visual information on the macroscopic appearance of the liver (Fig. 11.1), its size, the nature of its surface nodularity and the presence of portal hypertension and splenomegaly. At the same time, it increases the scope for multiple biopsies of both the diseased hepatic parenchyma and any suspect lesions. Apart from the targeted nature of the biopsy, bleeding, which may complicate the procedure particularly in patients with advanced chronic liver disease with impaired clotting function and thrombocytopenia, is easily dealt with by compression and the use of electrocoagulation whenever necessary. In this respect there is no doubt that laparoscopic biopsy is safer and has a higher diagnostic yield than the blind percutaneous procedure. The combined visual appearance of the liver, together with histological examination of the liver biopsies, results in a firm diagnosis in virtually all patients.

Laparoscopy is of particular value in patients with ascites (Fig. 11.2). The nature of the ascitic fluid—serous, bile-stained, chylous or haemorrhagic—its

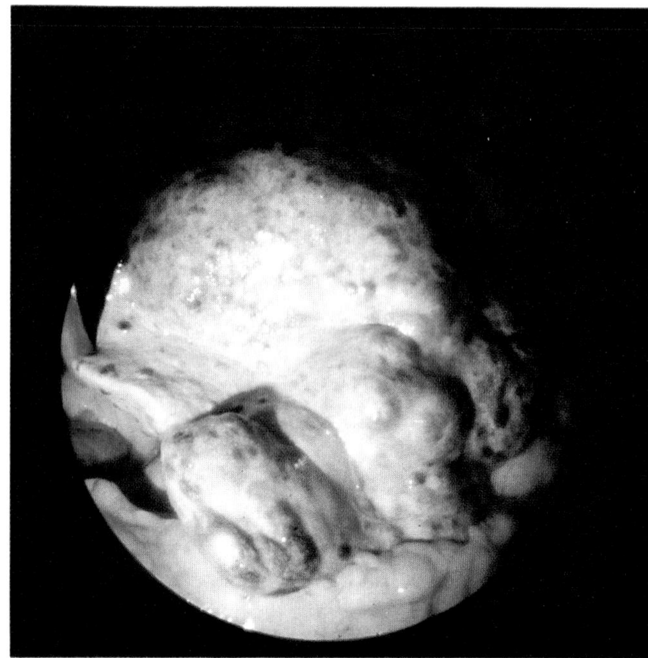

Fig. 11.1 Haemochromatosis in Wilson's disease.

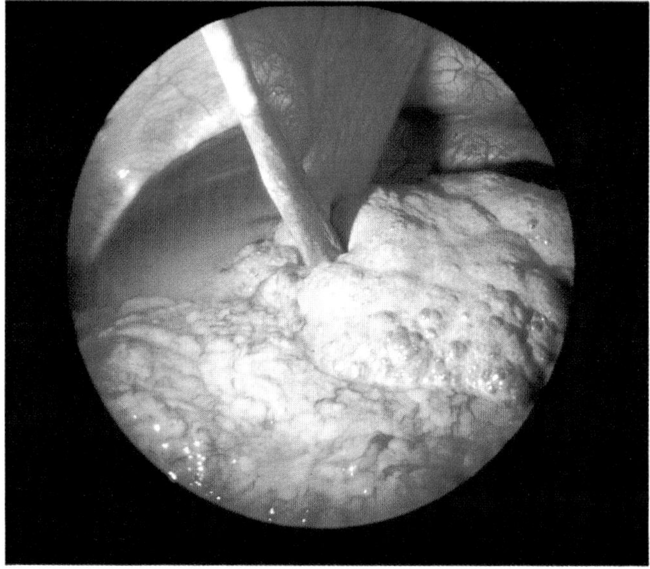

Fig. 11.2 Chylous ascites in a cirrhotic patient.

cellular composition and the state of the peritoneal lining (inflammation or nodular deposits) obtained by laparoscopy help to establish the exact cause in the individual patient. There is one practical point which needs stressing in patients undergoing diagnostic laparoscopy for ascites: the air-filled small bowel loops float on the surface of the ascitic fluid and thereby become closely opposed to the anterior abdominal wall (Fig. 11.3). This enhances the risk of bowel injury by the Veress needle during the creation of the pneumoperitoneum unless special precautions are taken. One way around this problem is the use of open laparoscopy. The alternative is the careful insertion of the Veress needle unconnected to any tubing and with the tap

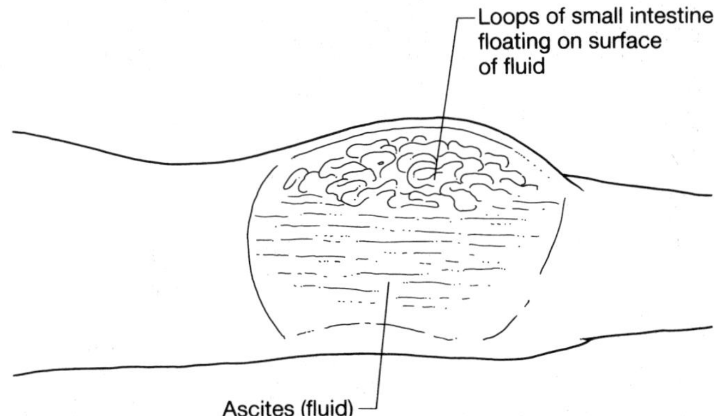

Fig. 11.3 In patients with gross ascites, the air-filled small bowel loops float on the surface of the ascitic fluid and thereby become opposed to the anterior abdominal wall. This enhances the risk of bowel injury by the Veress needle during the creation of the pneumoperitoneum.

opened. In this way, ascitic fluid will spurt out as soon as the tip of the Veress needle enters the peritoneal cavity. Enough ascitic fluid (1.0–2.0 l) should be released to reduce the intra-abdominal pressure and fluid volume, before insufflation is started and the trocar/cannula inserted. During laparoscopic inspection, more fluid may need to be aspirated to ensure a thorough examination of the peritoneal cavity and its contents.

In patients with chronic liver disease and suspected obstruction of the biliary tract, laparoscopic cholangiography—transhepatic or through the gallbladder—can be performed during the same operation [11–13].

Hepatic malignancy

Laparoscopy is extremely valuable in the diagnosis, assessment and histological confirmation of both primary and secondary hepatic tumours.

In primary liver tumours information is gained on the state of the hepatic parenchyma (normal or cirrhotic), the exact location, size, sectorial involve-

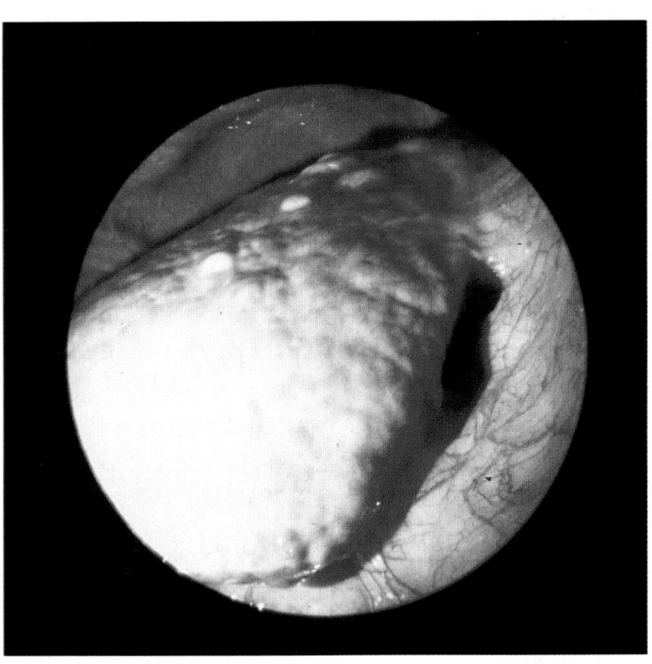

Fig. 11.4 Multicentric hepatoma (small white nodules) in a cirrhotic liver (from Moosa *et al.* (eds) *Comprehensive Textbook of Oncology*. © 1991, the Williams & Wilkins Co., Baltimore, with permission).

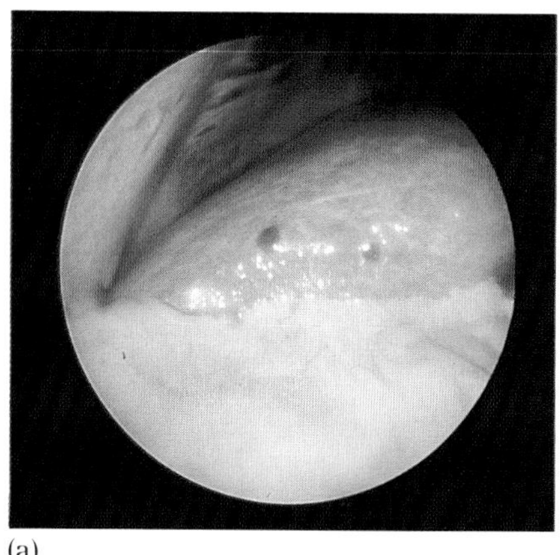
(a)

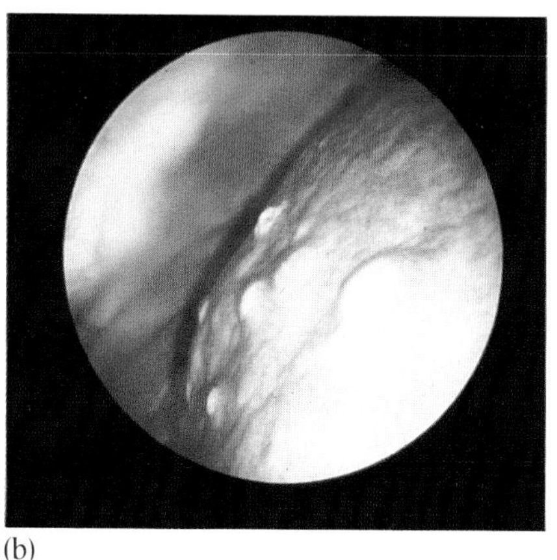
(b)

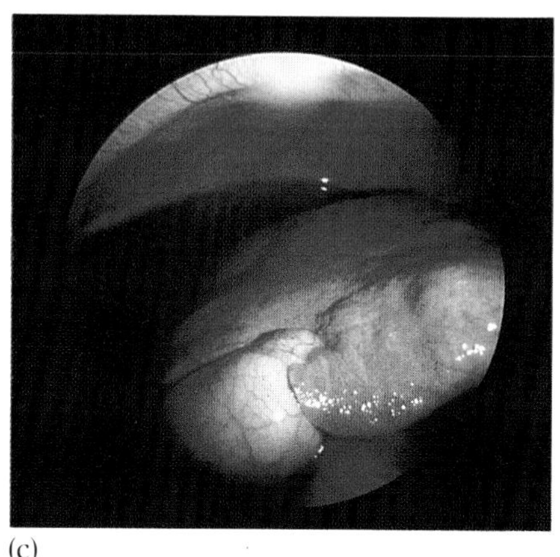
(c)

Fig. 11.5 Secondary deposits. (a) Two small deposits from primary melanoma of the trunk. (b) Multiple deposits from cancer of the sigmoid colon. (c) Large deposit on the anterior margin from primary cancer of the gallbladder. (From Moosa *et al.* (eds) *Comprehensive Textbook of Oncology*. © 1991, the Williams & Wilkins Co., Baltimore, with permission.)

ment, invasion of the diaphragm and the presence or absence of satellite lesions (Fig. 11.4). The operability by liver resection is ascertained from this information.

In patients with secondary tumour deposits (Fig. 11.5a–c), the size, number, extent and bilateral involvement of the liver will determine whether treatment is indicated, and if so, its nature. Apart from providing this information, it should be possible to treat small scattered lesions by cryotherapy [14] delivered through the laparoscopic route in the near future and such a cryoprobe is currently undergoing clinical trials.

Biopsy and cytology

Cytology and biopsy procedures considerably enhance the diagnostic yield of laparoscopy and are necessary, as it is unsafe to rely on macroscopic appearances alone.

Cytology

There are three cytological techniques which are used in laparoscopic work: lavage cytology, brush cytology and fine-needle aspiration cytology (FNA). Lavage cytology is performed for the detection of free neoplastic cells in the peritoneal gutters, and is an integral part of the staging of ovarian cancer, but is also used in the staging of gastric, colorectal and pancreatic cancer. Some 100 ml of saline are injected through an irrigation cannula into the relevant peritoneal gutter. After swilling, the fluid is aspirated, then centrifuged and submitted for cytological examination. Even in the absence of visible peritoneal spread, a positive cytological lavage indicates advanced disease and the need for systemic therapy after resection.

Brush cytology is useful for surface lesions. Standard endoscopic brush cytology sheathed devices are used. These are inserted and guided through a 5.0 mm metal Steptoe cannula.

Laparoscopic fine-needle aspiration cytology is best performed using a long lumbar-puncture needle (gauge 22) inserted percutaneously at the

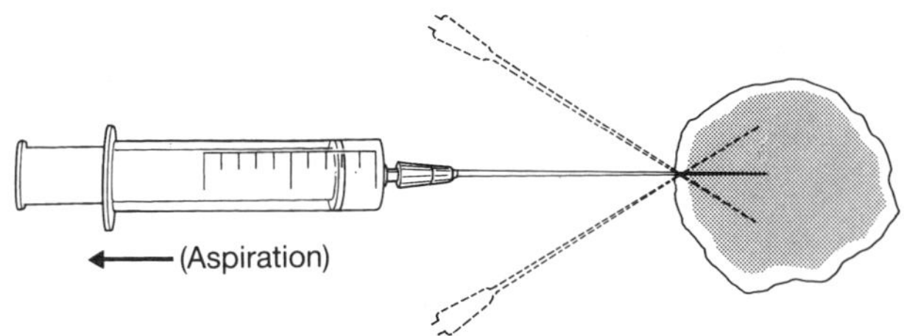

Fig. 11.6 The needle direction is changed without complete extrusion of the tip of the needle from the mass, to sample various regions of the lesion.

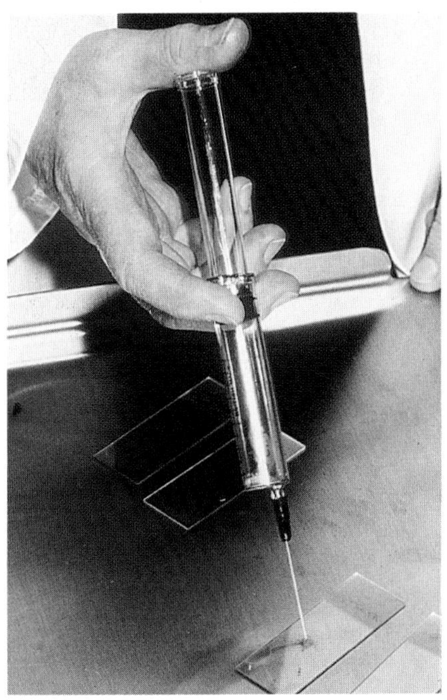

Fig. 11.7 The needle is detached from the syringe and the barrel of this withdrawn before it is reapplied to the needle. The aspirate is then squirted on to the centre of a previously marked glass slide.

appropriate site as determined by the finger depression test, and then guided to the lesion under vision. The cell yield is considerably enhanced if the lumen of the needle is previously wetted with heparinized solution. This is achieved by aspirating a few millilitres of heparinized saline (1:10 000) and then emptying the syringe completely. If the lesion is in surface view, it is impaled by the needle and aspiration maintained for several seconds. The needle direction is changed without complete extrusion of the tip of the needle from the mass, to sample various regions of the lesion (Fig. 11.6). A small bleb of blood-stained fluid should appear in the hub of the syringe before the aspiration is released and the needle withdrawn. The objective is to retain most of the cellular aspirate inside the needle shaft and, for this reason, it is important that aspiration is stopped before the needle is withdrawn from the mass, as this will dissipate the cellular aspirate inside the syringe, with a substantial loss of the cell yield. If, during aspiration of the mass, pure blood is obtained, the needle is withdrawn and pressure applied with a blunt probe for several seconds. The needle is then introduced into another area of the mass. If the lesion is situated behind the stomach or duodenum (e.g. a pancreatic mass), the lumbar-puncture needle can be inserted into the mass with complete safety transduodenally or transgastrically.

Once the aspirate is obtained, the needle is detached from the syringe and the barrel of this withdrawn before it is reapplied to the needle. The aspirate is then squirted on to the centre of a previously marked glass microscopy slide. A squash preparation is made by the use of a second slide (Fig. 11.7). One of the glass slides is air-dried and submitted to immediate cytological examination using the haematological Diff-Quik stain; the other is fixed by immersion in a solution of carbowax. Immediate cytological examination of the aspirate is extremely important as it tells the surgeon whether a satisfactory sample capable of cytological interpretation has been obtained, and if this is not the case, the procedure should be repeated. Often, the immediate cytological examination provides a definite diagnosis (Fig. 11.8), but in some cases this has to await further scrutiny of the fixed aspirate.

Biopsy

Whenever possible, biopsy is preferable to cytology. The instrument used for this purpose varies with the surface characteristics and size of the lesion. The golden rule is that no lesion should be biopsied before it has been carefully inspected close up and palpated. In this fashion catastrophic bleeding from puncture of haemangiomas and other vascular malformations (Fig. 11.9), or spilling the contents of a malignant cystic lesion, are avoided.

There is no doubt that small surface nodules and exophytic or ulcerative lesions are best biopsied using the cup biopsy forceps (Fig. 11.10). The technique is important: when the lesion is reached, the instrument is rotated such that the opened cups straddle the lesion (Fig. 11.11). The opened jaws are then depressed to lift the lesion to the centre of the cups opposite the central prong. The cups are then closed in the depressed position and the biopsy forceps is gently rotated from side to side until the enclosed fragment is detached. It is helpful to keep pressure on the biopsied area for a few more seconds before the forceps containing the specimen is removed. This will reduce bleeding, especially during the biopsy of hepatic lesions. Any haemorrhage from the biopsy site is controlled by electrocoagulation, either with the Berci spatula or with argon spray coagulation.

The best instrument for biopsy of the liver parenchyma and large surface lesions of the liver is the Biopty device (Fig. 11.12) or equivalent. This

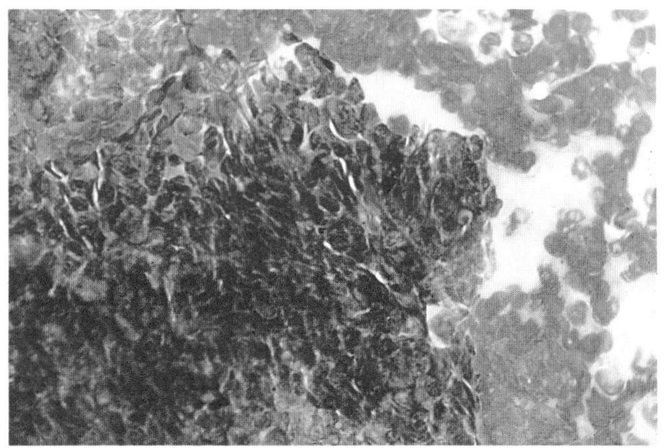

Fig. 11.8 Malignant aspirate from laparoscopic fine-needle aspiration of a mass in the body of the pancreas.

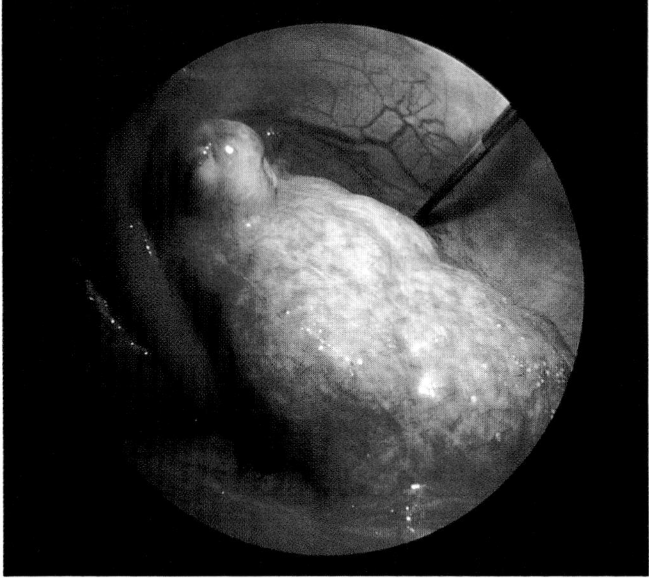

Fig. 11.9 Large venous malformation in a young patient with Budd–Chiari syndrome.

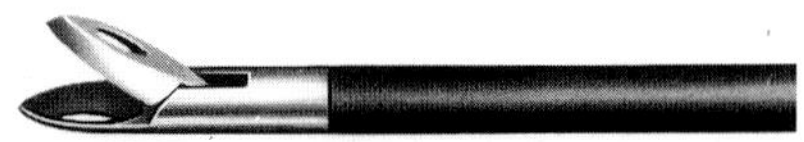

Fig. 11.10 Cup biopsy forceps.

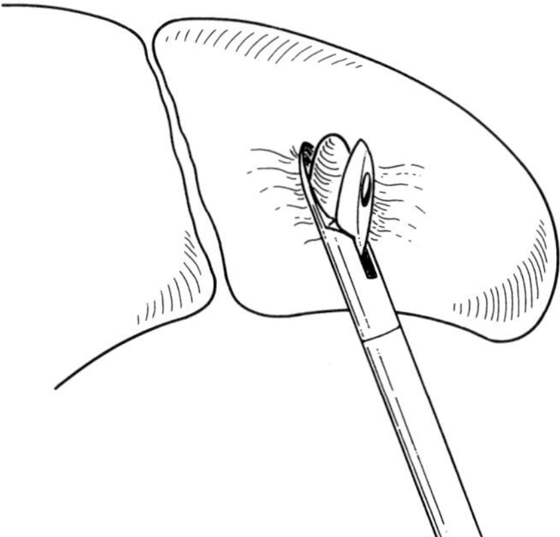

Fig. 11.11 Technique of biopsy of small lesions. When the lesion is reached, the instrument is rotated so that the opened cups straddle the lesion. The opened jaws are then depressed to lift the lesion to the centre of the cups opposite the prong. The cups are then closed in the depressed position and the forceps is gently rotated from side to side until the enclosed fragment is detached.

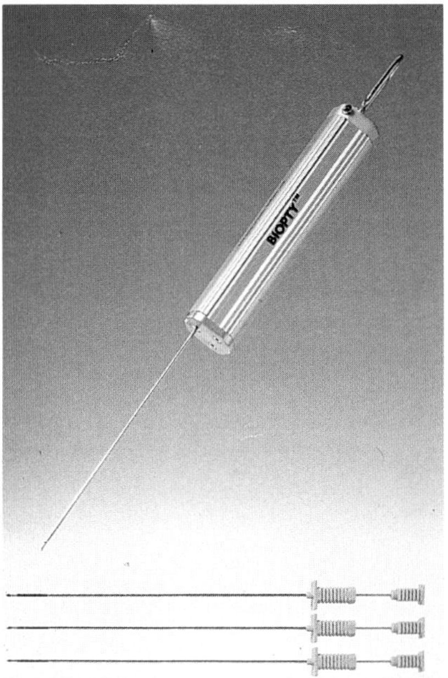

Fig. 11.12 Biopty spring-loaded device for core-needle biopsies.

consists of a spring-loaded Trucut-type needle which, when fired, obtains a needle-core biopsy. It is also useful for the biopsy of pancreatic lesions. When the mass is situated in the head of the pancreas, the needle is introduced transduodenally. After the biopsy has been taken, the small perforation in the anterior wall of the duodenum is closed by a single interrupted suture. Lesions of the body of the pancreas are best exposed either supra- or infragastrically (Chapter 10) before being biopsied by the Biopty device under direct vision. Contrary to fine-needle aspiration, this instrument should not be applied through the stomach as the perforation of the posterior gastric wall cannot be sutured laparoscopically.

Laparoscopic ultrasound scanning

Ultrasound scanning with probes (5–7 MHz) which are introduced through 10.0 mm cannulae is used in the examination of the biliary tract, liver, pancreas and other organs. Linear array probes are preferred to sector ones as they outline the anatomy in greater detail and provide useful information on the parenchyma of solid organs and on the mural structure of hollow viscera. The facility for colour Doppler imaging adds considerably to the diagnostic yield and in the interpretation of the anatomy of the liver. In any event, a good-quality high-resolution machine is needed.

Laparoscopic ultrasound examination is useful in the evaluation of gallbladder disease. Direct-contact scanning of the gallbladder is indicated in those patients with symptoms referable to disease in this organ, where the usual preoperative work-up is equivocal, such as the suspicion of small calculi, polyps and other intramural pathology. Laparoscopic scanning of the extrahepatic bile ducts for the detection of ductal calculi is currently under investigation in a number of centres. Although early results are encouraging, it is doubtful whether it has the potential for providing the detailed anatomical information which is elicited by intraoperative cholangiography (IOC), and for this reason it is unlikely to replace this contrast examination. However, laparoscopic biliary ultrasonography may be a substitute for IOC in easy straightforward cases as a quick method for excluding unsuspected ductal calculi. If positive or suggestive, it would need confirmation by IOC. Another useful role for laparoscopic ultrasonography with colour Doppler is the difficult cholecystectomy, where it can be used to identify vascular structures, including the common hepatic artery and its branches.

Laparoscopic ultrasound examination of the liver is invaluable in the detection of secondary deposits and other focal lesions in the liver. The technique is similar to that used in open surgery. The examination starts by identifying the vena cava above the liver, and subsequently the three hepatic veins which form the boundaries of the four parenchymatous sectors of the liver. The liver substance of each sector is scanned from the vena cava downwards to the free margin of the liver.

Although there have been no published reports, it is likely that laparoscopic ultrasound examination of the pancreas and stomach will provide very precise and useful information on the size and stage of tumours arising in these organs.

Deroofing of simple (non-parasitic) hepatic cysts

Simple hepatic cysts are generally considered to be congenital malformations. By definition they do not communicate with the biliary tree, are lined by a single layer of cuboidal or columnar epithelium, and contain clear serous fluid. They occur predominantly in the right lobe of the liver and may be uni- or multilocular. The majority of these cysts are asymptomatic and are usually discovered accidentally by hepatic imaging for some other condition. Nonetheless, a few become large and cause symptoms, commonly in elderly females. The manifestations include a dull ache, upper abdominal discomfort, dyspepsia and a palpable mass, usually in the right subcostal region. Less frequently, acute pain and jaundice may be encountered. This was associated in one 72-year-old female in the authors' series of 15 patients, with intracystic haemorrhage and external compression of the common duct by a tense large cyst, which extended behind and lifted the gallbladder and the structures of the porta hepatis in front of it.

The investigation of these symptomatic patients must include ultrasonography, CT scanning of the liver and alpha-fetoprotein to exclude malignancy, particularly cystic adenocarcinoma of the liver. The typical findings on ultrasound and CT examination reveal a uniform uni- or multilocular cystic lesion, usually to the right of the gallbladder, which is often displaced anteromedially (Fig. 11.13a,b). The features which should raise the possibility of malignancy are septation and calcification.

The more usual surgical management of these symptomatic cysts is suction drainage and partial excision of the dome of the cyst (deroofing). This is preferred to total excision, as this can be difficult because the interface between the intrahepatic portion of the cyst and the liver parenchyma is

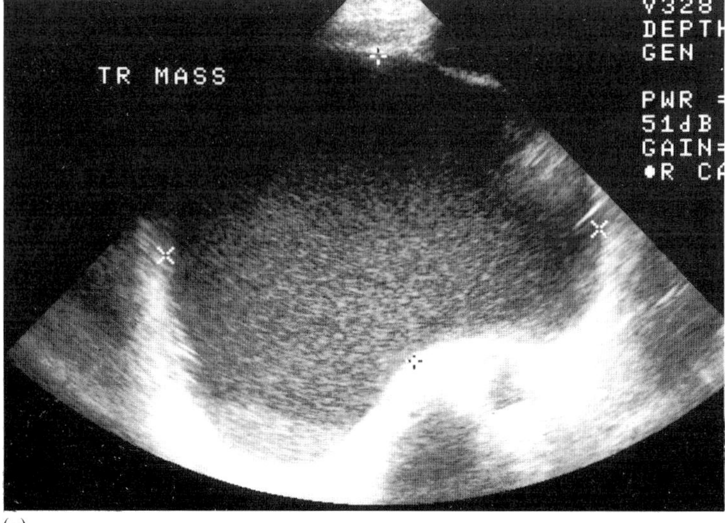

(a)

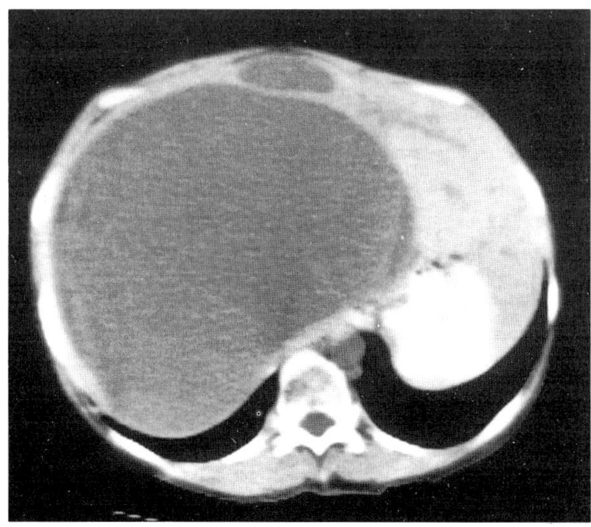
(b)

Fig. 11.13 (a) Ultrasound and (b) CT appearance of a giant benign hepatic cyst.

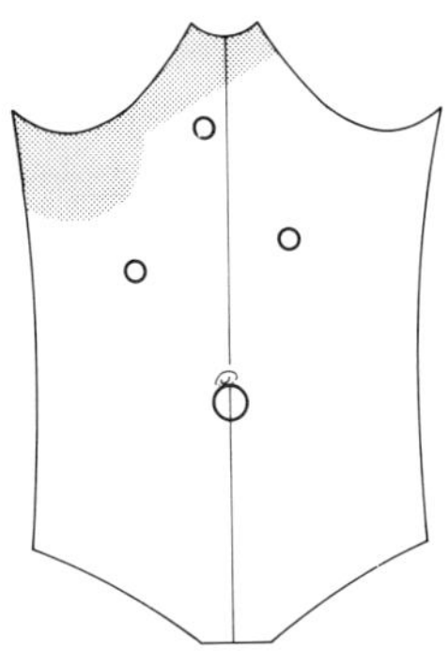

Fig. 11.14 Sites of trocar/cannulae used in laparoscopic deroofing of benign hepatic cysts.

usually ill-defined, and dissection of this plane is attended by bleeding and the risk of bile-ductal damage with subsequent biliary fistula [15,16].

The deroofing of simple non-parasitic hepatic cysts can be undertaken laparoscopically with complete safety and excellent results. The procedure has been performed on three patients in the authors' hospital, and others have reported similar laparoscopic interventions [17].

Technique

The exact position of the trocar/cannula depends on the location and size of the cyst. For the typical right-lobe lesion, the desired siting is shown in Fig. 11.14: umbilical 11.0 mm for the telescope, 5.5 mm midclavicular below the lower margin of the cyst, 5.5 mm left paramedian. Occasionally another cannula (right subxiphoid) may be necessary for retraction.

Confirmation of the diagnosis

After the creation of the pneumoperitoneum and insertion of the laparoscope, the cyst is identified as a dark yellowish-brown swelling, with fine vessels traversing its transparent wall. The remainder of the liver is inspected for other cysts. The first step consists of sampling the cyst fluid. This can be carried out with a lumbar-puncture needle inserted percutaneously and preferably through the edge of the right lobe of the liver (Fig. 11.15). The fluid is inspected macroscopically and a specimen is sent for immediate cytological examination using the Diff-Quik stain. The fluid is normally yellow and serous. Suspicions of malignancy should be entertained if the fluid is turbulent, blood-stained, or contains atypical cells.

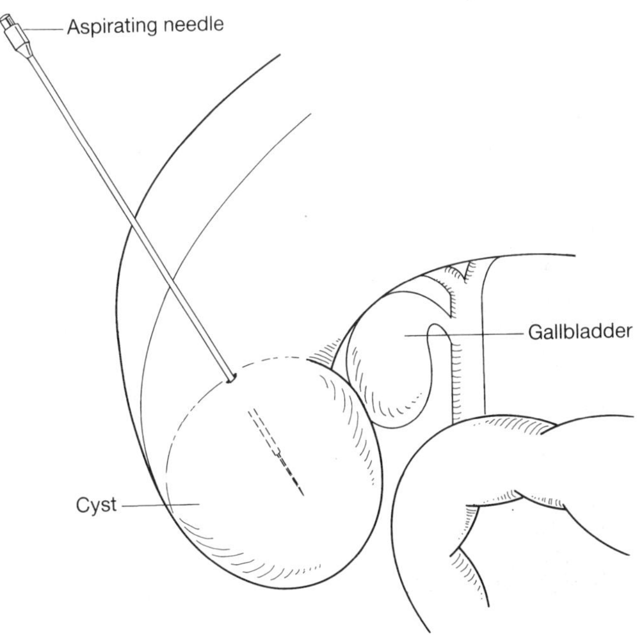

Fig. 11.15 Sampling the cyst fluid. This can be carried out with a lumbar-puncture needle inserted percutaneously, and preferably through the edge of the right lobe of the liver.

Aspiration of cyst fluid

After the benign nature of the lesion has been confirmed, the suction device is placed near the summit of the cyst and a small incision is made with scissors or a retractable diamond knife, large enough to admit the sucker tip, which is then introduced into the cyst cavity and the fluid aspirated as completely as possible.

Deroofing of cyst

The redundant wall is then grasped by an atraumatic forceps and excised by the electrosurgical hook knife using a blender current (Fig. 11.16). The excised cyst wall is sent for histology. Once the partial excision is completed the telescope is introduced further into the cyst for a more complete inspection of the interior, in addition to evacuation of any residual fluid. This is helped by changing the position of the patient to a head-up tilt and slightly to the left. The insertion of a drain is unnecessary unless the cyst is multiloculated and very large, so that aspiration of the fluid content is considered to have been incomplete.

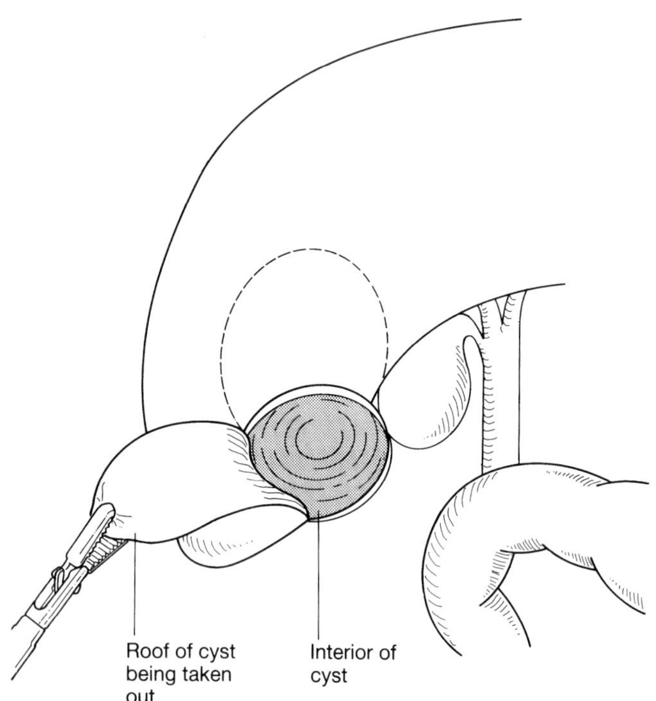

Fig. 11.16 The redundant wall is then grasped by an atraumatic forceps and excised by the electrosurgical hook knife, using a blender current.

Laparoscopic treatment of infected simple cysts and abscesses

Infected simple cysts

These become adherent to surrounding organs, especially the hepatic flexure and duodenum. When located in the posterior segments of the right lobe,

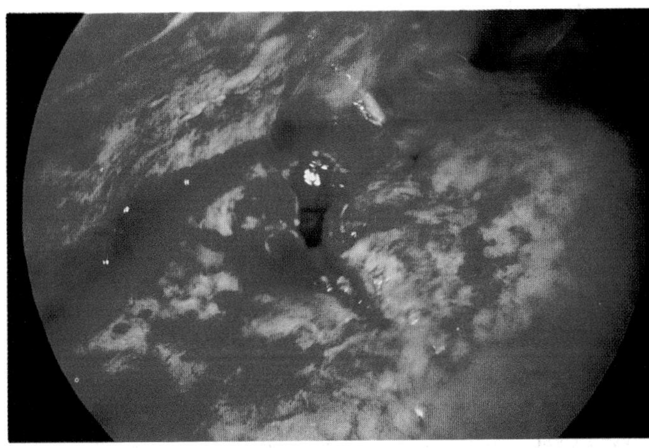

Fig. 11.17 A small portion of the cyst wall is then excised and sent for histological examination.

they become stuck to the diaphragm. The laparoscopic treatment begins by freeing enough superficial wall of the cyst or abscess from the adherent structures. This is followed by aspiration, preferably with the Veress needle with intervening trap attached to a suction line. When the cyst or abscess is emptied, the suction line is disconnected from the Veress needle and saline is injected slowly by syringe into the cyst cavity and then aspirated. This is repeated until the returning fluid is clear. A small portion of the cyst wall is then excised and sent for histological examination (Fig. 11.17). After inspection of the interior of the cyst, a silicon drain is placed inside its cavity. The purulent fluid is examined immediately by microscopy after Gram staining, and a specimen is sent for culture and sensitivity tests. Thorough lavage with saline or Hartmann's solution is performed before desufflation and removal of the cannulae.

Hepatic and subphrenic collections and abscesses

Provided access can be obtained—which is the case in the majority of these patients—pathological purulent collections can be dealt with laparoscopically. As in many instances the pus is under tension; a sucker placed near the summit of the abscess must be ready for activation as soon as the swelling is needled. As the walls of these collections are soft, gentle pressure by the sucker tip over the perforation caused by the sampling needle often results in entry of the sucker into the abscess cavity when the contents are aspirated. Following evacuation, irrigation and aspiration of the cavity is undertaken until all necrotic debris has been removed. A drain is then placed into the abscess cavity and the peritoneal gutters are lavaged with a clean irrigating/suction cannula.

Cholecystoduodenal fistula

This complication of gallstone disease may or may not be accompanied by gallstone ileus. When encountered during elective cholecystectomy, laparoscopic repair is possible in the majority [18], provided the surgeon has experience with endoscopic suturing. The best approach in these patients is to divide the adhesions to outline the exact anatomy and configuration of the fistulous communication. The fistula is then disconnected, preferably with scissors or a retractable diamond knife. The hole in the gallbladder is closed with an endoloop (Fig. 11.18). The duodenal perforation is sutured with two or three interrupted sutures using 3/0 polyamide or silk with internal microsurgical knotting (Fig. 11.19). The cholecystectomy is then carried out. It is the authors' practice to put these patients on a 5-day course of antibiotics.

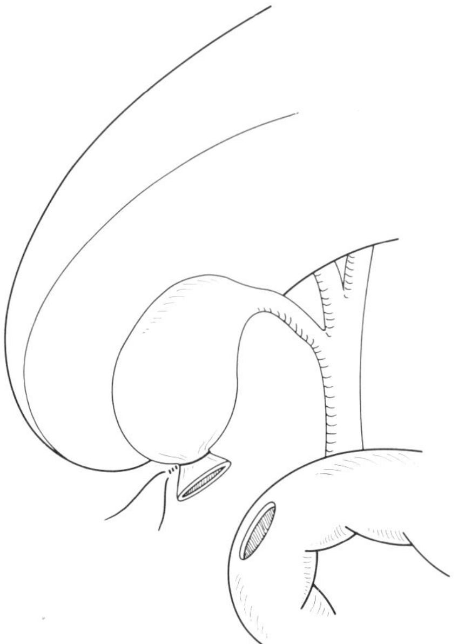

Fig. 11.18 The hole in the gallbladder is closed with an endoloop.

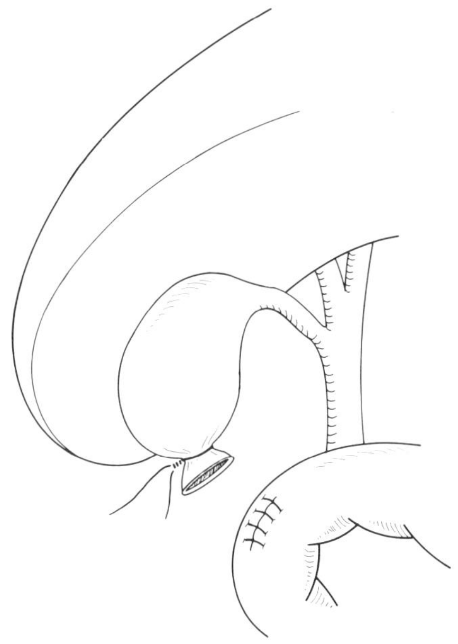

Fig. 11.19 The duodenal perforation is sutured with two or three interrupted sutures using 3/0 polyamide or silk, with internal microsurgical knotting.

References

1 Lightdale CJ. Clinical application of laparoscopy in patients with malignant neoplasms. *Gastrointest Endosc* 1982; **28**: 99–102.

2 Shandall A, Johnson C. Laparoscopy or scanning in oesophageal and gastric carcinoma? *Br J Surg* 1985; **22**: 449–451.

3 Possik RA, Franco EL, Pires DR *et al.* Sensitivity, specificity and predictive value of laparoscopy for the staging of gastric cancer and for the detection of liver metastases. *Cancer* 1986; **58**: 1–6.

4 Warshaw AL, Tepper JE, Shipley WU. Laparoscopy in the staging and planning of therapy for pancreatic cancer. *Am J Surg* 1986; **158**: 76–80.

5 Cuschieri A. Laparoscopy for pancreatic cancer: does it benefit the patient? *Eur J Surg Oncol* 1988; **14**: 41–44.

6 Berci G, Cuschieri A. *Practical Laparoscopy*. Baillière Tindall, London, 1984.

7 Shandall A, Johnson C. Laparoscopy or scanning in oesophageal and gastric carcinoma? *Br J Surg* 1985; **72**: 449–451.

8 Friedman IH, Woeff WI. Laparoscopy. A safe method for liver biopsy in the high risk patient. *Am J Gastroenterol* 1977; **67**: 319–323.

9 McCallum RW, Buci G. Laparoscopy in hepatic disease. *Gastrointest Endosc* 1970; **23**: 20–24.

10 Beck K. *Colour Atlas of Laparoscopy*. WB Saunders, Philadelphia, 1984.

11 Berci G, Morgenstern L, Shore JM, Shapiro S. A direct approach to the differential diagnosis of jaundice. Laparoscopy with transhepatic cholecystocholangiography. *Am J Surg* 1973; **126**: 372–378.

12 Cuschieri A. Value of laparoscopy in hepatobiliary disease. *Ann Roy Coll Surg Eng* 1975; **57**: 33–38.

13 Irving AD, Cuschieri A. Laparoscopic assessment of the jaundiced patient. *Br J Surg* 1978; **65**: 678–680.

14 Ravikumar TS, Kane R, Cady B *et al.* Hepatic cryosurgery with intraoperative ultrasound monitoring for metastatic colon carcinoma. *Arch Surg* 1987; **122**: 403–409.

15 Doty JE, Tompkins RK. Management of cystic disease of the liver. *Surg Clin North Am* 1989; **69**: 285–295.

16 Lai ECS, Wong J. Symptomatic non-parasitic cysts of the liver. *World J Surg* 1990; **14**: 452–456.

17 Z'graggen K, Metzger A, Klaiber C. Symptomatic simple cysts of the liver: treatment by laparoscopic surgery. *J Surg Endosc* 1991; **5**: 224–225.

18 Velez M, Mule J, Brandon L, Kannegieter L. Laparoscopic repair of cholecystoduodenal fistula. *Surg Endosc* 1991; **5**: 221–223.

Index

Page numbers in **bold** refer to tables, those in *italic* refer to figures.